s dedicated, with affection and gratitude, to the
e late Dr Joseph Earle Moore, of Baltimore, to
all who work in the subject owe so much

This book i
memory of th
whom we and

VENEREAL DISEASES

FOURTH EDITION

AMBROSE KING, TD, KSG, MB, BS(LOND), FRCS(ENG)

Honorary Consulting Venereologist to the London Hospital; Member of the Expert Advisory Panel on Venereal Infections and Treponematoses, WHO; Past President and Member of the Council of the Medical Society of Venereal Diseases; Consultant and Past President of the International Union against the Venereal Diseases and the Treponematoses; Formerly Consultant Adviser in Venereology to the Department of Health and Social Security; Senior Physician, Whitechapel Clinic, The London Hospital; Lecturer on Venereal Diseases, The London Hospital Medical College; Honorary Consultant Venereologist to the British Army

CLAUDE NICOL, CBE, TD, MD(LOND), FRCP(LOND)

Formerly Physician-in-Charge, Venereal Diseases Department, St Thomas's Hospital, London; Consultant Adviser in Venereology to the Department of Health and Social Security; Recognized Teacher in the University of London; Member of the Expert Advisory Panel on Venereal Infections and Treponematoses, WHO; Past President and Member of the Council of the Medical Society for the Study of Venereal Diseases; Vice-President of the International Union against the Venereal Diseases and the Treponematoses; Honorary Consultant Venereologist to the British Army

PHILIP RODIN, MB, BS(LOND), FRCP(LOND)

Consultant Venereologist to the London Hospital; Recognized Teacher in the University of London; Past Editor of the British Journal of Venereal Diseases; *Past Member of the Council of the Medical Society for the Study of Venereal Diseases*

BAILLIÈRE TINDALL · LONDON

A BAILLIÈRE TINDALL book published by
Cassell Ltd.
35 Red Lion Square, London WC1R 4SG

and at Sydney, Auckland, Toronto, Johannesburg

an affiliate of
Macmillan Publishing Co. Inc.
New York

© 1980 Baillière Tindall
a division of Cassell Ltd.

First published 1964
Third edition 1975
Fourth edition 1980

ISBN 0 7020 0816 8

French edition (Librarie Maloine, Paris) 1965

Printed in Great Britain by The Whitefriars Press Ltd,
London and Tonbridge

British Library Cataloguing in Publication Data

King, Ambrose
   Venereal diseases.
   1. Venereal diseases
   I. Title   II. Nicol, Claude
   III. Rodin, Philip
   616.9'51   RC200

   ISBN 0-7020-0816-8

Contents

Colour Plates

Preface

It is now 16 years since the first edition of this book appeared in 1964, to be followed by a second edition in 1969 and a third in 1975. This is a considerable period in modern medicine and developments in knowledge, experience and practice have been very great, not least in the subject of venereology. Hopes that new remedies and improved methods would abolish, or at least greatly diminish, the problem have been abandoned long since and perhaps, in retrospect, this is not surprising with these contagious diseases, the spread of which is so closely related to social circumstances and human behaviour. During this time habitual promiscuity has been widespread, particularly among young people, so many of whom lack the discipline, care and affection of a satisfactory home life. But this is only one of a number of factors concerned, as our discussion of the problem in Chapter 29 makes clear. There have been considerable efforts to give the general public, and young people in particular, more information about these diseases and their dangers; but such instruction is hardly likely to be successful while so many of those who give advice in schools and elsewhere concentrate on the importance of avoiding pregnancy and take comparatively little account of the need for restraint and discipline and the dangers of venereal disease.

Those who like to rely on the letter of the law point to the fact that the venereal diseases, as legally defined, include only syphilis, gonorrhoea and chancroid. But this definition was made in 1917 when knowledge of the subject was rudimentary. Over the years there has been overwhelming evidence relating the spread of non-gonococcal urethritis, trichomoniasis, herpes genitalis and some other conditions to sexual intercourse. So important are these diseases now considered to be, that for some years the preponderance of effort in research has been directed to them.

Thus, in the fourth edition we retain the original title, *Venereal Diseases*, because it is time-honoured and, apart from an outdated legal definition, is accepted as embracing all the sexually transmitted diseases. The description, genitourinary medicine, used by some would be, in our opinion, a misleading title for this book for it would imply coverage of a number of important conditions which do not come within the field of venereology. Nevertheless, we have continued to give some description of various non-venereal conditions, including the tropical disease yaws, for which the differential diagnosis from venereal diseases may give rise to difficulties.

Whatever the diseases are called, they remain throughout the world a problem which advances in knowledge and considerable efforts have failed to resolve. Although in some respects the patterns of disease have changed the difficulties in diagnosis, treatment and epidemiological control have not lessened.

Because of the passage of time, the authors of earlier editions decided that it was now important to introduce younger ideas associated with the right blend of wisdom, experience and clinical ability. At the risk of causing some embarrassment to a talented colleague, they would like to place on record their belief that their judgement in the matter has been more than vindicated.

Many sections of the book have been re-written entirely, especially those on the 'minor' diseases which have attracted so much more attention in recent years. A good deal of new information has been added and, of course, the treatment of all the diseases has been brought up to date. A new chapter has been introduced on the psychological aspects of venereal disease. The best of the illustrations used in former editions remain, but others have been replaced, when improvement seemed necessary, and some have been added. In the past it has been our policy to provide references but not an exhaustive bibliography. In several chapters the lists of references have now been expanded to a point at which, although not complete, we believe they are likely to be of value even to a research worker.

We thank Miss N. Philcox, who has done most of the typing, and our publishers, Baillière Tindall, for their unfailing understanding and support.

April 1980

AMBROSE KING
CLAUDE NICOL
PHILIP RODIN

1

Syphilis

Syphilis was defined by Stokes as an infectious disease; due to *Treponema pallidum*; of great chronicity; systemic from the outset; capable of involving practically every structure of the body in its course; distinguished by florid manifestations on the one hand and years of completely asymptomatic latency on the other; able to simulate many diseases in the fields of medicine and surgery; transmissible to offspring in man; transmissible to certain laboratory animals; and treatable to the point of presumptive cure.[1]

HISTORY

There are two theories concerning the origin of syphilis. Some believe that it first appeared in the tropics as a primitive treponemal disease, usually transmitted by chance contact between individuals, especially children, and thus closely resembling the tropical treponematoses of the present day, such as yaws. The suggestion is that as the disease spread to more temperate climates, where more clothing was worn, and affected more advanced communities with better hygienic standards, transmission by sex contact became the usual method of spread of the disease. In the past, forced emigration of negro races, in the course of the slave trade, may have speeded dissemination of infection. The facts that the treponemes of syphilis and yaws are morphologically indistinguishable, that the same blood tests are positive in both diseases and both respond to the same treatment are points in favour of this theory.

A larger body of opinion affirms that there are no descriptions of any disease that can be identified as syphilis in Egyptian, Greek or Arabic treatises on medicine. Syphilis was not known in Europe before the end of the fifteenth century. On the other hand evidence of bone syphilis has been reported in the skeletons of American Indians who lived before this time. It is known that after Columbus discovered the New World members of his crews mixed freely with the local Indian inhabitants, and these are believed to have been the source of the new infection. Columbus arrived back in Spain in 1493, landing at Palos; his crews were later disbanded and some members who were in the pay of King Ferdinand of Aragon were sent to help in the siege of Naples in 1494. This city had been invested by the armies of Charles VIII of France following his invasion of Northern Italy. Warfare in the fifteenth century was such that sexually transmitted infection could spread easily among the soldiers and camp followers of the opposing forces of besiegers and besieged. There is no doubt that a great epidemic broke out at Naples that year and that this was what was later called syphilis, although at this time the Italians called it the 'French disease' and the French, the 'Italian disease'. In 1521 Fracastorius wrote his famous poem 'Syphilis sive Morbus Gallicus' and gave the disease its name. By this time syphilis had been spread all over Europe by soldiers and mercenaries returning from the wars, and had been carried by Portuguese sailors to India and the Far East.

Because of its long incubation period it was not at first appreciated that syphilis was a venereal disease; nor was it realized that its late manifestations resulted from infection so many years previously. In the sixteenth century, however, the famous French surgeon, Ambroise Paré, attributed aortic aneurysm to syphilis. In the same century, in Germany, Ulrich von Hutton described treatment of the disease with mercury and guaiacum; in the seventeenth century the British physician, Sydenham, used mercury in the form of inunctions.

In the eighteenth century it was known that syphilis and gonorrhoea were transmitted by sexual intercourse, but many believed them to be manifestations of the same infection. In London, John Hunter supported the view that they were the same disease, and it has been commonly supposed that to test the validity of this theory he inoculated himself with gonococcal pus. This suggestion was first made by d'Arcy Power in a Hunterian Oration in 1925,[2] and was generally believed. Qvist[3] has recently re-examined the evidence and concluded that there is no reason to suppose that Hunter suffered from syphilis, and that his famous inoculation experiment was performed not on himself but on another subject. However, Weimerskirch and Richter[4] have drawn attention to what appears to be a verbatim transcript of Hunter's lectures on venereal disease, held in the Edward G. Miner Library of the Rochester (N.Y.) School of Medicine and Dentistry, in which the following appears:

It has often been disputed whether the matter of a chancre and gonorrhoea essentially differ—or whether they are the same, but as I have produced in myself a chancre by matter from a gonorrhoea that point is now settled. I am led to conclude that there is no difference. . . .

Unfortunately for medical progress the patient from whom he obtained the inoculum was also suffering from syphilis. The person inoculated, whether himself or another, contracted both diseases, which naturally convinced Hunter, and many other people, that he was right. It was not until 1793 that Bell of Edinburgh maintained the view that syphilis and gonorrhoea were different diseases. This was finally established in 1838 by Ricord who carried out over a thousand inoculations in human subjects. The fact that tabes dorsalis and general paralysis are related to syphilis was first pointed out by Jean-Alfred Fournier of Paris during the period 1876 to 1894. In the nineteenth century also, Roux and Neisser were able to demonstrate the transmission of syphilis to apes.

The most important contributions to knowledge of the disease were made in the present century. In 1905 Schaudinn and Hoffmann of Hamburg discovered that syphilis was caused by a spirochaete which they called, at first, *Spirochaeta pallida*. Later they changed the name to *Treponema pallidum*, but, because the first name had been widely accepted, both are now regarded as correct. In the following year (1906) Wassermann of Berlin described a diagnostic blood test, the Wassermann reaction (WR). These discoveries were followed by important advances in treatment. In 1909 Ehrlich of Frankfurt produced an organic arsenical preparation which was effective when given intravenously. It was his 606th experiment with drugs of this group, and he called it '606', or Salvarsan. Its generic name is arsphenamine. Some years later, in his 914th experiment, he produced neo-arsphenamine. In 1921, in France, Sazerac and Levaditi introduced intramuscular injections of bismuth as a less toxic and more effective substitute for mercury. The next major advance in treatment was in 1943 when penicillin, which had been discovered by Fleming and developed by Florey and his colleagues, was successfully used in the treatment of syphilis by Mahoney and his colleagues in New York. A more recent important advance was in serological diagnosis when, in Baltimore in 1948, Nelson and Mayer introduced the first specific blood test for syphilis, the *Treponema pallidum* immobilization (TPI) test.

EPIDEMIOLOGY

Moore[5] collected evidence of a progressive decline in the morbidity of syphilis in Western countries since 1860, punctuated by transitory increases of almost epidemic character associated with war, political unrest, and movements of populations. He believed that this decline was probably not due to the control of syphilis (including treatment) but to general improvement in socio-economic conditions brought about by the Industrial Revolution. The number of cases of syphilis in all stages and the number of cases of early infectious syphilis reported from the treatment centres in England and Wales from 1940 to 1977 are shown on p. 4. There was a marked decline in cases of infectious syphilis in the decade following the peak incidence in 1946, possibly partly due to the widespread use of penicillin whereby

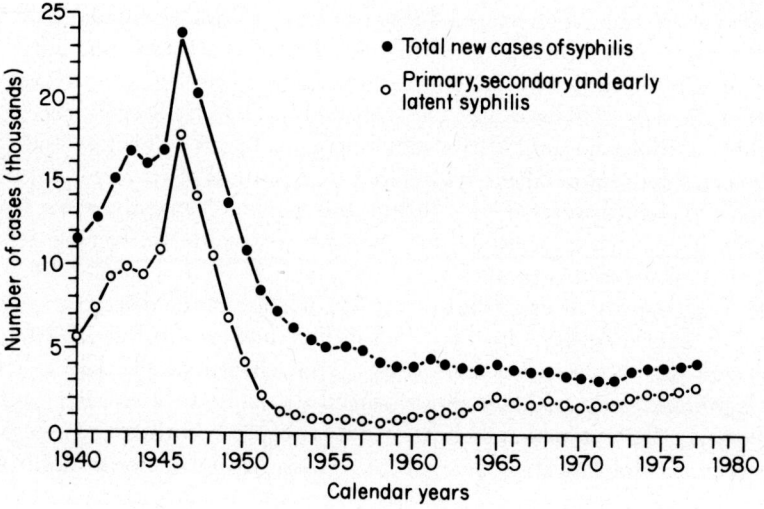

Syphilis in England and Wales, 1940–1977.

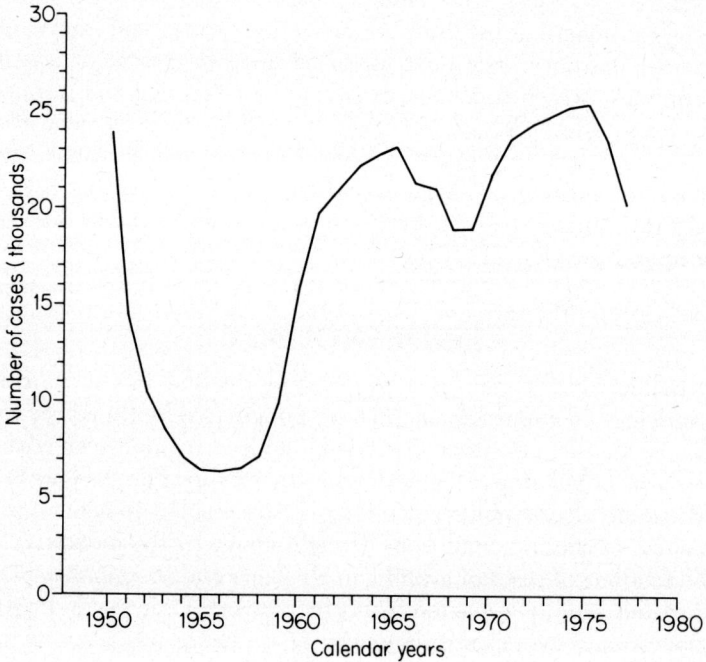

Primary and secondary syphilis in the United States of America, 1950–1977.

patients who had undiagnosed syphilis were rendered non-infectious by chance (so-called 'happenstance' treatment). Since then there has been some increase in infectious syphilis, but the disease still seems to be well under control in the United Kingdom. In the year ending 30 June 1977[6] the number of reported cases of primary and secondary syphilis in England was 1735. These comprised 1486 men and 249 women and the rate per 100,000 population was 3·74. Certain other countries have experienced a greater increase in the incidence of infectious syphilis. The number of reported cases of primary and secondary syphilis in the United States from 1950 to 1977 is shown. The rate per 100,000 population was 3·4 in 1956 and 9·5 in 1977,[7] there being 15,207 men and 5155 women affected in 1977. Because of the large number of cases which are not reported,[8] the true incidence of infectious syphilis in the United States has been estimated to be nearly four times that reported. A large proportion of these infections is now contributed by homosexuals. A survey done in 1971[9] showed that in the United Kingdom 42·4 per cent of cases of primary and secondary syphilis were acquired homosexually. In London the percentage was 62·1. It is probable that much syphilis is suppressed, but not necessarily cured, by the widespread and not always discriminating use of antibiotics.

BACTERIOLOGY

The order Spirochaetales comprises the families Spirochaetaceae and Treponemataceae; the latter is of importance to man and consists of the following genera:

1. Treponemata
   a. Pathogenic; *b*. Saprophytic; *c*. Special Strains
2. Borrelia
3. Leptospira

Treponemata

Those *pathogenic* to man cause syphilis, yaws, bejel, pinta, and various locally occurring treponematoses, such as dichuchwa in Africa. These organisms are morphologically and serologically identical. It is not possible to grow them in artificial media.

Saprophytic treponemes are found in the mouth, particularly in patients with dental sepsis. They include *T. microdentium* and *T. macrodentium*.

Certain *special strains* have been studied for many years. One of these is the Nichols strain, which is pathogenic and has been maintained in animals. The non-pathogenic Reiter strain has been preserved for many years in artificial culture media.

Borrelia

Various organisms of this group, such as *B. gracilis*, *B. refringens* and *B. balanitidis*, are commonly found in subpreputial discharges.

Leptospira

The only pathogenic organisms of this type found in Great Britain are *L. icterohaemorrhagiae*, the cause of Weil's disease, and *L. canicola*.

TREPONEMA PALLIDUM[10]

Morphology

The morphological characteristics of *T. pallidum* can be studied microscopically. In clinical work the usual method employed is that of darkground illumination (DG) (Fig. 1), but both the phase-contrast and the electron microscopes have been used for research on the organism.

  T. pallidum is a close-coiled, slender, regular spiral organism varying in length from 6 to 15 μm and consisting of from 8 to 24 coils; its width is seldom more than 0·25 μm. The organism is so narrow and the volume of protoplasm so small that it is extremely difficult to see by direct illumination in an unstained preparation. The electron microscope shows an axial bundle. This is surrounded by a number of spirally wound filaments which, when they have become detached from the axial bundle, have been misinterpreted as flagella.[11, 12] There is probably a 'periplast' or capsular structure. There is no evidence of a life cycle in virulent *T. pallidum*, although such a cycle has been demonstrated in the non-virulent strains of treponemes. There is evidence that *T. pallidum* multiplies by transverse fission and that in an active phase this probably occurs about every 30 hours.[13]

Motility—Microscopic Identification

The movements of *T. pallidum*, as seen by DG examination, may be divided into those of locomotion and those of change of shape. Locomotion consists of rotation and propulsion, the speed of the corkscrew movement of rotation varying with the viscosity of the surrounding medium. Propulsion is slow and regular rather than spasmodic; when examined with the 2 mm oil-immersion objective of the microscope the organism stays within the field of vision for a considerable time. Movements of change of shape are angulation, buckling, undulation, coil compression and expansion, and looping; of these, angulation, in which the organism bends on itself at an acute or obtuse angle, is most typical. In buckling, as when a coil spring is compressed at each end, central coils resist the movement and spring out of line. In coil expansion the organism increases in length. Occasionally, looping in the form of a U may be seen.

Identification

The usual method is by DG examination of serum obtained from lesions in cases of early syphilis. This may be difficult in the presence of blood or pus, when centrifugation of the specimen in a sealed capillary tube may help.

Ordinary staining methods have seldom proved satisfactory. Treponemes are easily stained with dyes, but the organisms are very small and the contrast with the staining of the host tissues is minimal. Various techniques using silver impregnation have been used with moderate success (see Fig. 77, p. 107). In recent years immunofluorescent staining techniques have proved of value.[14]

Although virulent *T. pallidum* has never been cultured in artificial medium, it can be kept alive and mobile for a short time in a special survival medium (see TPI test, p. 137). On the other hand the non-virulent (Reiter) treponemes can easily be grown and maintained in artificial medium (see RPCF test, p. 138).

Animal Inoculation

Infection of the larger apes with syphilis can produce clinical signs similar to the human disease. In other animals the disease takes a different course, but it can be produced in rabbits fairly easily by intratesticular or intradermal inoculation, with inflammatory response and antibody formation.

Inoculation of mice with *T. pallidum* produces no tissue reaction but infectivity can be shown by passage back to rabbits. It has also been shown that hamsters can be infected and therefore used as laboratory animals in the study of treponemal diseases.

Typing

There is no known method of typing *T. pallidum*. It has been suggested that some treponemes are 'neurotropic', on the grounds that neurosyphilis is frequently found in husband and wife, but the evidence for the existence of special strains with a predilection for the nervous system is slender.

Viability

T. pallidum is rapidly destroyed by drying, by heat and by antiseptics. Rubber gloves provide protection against contact infection, but even if chance contamination does occur, washing the hands with soap and water effectively destroys all treponemes. The application of an antiseptic solution or cream to early lesions is likely to destroy all surface treponemes and make diagnosis difficult. This applies particularly to creams or lotions containing penicillin, chloramphenicol or tetracyclines. Experimental evidence suggests that lotions or ointments containing steroid drugs will, if anything, cause an increase in the number of treponemes in a lesion.

T. pallidum will not survive for more than a few days in blood stored at ordinary refrigeration temperatures. It can, however, be preserved for several years at $-78°C$.

Immunity

Experimental work on rabbits inoculated intradermally with virulent *T. pallidum*, previously incubated with serum from patients with syphilis, has shown the existence of protective antibodies.

Antibodies are those directed specifically against pathogenic *Treponema pallidum* and those directed against the protein antigen group common to various spirochaetes. Jakubowski and Manikowska-Lesinska[15], using an immunofluorescent technique, have shown that antibodies directed against the group antigen in cases of early syphilis are mainly among the immunoglobulins IgG and IgA. The proportion of non-specific antibodies associated with IgG immunoglobulin falls considerably in later stages of syphilis. Specific antibodies produced in response to pathogenic *Treponema pallidum* in the early stages of syphilis are found chiefly in the IgM immunoglobulins. In the later stages of syphilis their numbers diminish. The percentage of non-specific IgA antibodies increases significantly in the course of untreated syphilis.

Humoral immunity seems to play only a minor role in protection against syphilis. The importance of cell-mediated immunity has received more attention in recent years. There is evidence of a state of immunosuppression in the early stages of human and experimental rabbit syphilis and Levene et al.[16] found a factor in serum from patients with secondary syphilis that inhibits the transformation of normal lymphocytes by phytohaemagglutinin. In the later stages of the disease there is generally evidence of active cellular immunity. The matter has been discussed by Wright and Grimble[17] and more recently by Pavia et al.[18]

In the human subject, treponemes inoculated at new sites during the incubation period of experimental infection, will multiply and produce lesions. After the primary stage has appeared, no later inoculation is likely to produce tissue response. Superinfection may, however, occasionally occur in cases of late acquired or congenital syphilis, provided that the inoculum is large enough, and this has also been demonstrated in rabbit syphilis. Re-infection is possible if early and successful treatment of the first attack of the disease has been achieved. It is possible, too, for a patient who has suffered from another treponemal disease, such as yaws, in childhood to acquire syphilis in later years.

CLASSIFICATION OF SYPHILIS

Acquired Syphilis

EARLY INFECTIOUS PHASE (diagnosed in first two years of infection). Primary stage; secondary stage; recurrent stage (sometimes of primary but usually of secondary type); early latent stage.

LATE NON-INFECTIOUS PHASE (diagnosed after the end of second year of infection). Late latent stage; tertiary stage: (*a*) Covering structures of the body (skin and mucous membrane, subcutaneous tissues); (*b*) Supporting structures of the body (bones, joints, muscles, etc.); (*c*) Viscera.

CARDIOVASCULAR SYPHILIS AND *NEUROSYPHILIS* present special problems. They are regarded by some as manifestations of tertiary syphilis; by others, as 'quaternary' syphilis.

Congenital Syphilis

There is no stage analogous to the primary stage in the acquired form of the disease. Lesions of congenital syphilis may be:

1. *EARLY*: Within the first two years of life. In general these are the infectious lesions, and many of them resemble those of the secondary stage of acquired syphilis.

2. *LATE*: These occur from the beginning of the third year of life onwards. They include gummata which are identical with those of the tertiary stage of acquired syphilis.

The division between *early* and *late* is arbitrary but in practice reasonably satisfactory.

3. *THE STIGMATA*: These are the scars and deformities of lesions, early or late, which are no longer active. Many of them are characteristic.

PATHOLOGY OF SYPHILIS

Early Phase

In cases of acquired syphilis *T. pallidum* is inoculated into the tissues, possibly through a small abrasion, usually as a result of sex contact. The organisms then multiply and the incubation period probably varies with the size of the original inoculum. The host tissues react to the presence of treponemes as they multiply, and the tissues become infiltrated with small lymphocytes and plasma cells which are concentrated particularly in the perivascular lymphatics and involve the vessel walls. An electron microscopic study of sections from a syphilitic chancre[19] showed proliferating small vessels surrounded by treponemes and inflammatory cells, including plasma cells. The organisms were seen between the capillary endothelium and the surrounding perivascular tissue. The appearances suggested that

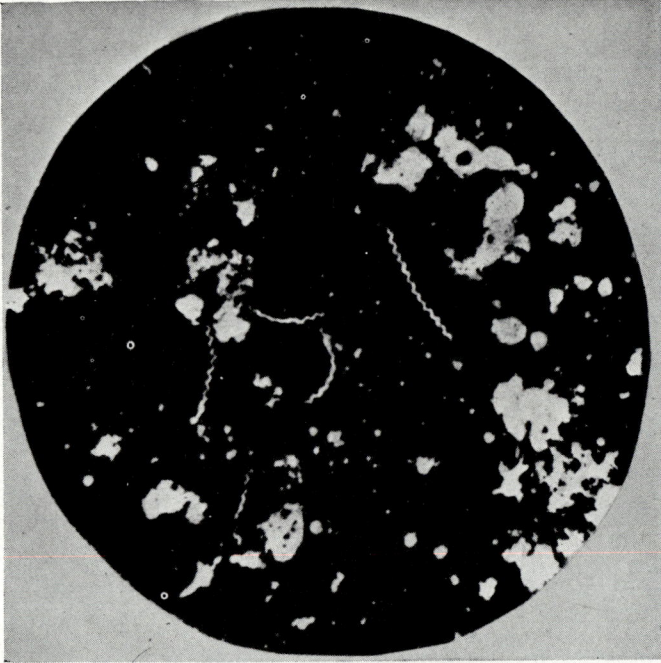

Fig. 1. *T. pallidum* seen by dark-ground illumination method.
(*Magnification* × 1000.)

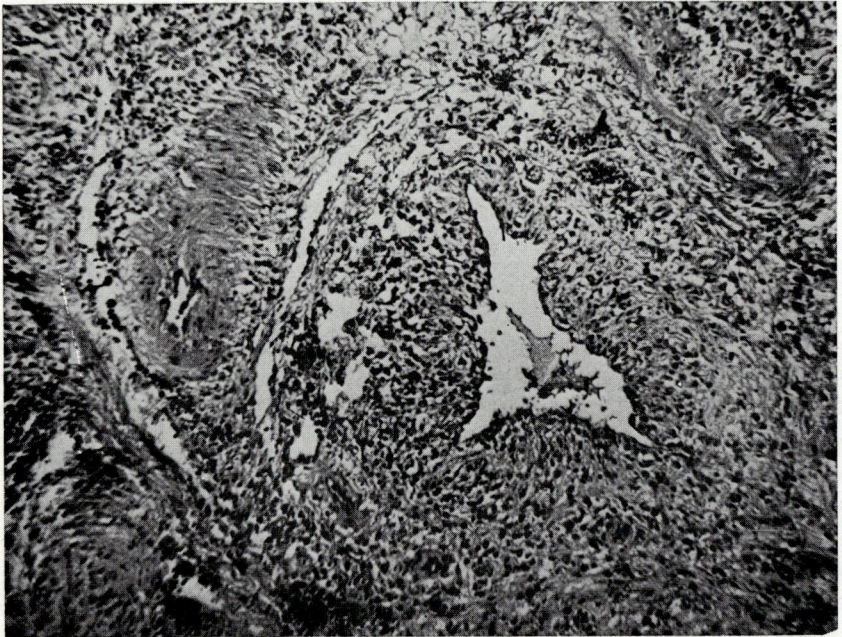

Fig. 2. Section of syphilitic chancre showing round-cell infiltration, especially
around the blood vessels. (*Magnification* × 100.)

these were the sites of proliferation. Endarteritis of the small blood vessels produces hypertrophic changes in the endothelium which may obliterate the lumen (endarteritis obliterans) (Fig. 2). Loss of blood supply results in erosion of the surface of the lesion. Before the primary lesion has appeared, however, treponemes have reached the regional lymph nodes by way of the lymphatics, and there they multiply. The tissue response is similar and results in characteristic enlargement of the nodes. At the same time treponemes have found their way into the blood stream and have been disseminated to all the tissues of the body. Multiplication is followed by reaction in the tissues which produces the secondary stage, perhaps six to eight weeks after the beginning of the primary stage. The primary lesion slowly heals as the local treponemes diminish in number; fibroblasts appear; and finally healing occurs by scar formation. In the same way the secondary lesions slowly regress and disappear but evident scarring is rare. They are likely to be followed by fresh lesions, and final disappearance may take as long as nine months. The patient is now in a stage of latency with no signs or symptoms of the disease, yet infection is still present and active. As an example of this, it is not uncommon for a pregnant woman in this stage of early latency to give birth to an infant suffering from congenital syphilis. Sometimes the immunity processes fail to control the infection and treponemes again multiply at the site of the primary lesion, producing a recurrent lesion, or the treponemes disseminated through the tissues produce a similar reaction resulting in recurrent lesions of the secondary type; the latter is more common than the former. Infectious lesions may appear and reappear on several occasions, but usually not after the end of the second year of the disease. It should be added that in some cases the tissue reactions in early syphilis are so slight that they escape notice.

Late Phase

The latent stage may continue for many years, with treponemes apparently lying dormant and producing no evident tissue reaction. Nevertheless antibodies continue to be present in the patient's serum. For reasons which remain obscure, the balance between organisms and tissues may suddenly be altered. Trauma appears to be one factor which may precipitate a gummatous reaction of the tertiary stage. Although it may not be possible to demonstrate T. pallidum in the tissues involved, except by animal inoculation, a severe reaction occurs which may affect one or more areas and may vary considerably in size. The area of involvement is infiltrated with small lymphocytes and plasma cells, with endarteritis of the small vessels resulting in necrosis of central or surface tissue which is apt to be severe and very destructive (see Figs. 36 and 37). The original lesion heals slowly with the formation of fibrous tissue, but new lesions may appear peripherally, and these tertiary lesions may continue to spread over a period of many years. After varying intervals of latency they may appear at other sites. The first lesion is often found from three to ten years after infection but may be delayed for much longer periods. Treponemes reaching the cardiovascular and nervous systems early in the disease produce a similar chronic cellular reaction, but gross tissue necrosis is rare and progression is apt to be so slow that destruction of tissue, scarring and degenerative changes may take many years to produce clinical effects. Past experience has suggested that patients with gummatous syphilis seldom develop late lesions of the nervous and cardiovascular systems and that the reverse is also true. However, this view is not borne out by Gjestland's[20] study of untreated patients in Oslo in which it was found that those with and without gummatous syphilis showed the same proportions of cardiovascular syphilis and neurosyphilis.

In about two-thirds of the cases the latent stage continues for the rest of the patient's life without the development of any clinical lesions. In a number of these, however, there is evidence of syphilis at autopsy; but it is difficult to estimate the exact proportion, because criteria for the diagnosis of syphilitic tissue reaction vary considerably between different pathologists, and *T. pallidum* is difficult to find in the late stages of the disease.

INCIDENCE: RACE AND SEX

The incidence of various types of syphilis varies in the white and negro races. In negroes, cutaneous, osseous and cardiovascular lesions are commoner than in whites. The reverse is true of the incidence of neurosyphilis.

Syphilis often appears to be a milder disease in women. This may be due to the fact that pregnancy modifies the course of the disease. Women who become pregnant in the early stages of syphilis commonly lose the signs of infection and are likely to be spared the late serious effects. (See p. 104.)

METHODS OF DIAGNOSIS IN THE VARIOUS STAGES

Diagnosis depends on: 1. clinical history and examination; 2. dark-ground examination for *T. pallidum*; 3. blood tests for syphilis, that is (a) reagin tests and (b) specific tests; 4. tests of the cerebrospinal fluid; 5. radiological and other accessory methods.

Sometimes diagnosis can also be aided by examination and tests of the patient's family and of any known sex contacts.

Clinical Examination

The symptoms and signs of syphilis in its various stages will be described in the ensuing chapters. They are absent in the periods of latency.

Dark-ground Examination

Identification of the organism by this method is only possible in cases of early infectious syphilis when surface lesions are present on skin or mucous membrane, or at mucocutaneous junctions, or when accessible regional lymph nodes are enlarged in the primary, secondary and recurrent stages.

Blood Tests for Syphilis

REAGIN TESTS are either complement-fixation tests, such as the cardio-lipin Wassermann reaction (CWR), or flocculation tests, such as the VDRL (Venereal Disease Research Laboratory) slide test, the Rapid Plasma Reagin Test and the Automated Reagin Test. They are not specific and indicate the presence of an antibody-like substance called 'reagin' which may also be present with other diseases (see p. 133). The tests are negative in the incubation period and for a short period in the primary stage, but in most cases they are positive within 7 to 14 days after the appearance of the syphilitic chancre. Occasionally they remain negative for some weeks. The reagin tests are virtually always positive in the secondary and recurrent stages and in the early latent stage. They are also positive in the majority of cases in the late latent stage of the disease. It is open to question whether, with modern techniques, the tests are ever negative in the presence of active gummata, but in cases of late cardiovascular syphilis and late neuro-syphilis they are negative in a proportion of the cases (see p. 67 and p. 102).

SPECIFIC TESTS (see p. 137) include the *Treponema pallidum* immobiliza-tion (TPI) test, the fluorescent treponemal antibody (FTA) test, and the *Treponema pallidum* haemagglutination (TPHA) test in which virulent *T. pallidum* is used as antigen. These tests are usually negative at the begin-ning of the primary stage of syphilis; the FTA test tends to become positive early but the TPHA and TPI tests usually become positive later. The specific tests are positive in all stages of untreated late syphilis, with rare exceptions. The Reiter protein complement-fixation (RPCF) test, which employs an extract of cultivable treponemata sharing a common antigenic component with *T. pallidum*, is only group specific and therefore less reliable as a con-firmatory test.

Tests of Cerebrospinal Fluid

These are essential to the diagnosis and exclusion of neurosyphilis. They are described in the section on that subject (see p. 81).

Radiological Methods

These methods are valuable in the diagnosis of certain late manifestations of syphilis, and are described in the appropriate sections.

REFERENCES

1. STOKES, J. H., BEERMAN, H. and INGRAHAM, N. R. (1945) *Modern Clinical Syphilology*, 3rd ed., p. 1. Philadelphia and London: W. B. Saunders.

2. POWER, d'A. (1925) Hunterian Oration 'John Hunter: a Martyr to Science'. In: *Selected Writings*, 1877–1930, p. 1. Oxford: Clarendon Press, 1931.

3. QVIST, G. (1977) *Ann. R. Coll. Surg.*, **59**, 205.

4. WEIMERSKIRCH, P. J. and RICHTER, G. W. (1979) *Lancet*, **1**, 503.

5. MOORE, J. E. (1951) *Lancet*, **1**, 699.

6. *A.R. Med. Offr Dept Hlth* (Lond.) (1977) H.M.S.O. 1978.

7. *S.T.D. Statistical Letter* (1978) U.S. Department of Health, Education and Welfare, Public Health Service, Center for Disease Control, Atlanta, Georgia.

8. FLEMING, W. L., BROWN, W. J., DONOHUE, J. F. and BRANIGAN, P. W. (1970) *J. Am. med. Ass.*, **211**, 1827.

9. British Cooperative Clinical Group (1973) *Br. J. vener. Dis.*, **49**, 329.

10. WILLCOX, R. R. and GUTHE, T. (1966) *Treponema pallidum. Bull. Wld Hlth Org.*, Suppl. 35.

11. OVČINNIKOV, N. M. and DELEKTORSKIJ, V. V. (1966) *Bull. Wld Hlth Org.*, **35**, 223.

12. OVČINNIKOV, N. M. and DELEKTORSKIJ, V. V. (1968) *Br. J. vener. Dis.*, **44**, 1.

13. TURNER, T. B. and HOLLANDER, D. H. (1957) *Biology of the Treponematoses*. Geneva: Wld Hlth Org. Monogr. Ser., **35**, 42.

14. WILKINSON, A. E. and COWELL, L. P. (1971) *Br. J. vener. Dis.*, **47**, 252.

15. JAKUBOWSKI, A. and MANIKOWSKA-LESINSKA, W. (1970). *Br. J. vener. Dis.*, **46**, 383.

16. LEVENE, G. M., TURK, J. L., WRIGHT, D. J. M. and GRIMBLE, A. G. S. (1969) *Lancet*, **2**, 246.

17. WRIGHT, D. J. M. and GRIMBLE, A. S. (1974) *Br. J. vener. Dis.*, **50**, 45.

18. PAVIA, C. S., FOLDS, J. D. and BASEMAN, J. B. (1978) *Br. J. vener. Dis.*, **54**, 144.

19. AZAR, H. A., PHAM, J. D. and KURBAN, A. K. (1970) *Archs Path.*, **90**, 143.

20. GJESTLAND, T. (1955) *Acta derm.-vener.* (Stockh.), **35**, Suppl. 34.

2

Early Acquired Syphilis

Syphilis is an extremely variable disease and clinical description of its different stages can only cover the likely course in the majority of cases.

The incubation period may vary between 10 and 90 days, the usual time being two to four weeks. The local tissue reaction to the inoculation of treponemes is termed the *primary stage* and usually lasts for from three to eight weeks.

Six to eight weeks after the beginning of the primary stage the first symptoms and signs of the *secondary stage* may appear; but sometimes they appear sooner, and occasionally they are delayed, even for a year or more. They result from the general tissue reaction to the dissemination of treponemes, and manifestations are apt to come and go over periods varying from three to nine months. It should be emphasized, however, that both the primary and secondary stages may be so inconspicuous and so transient that they are not noticed by the patient. About 25 per cent of patients diagnosed in the secondary stage give no history of a primary lesion and show no signs of it. In some cases the absence of history may be due to the fact that the primary lesion is hidden from sight, an occurrence common with women.

When the signs of the secondary stage have gone the patient has reached the *early latent stage*, which may persist up to the end of the second year of infection. At this time there are no symptoms or signs of infection, which nevertheless is still present in the tissues.

In some cases, in the absence of treatment or if treatment is inadequate, the disease undergoes a *recurrent phase*, in which reappearance of lesions of the secondary type may alternate with periods of latency. Recurrences of this kind do not usually occur after the end of the second year of infection. Surface infection is likely to be contagious in the primary, secondary and recurrent stages.

PRIMARY SYPHILIS

In most cases the initial lesion is single, but sometimes multiple syphilitic chancres are seen, appearing simultaneously or within a few days of each other. The lesion begins as a dull-red macule which becomes papular. The papule varies in size, but is commonly about the size of a pea. The surface soon becomes eroded, giving rise to an ulcer which is rounded, regular and clearly defined in outline. The floor consists of dull-red, clean-looking granulation tissue which may be covered by a thin pellicle of yellowish slough or a greyish scab due to dried secretion. Occasionally the scab contains altered blood and may then be black or dark red in colour. On palpation, the base can be felt to be indurated, sometimes to the extent that it feels like a button in the tissue, but induration is not invariable. Manipulation of the ulcer or friction of its surfaces produces serous exudate, usually without blood. The exudate contains numerous treponemes and is very infectious.

The syphilitic chancre is indolent, taking a slow course and healing spontaneously, if untreated, in three to ten weeks. It leaves a thin, atrophic scar which may be very inconspicuous and may well be missed in later examinations. The lesion is practically painless, unless secondary pyogenic infection has occurred, in which case both the sore and the regional lymph nodes may become tender. Considerable firm oedema of the tissues in the proximity of a primary chancre is not uncommon, but there are no signs of acute inflammation. In the majority of cases the regional lymph nodes become enlarged within a week of the appearance of the primary sore. They are discrete, painless and of a firm, rubbery consistency. With syphilitic chancres on the genitalia, enlargement is often bilateral but with extra-genital lesions it may be unilateral.

The primary stage is likely to be absent in cases of infection resulting from deep inoculation of treponemes, as from puncture wounds with needles or blood transfusion with infected blood. This is sometimes called 'syphilis d'emblée'. The presenting signs and symptoms are those of the secondary stage.

Most syphilitic chancres occur on the genitalia; extragenital lesions are found on the lip, the tongue, the tonsils, the finger, the eyelid, the nipple—a common hazard in the days when wet nurses were employed—the anus and anal canal, or on any part of the surface of skin or mucous membrane. Anal chancres affecting passive homosexuals have been seen more often in recent years. In each site extragenital lesions may present difficulties in diagnosis, which will be discussed later.

Males

In males, the syphilitic chancre may occur on any part of the external genitalia (Plate I i and Figs. 3–9). The commonest site is the coronal sulcus

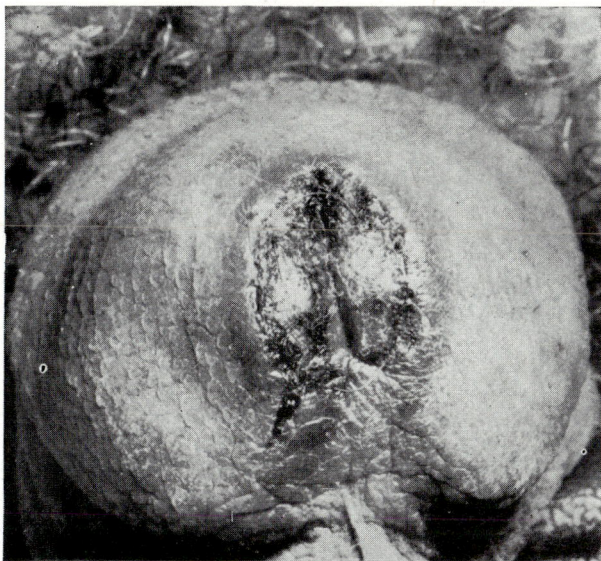

Fig. 3. Meatal syphilitic chancre in a male.

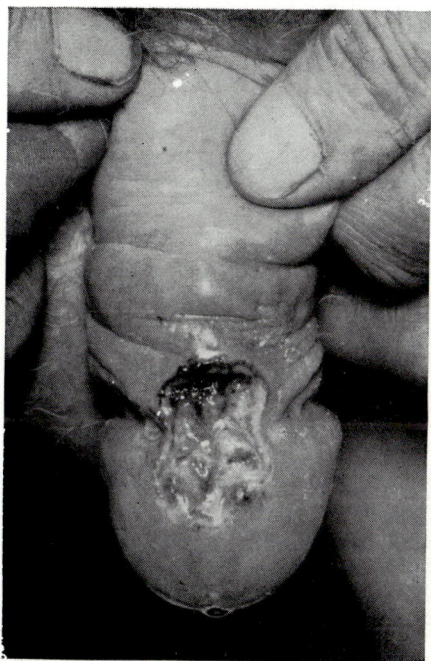

Fig. 4. Frenal syphilitic chancre with contact lesion on glans.

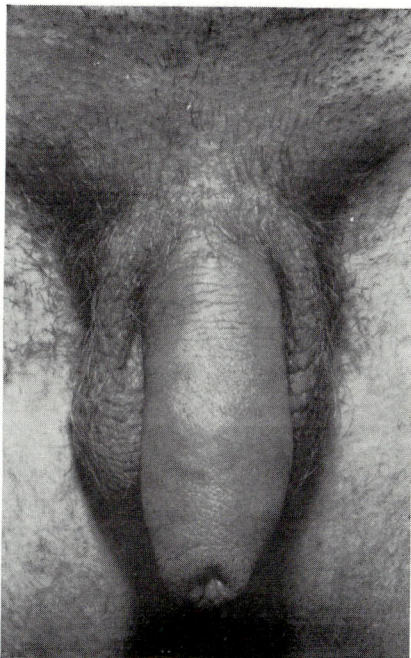

Fig. 5. Concealed syphilitic chancre with oedema of prepuce and enlarged inguinal nodes.

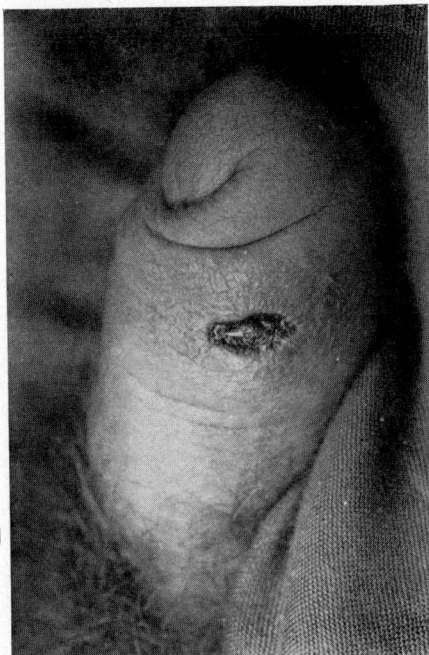
Fig. 6. Syphilitic chancre on external surface of the prepuce with oedema.

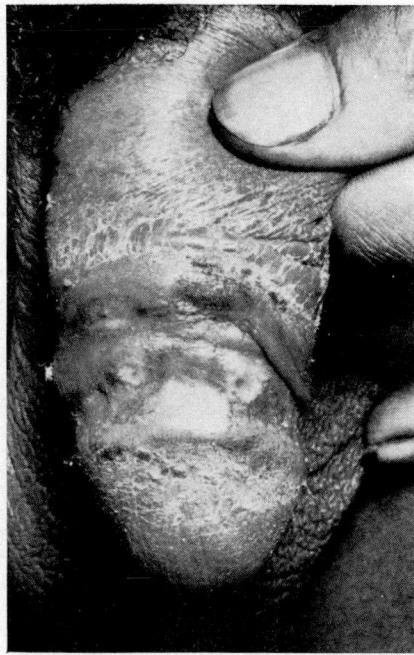
Fig. 7. Multiple syphilitic chancres.

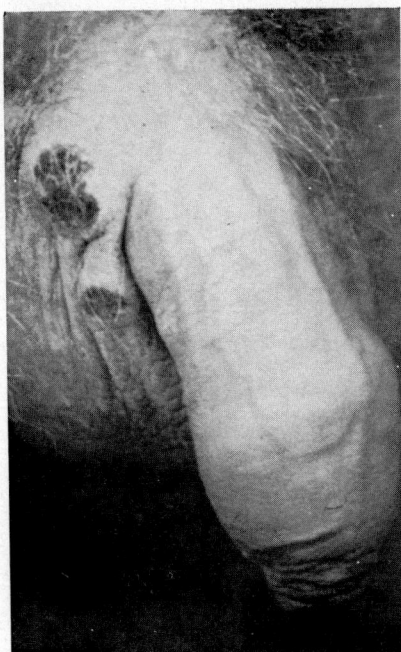
Fig. 8. Syphilitic chancres near root of penis ('condom chancres').

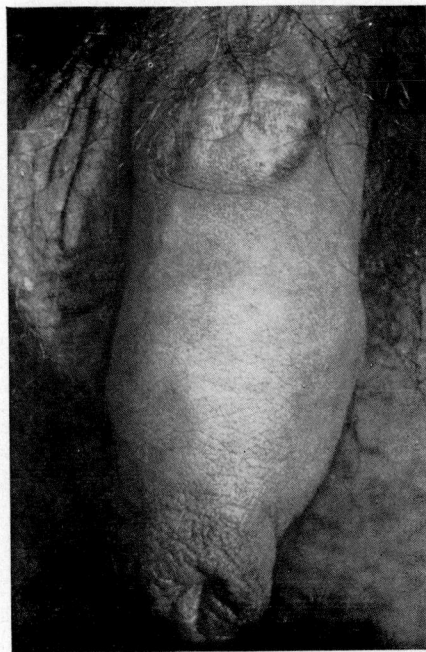
Fig. 9. Scar of syphilitic chancre on shaft of penis.

of the penis, but the glans penis, the prepuce, the frenum of the prepuce, the external urinary meatus or the skin of the shaft of the penis may be involved. Syphilitic chancre of the mucous surface of the prepuce often causes 'button' induration, so that on retraction the area flaps back in characteristic fashion, rather like the tarsal plate when the upper eyelid is turned backwards. The primary lesion may occur inside the urethra, the so-called intrameatal chancre, of which the only symptom may be scanty serous urethral discharge; the clinical diagnosis may be suggested by palpation or be evident on urethroscopy. A syphilitic chancre occurring under the prepuce may give rise to balanoposthitis with oedema and phimosis. In some cases in which the skin of the proximal shaft of the penis or of the pubes or groins is involved, the distal part of the penis may have been protected by a condom during sexual intercourse.

Females

Primary chancres in women may occur on the labium majus or minus, at the fourchette, on the clitoris, or near the urethral orifice; they may also be found on the cervix uteri or, rarely, on the vaginal wall (Plate I ii and Figs. 10–13). Syphilitic chancres on the vulva may be associated with considerable oedema of the labia, and this may be unilateral. During pregnancy the lesions may be larger and more indurated on account of the increased vascularity of the parts.

Diagnosis

Diagnosis is made by a combination of clinical and laboratory examinations but never on clinical evidence alone. In cases of primary syphilis the most certain method is by identifying *Treponema pallidum* in serous exudate from the ulcer by dark-ground examination. If negative at first, dark-ground examinations should be repeated daily for at least three consecutive days, and it may be necessary to search for a longer period. During the period of investigation the lesion should be bathed frequently in warm saline solution. In cases in which an antibiotic or other antiseptic lotion or cream has been applied, or in which the sore is healing or is hidden in the terminal portion of the urethra or under a phimotic prepuce, diagnostic puncture of lymphatic nodes is particularly useful. By this technique o·1 ml of sterile, normal saline is injected into an enlarged regional lymphatic node. The node is steadied between finger and thumb with the skin stretched over it. A hypodermic needle attached to a small syringe containing the saline is introduced through the skin along the long axis of the node and plunged well into its body. Movement of syringe and needle in various directions will confirm that the needle is in the correct position. The saline is then injected into the node and, after further movement of the needle to encourage flow of lymph, aspiration is performed. The fluid withdrawn is then examined by the dark-ground method.

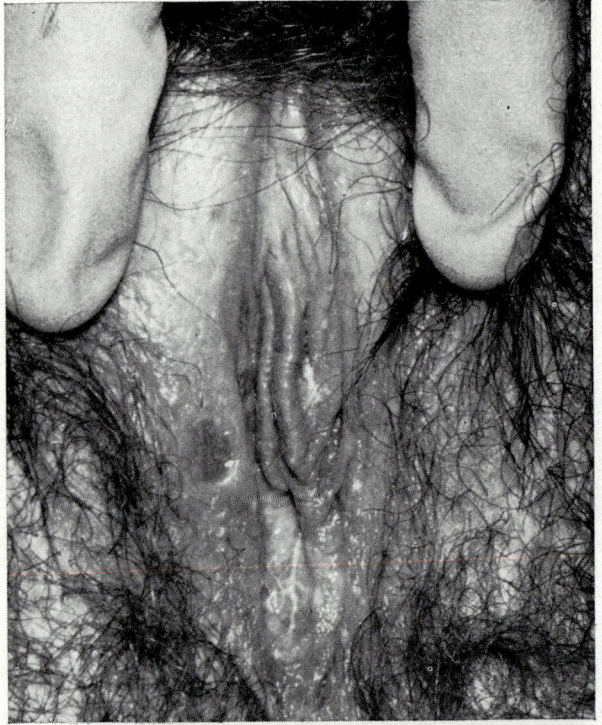

Fig. 10. Syphilitic
chancre of labium
majus.

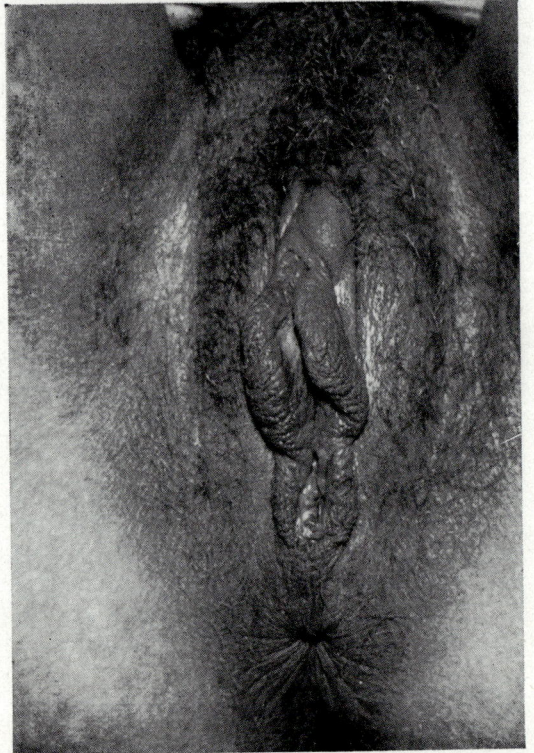

Fig. 11. Concealed
syphilitic chancre
causing oedema of the
labia minora.

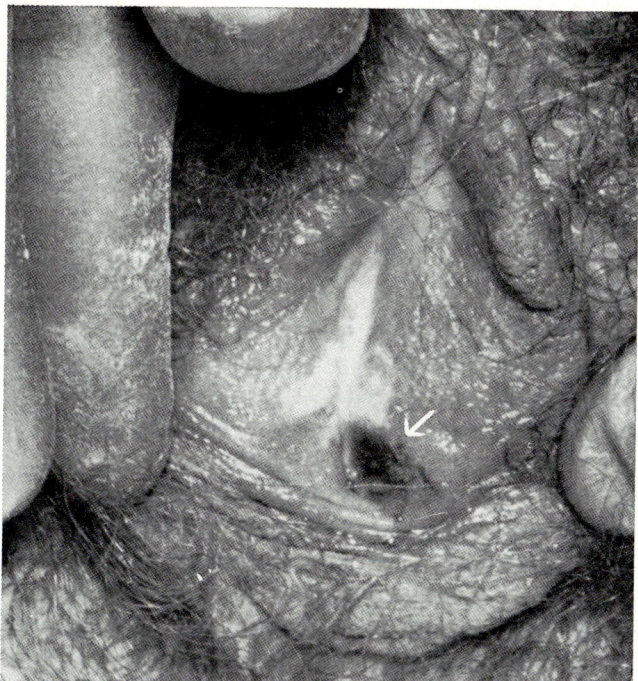

Fig. 12. Syphilitic chancre at the fourchette.

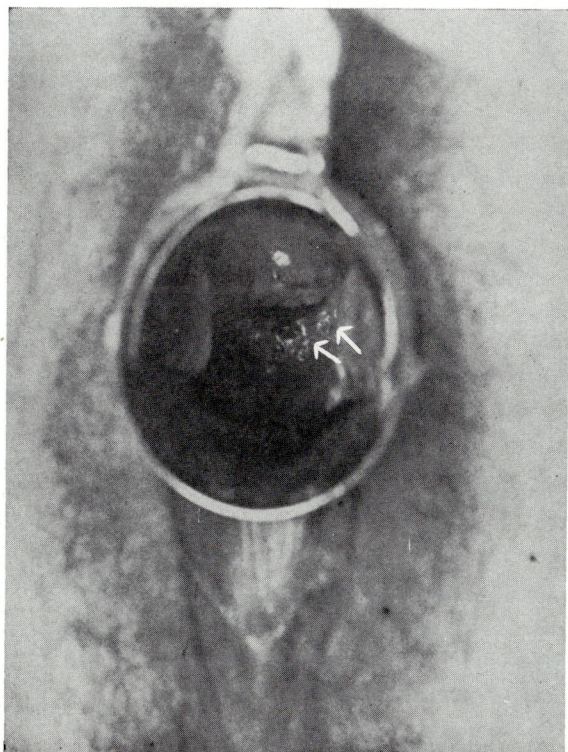

Fig. 13. Two syphilitic chancres on the cervix uteri seen through a speculum.

The value of the reagin tests in the diagnosis of primary syphilis is limited by the fact that the tests are likely to be negative in the early stages, or, if positive, the findings may be due to unrelated syphilis or some non-syphilitic cause. However, serological tests should always be done as a base line for further serological investigations. The fact that serological tests are at first negative but become positive on repetition is important evidence of primary syphilitic infection in the diagnosis of a suspected lesion. The FTA test is generally the first to become positive. One of the reagin tests should always be estimated quantitatively, as this information is useful for following the progress of the disease and for estimating the efficacy of treatment.

Differential Diagnosis

Genital Syphilitic Chancres

Lesions occurring on the genitalia which may be mistaken for primary syphilis include chancroid (soft sore), the ruptured vesicles of herpes genitalis, erosive balanitis, scabies with secondary infection, moist lesions of secondary syphilis, gummatous ulceration, and epitheliomata. Lympho-granuloma venereum, Behçet's disease, tuberculosis, herpes zoster involving the third sacral segment, granuloma inguinale, and traumatic ulcers may also occasionally have to be considered in the differential diagnosis. In temperate climates the incidence of chancroid is low, but in tropical and subtropical countries it is probably the main differential diagnosis. A full description of chancroidal ulceration is to be found on page 252, but the salient features are as follows: The lesions are usually painful, multiple, and destructive; they bleed easily and are not indurated; the inguinal lymphatic nodes, if involved, are enlarged, tender and matted together, with redness of the overlying skin. This inguinal swelling, often called the 'inflammatory bubo', is in contrast to the so-called 'indolent bubo' of primary syphilis. If untreated, the suppurative adenitis will break down and discharge pus, forming a chancroid in the groin. Dark-ground examinations are negative and serological tests for syphilis are likely to be so, unless the patient is also suffering from syphilis. The absence of induration helps to distinguish herpetic lesions, which are the commonest cause of genital ulceration in temperate climates. On close examination there may well be seen a collection of tiny ulcers representing the original group of vesicles. Cell culture from the lesions may identify herpesvirus. Scabies is likely to be associated with a history of nocturnal itching and other burrows may be found on the body in the typical distribution; a scraping from the genital lesions may demonstrate *Sarcoptes scabiei* or its ova. In all these cases, how-ever, it must be remembered that there may be a coincidental syphilitic infection, the initial lesion having afforded the necessary route of entry

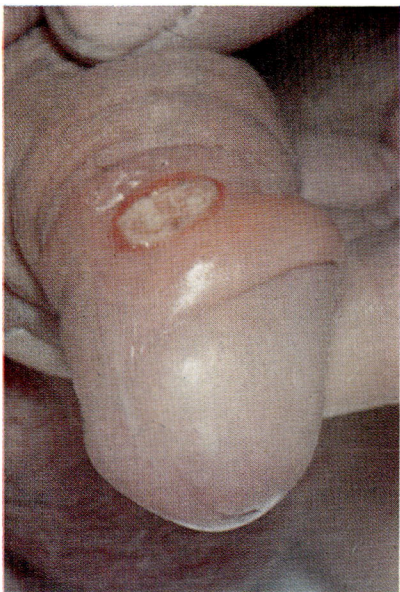

i Primary stage: typical penile chancre.

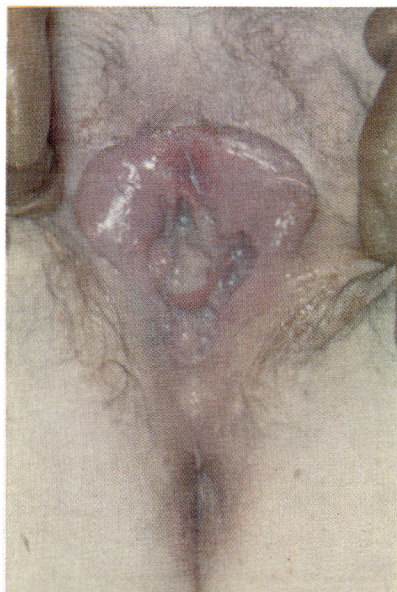

ii Primary stage: chancre at the urethral orifice, with chancroidal lesions below, in a female.

iii Secondary stage: roseolar macular rash on body, and primary chancre on lip.

iv Secondary stage: papular rash on body with some papulosquamous lesions.

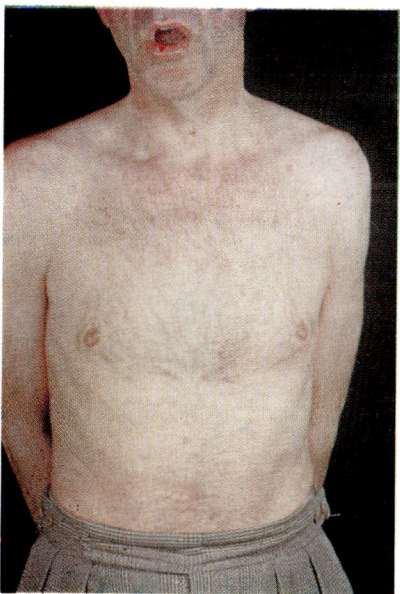

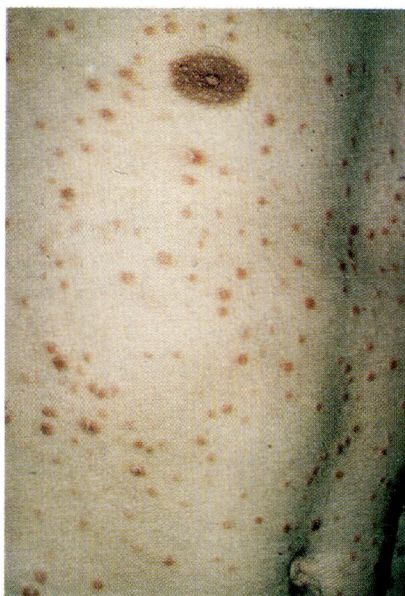

PLATE I: EARLY ACQUIRED SYPHILIS

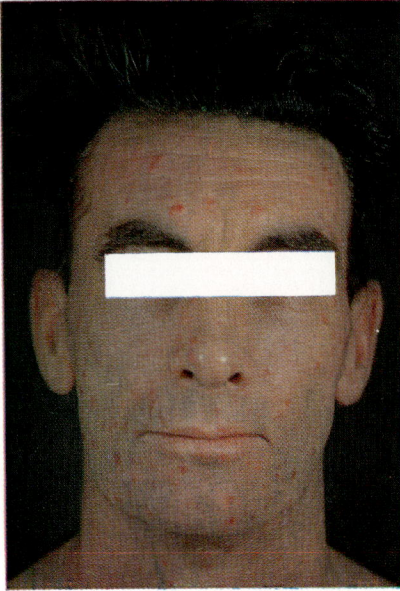

i Secondary stage: papular rash on face.

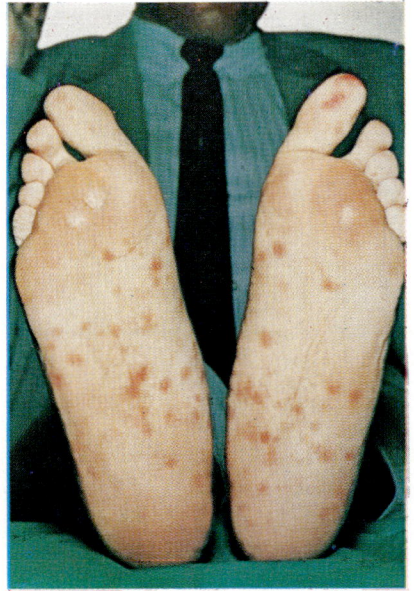

ii Secondary stage: plantar syphilide.

iii Secondary stage: mucous patch on
the upper lip.

iv Secondary stage: perianal and peri-
vulval condylomata lata.

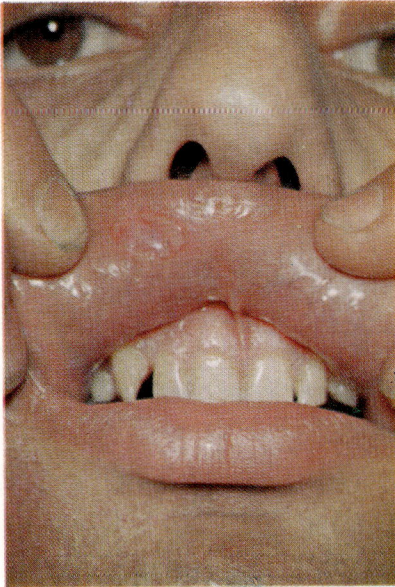

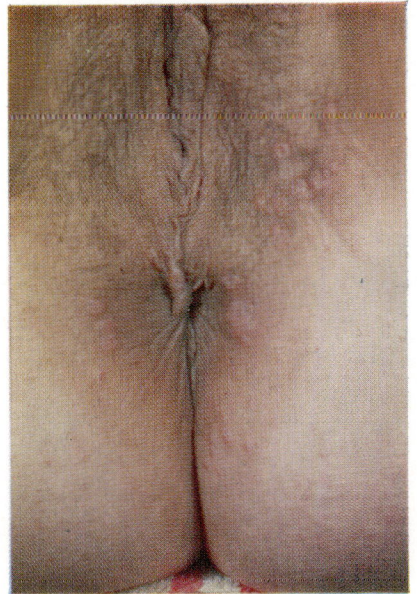

PLATE II: EARLY ACQUIRED SYPHILIS

for *Treponema pallidum*. Therefore, routine serological tests for syphilis should be carried out over a period of three months in all cases of genital sore.

In cases of secondary syphilis lesions are usually present elsewhere on the body. With gummatous ulceration of the genitalia the inguinal nodes are not involved, but serological tests for syphilis are positive; there may be other clinical evidence of late syphilis.

Epithelioma is more likely to be found in older patients. It has the typical raised, rolled, everted edge, and its mobility over the deeper tissues is likely to be impaired. The lesion may have been present for some time before advice is sought, and the hard enlargement of lymphatic nodes is a later development.

Extragenital Syphilitic Chancres (Plate I iii and Figs. 14–17)

A primary chancre of the lip or tongue must be differentiated from a mucous patch of secondary syphilis, from a gummatous lesion, an epithelioma, a primary tuberculous lesion, from herpes simplex with secondary pyogenic infection, from aphthous ulcers and from the oral ulceration of Behçet's syndrome. Primary syphilis of the tonsil might resemble Vincent's angina, diphtheria or lymphosarcoma. Syphilitic chancre of the nipple must be differentiated from Paget's disease. On the finger a primary chancre near the nail may be painful and may be mistaken for a simple paronychia. An epithelioma, sarcoma or anthrax pustule at this site rarely gives rise to difficulty in diagnosis. Syphilitic chancre of the eyelid must be distinguished from a stye. At the anal margin, a primary chancre may simulate a fissure, a thrombosed external pile, or Bowen's disease. The final diagnosis will rest on microscopical and serological findings and, if necessary, section after biopsy. Some difficulty may arise in the diagnosis of a lesion in the mouth or pharynx because certain treponemes, such as *T. microdentium*, are common saprophytes in the mouth; they may be found in the exudate and be mistaken for *Treponema pallidum*. Immunofluorescent staining for treponemes is helpful in these cases. Aspirate from puncture of regional lymphatic nodes may demonstrate *T. pallidum* by dark-ground examination; non-syphilitic treponemes are not found in these organs. If these examinations are negative, serological tests should be repeated frequently until the diagnosis is excluded by negative or confirmed by positive reactions. The early examination of the patient's sexual contacts may be of great value as an aid to diagnosis.

SECONDARY SYPHILIS

The interval between the appearance of the primary chancre and the onset of secondary manifestations is subject to variation, but is usually from

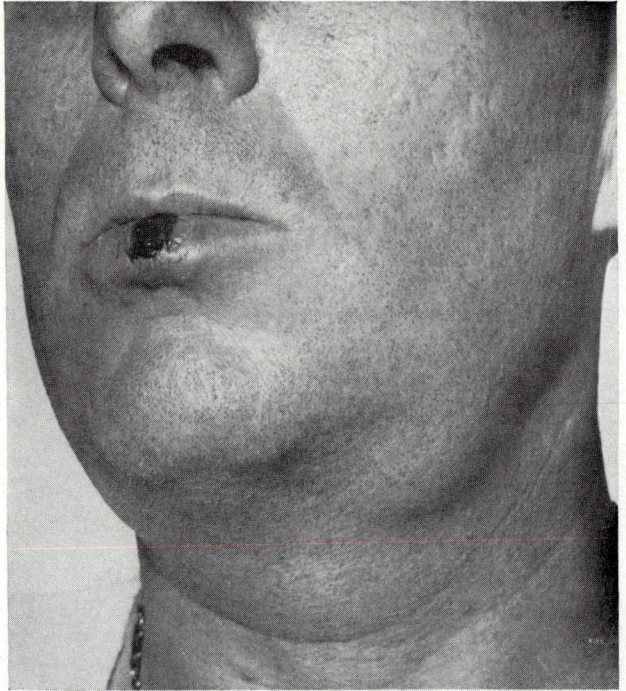

Fig. 14. Extragenital syphilitic chancre of the lip with enlargement of submaxillary nodes.

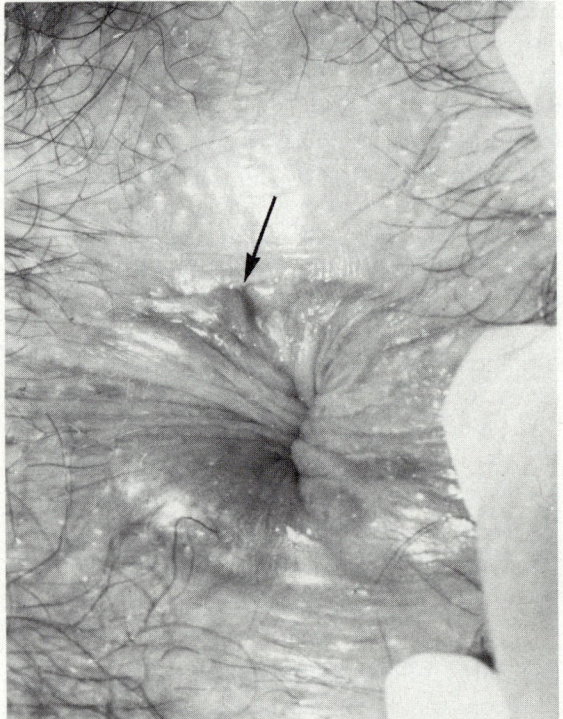

Fig. 15. Extragenital syphilitic chancre of the anus in a male passive homosexual.

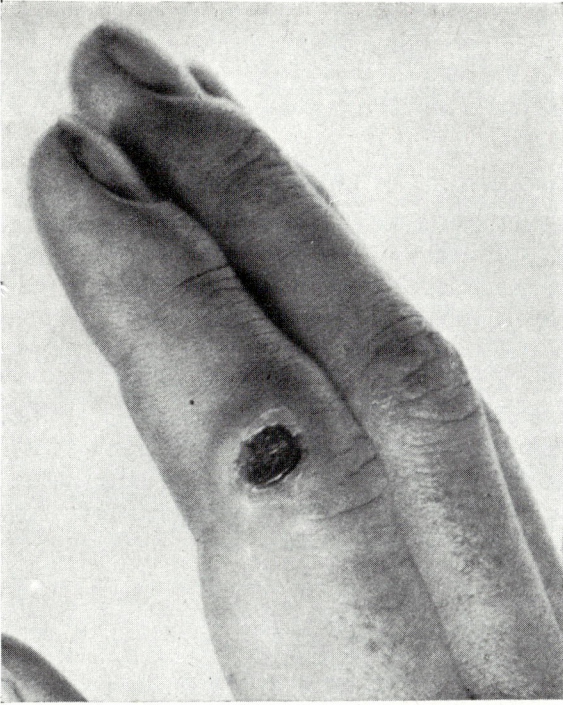

Fig. 16. Extragenital syphilitic chancre of a finger.

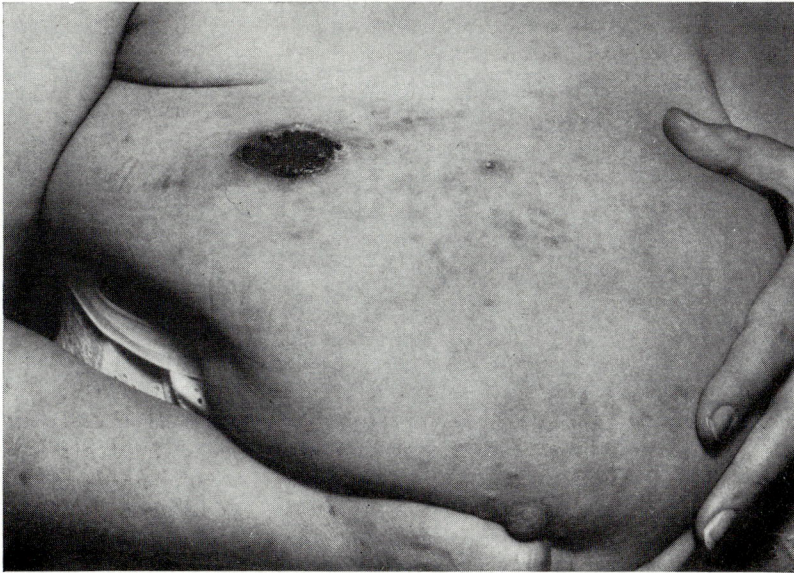

Fig. 17. Extragenital syphilitic chancre of the breast due to a bite.

six to eight weeks. In about a third of the cases the syphilitic chancre is still present and active when the secondary stage begins.

Constitutional Symptoms

These may precede or accompany the first signs of generalization. They may be slight or severe, but usually they are of moderate degree. There may be headache, malaise, anorexia and loss of weight. Low-grade fever is common and may be intermittent, continuous, or remittent. If there are lesions in the throat, the patient may complain of sore throat; if in the larynx, he may complain of hoarseness. There may be aching pain in the long bones, muscles and joints, and this may be worse at night. Waugh[1] has described the case of a patient who presented with persistent low backache as the first evidence of secondary syphilis. If the headache is severe and persistent it is most likely to be due to meningeal involvement. Patients may have noticed rashes on the skin, swelling of lymphatic nodes or other changes. Sometimes the initial complaint is of falling hair.

Signs

The signs of secondary syphilis are equally variable. Over three-quarters of the patients seen at this stage have lesions of the skin; about one-half have generalized enlargement of lymphatic nodes; about one-third have lesions of the mouth and throat; but less than one-tenth have lesions involving the osseous system, the nervous system, the eye or the abdominal viscera. Slight to moderate anaemia is fairly common.

Cutaneous lesions vary greatly and may resemble any generalized eruption which is not vesicular or bullous. Usually they do not irritate and are widespread and symmetrically disposed. The spots are rounded in outline and dull red in colour; they are more thickly distributed on flexor surfaces. Different types of spots are usually present in the same patient at the same time (polymorphism). The eruptions are usually indolent and may persist for weeks or months if untreated. On the other hand, in some cases, rashes may be inconspicuous and transient; often patients found to be suffering from late syphilis give no history of an illness resembling secondary syphilis. The rash may only become apparent as a manifestation of the Jarisch–Herxheimer reaction, which occurs within a few hours of the commencement of treatment with penicillin (see p. 158). The leucocyte count may be moderately raised with an increase in the lymphocytes. The erythrocyte sedimentation rate is usually raised, sometimes to over 100 mm in one hour (Westergren).

Types of Eruption

The eruptions of secondary syphilis can be divided into four main groups: a. macular or roseolar, b. papular, c. papulosquamous, and d. 'pustular'.

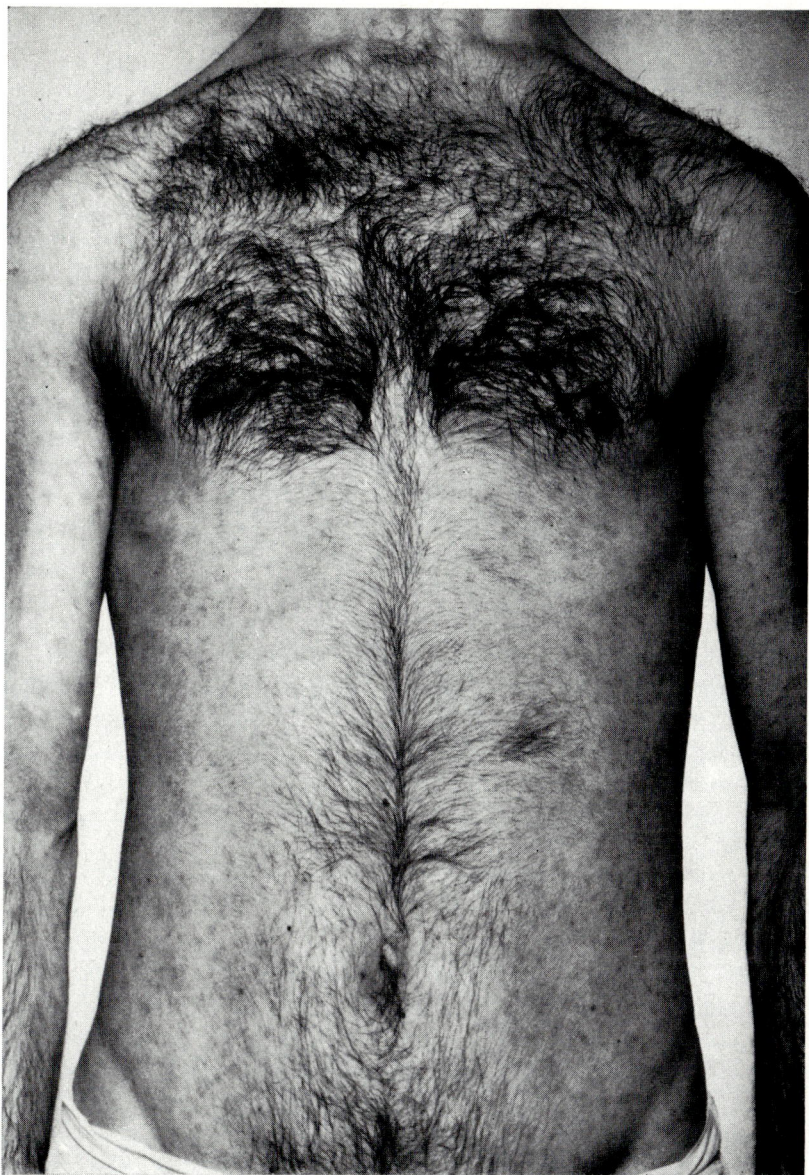

Fig. 18. Secondary stage: roseolar macular rash on body.

Macular or Roseolar Syphilide

The macular or roseolar syphilide (Plate I iii and Fig. 18) is usually the first
eruption to appear. The spots are rose-pink in colour, rounded in outline,
discrete, and 0·5–1 cm in diameter. As the name implies they are within
the skin and do not project above the skin. They are found chiefly on the
shoulders, chest, back, abdomen and flexor surfaces of the upper arms. The
colour may be so delicate as to be invisible in artificial light. The eruption
appears to be the first local reaction to the presence of *T. pallidum* in the
skin and the colour is due to engorgement of blood vessels without cellular
infiltration. On pressure with a glass slide the pink colour disappears. The
rash may last only for a few days and may be sparsely distributed. Occasionally it persists, changes colour, and develops into a papular syphilide.

Papular Syphilide

The papular syphilide (Plate I iv; Plate II i and ii; Fig. 19) is the commonest
and most characteristic of the secondary syphilitic eruptions. It consists
of dull-red papules which may be a quarter to one centimetre in diameter,
although lesions of the smaller size are more common. The papules are
rounded in outline, discrete and symmetrically distributed. Characteristically they are widely distributed over trunk, arms and legs, and are found on
the palms, soles, face and genitals. Sometimes a line of papules is seen on
the forehead, just below the hair line, and has been called the corona veneris.
On palpation with the finger tips the papules give a sense of localized induration in the skin. The rash is usually polymorphic, showing dull-red macules
and papules surmounted by scales. These are different stages of the same
process, but the rash is called by the name of the lesion which predominates.

Round the anus, between the buttocks, on the lateral surfaces of scrotum
and vulva (Plate II iv and Fig. 30), on the inner aspects of the upper thigh,
and in other warm and moist areas of the body where skin surfaces are
opposed, the papular lesions often become large and prominent, forming
fleshy-looking masses, rounded in outline, with broad bases and flat tops.
These are the 'broad condylomata', condylomata lata or 'syphilitic moist
papules'. They are dull red or dull pink in colour, but the surfaces may
become greyish-white due to necrosis. The surface slough is shed, leaving
a dull-red, eroded surface which oozes serum packed with treponemes.
They are the most infectious lesions of syphilis. They are occasionally found
in the axilla, under pendulous breasts, around the umbilicus and between
the outer toes. Because they are lesions of some size in a restricted area
they may become confluent. They are often seen independently of a skin rash.
Sometimes, especially on the skin of the face, dry papules may appear in
rings; central regression of a large papule may also give a ring formation.
These are called 'annular syphilides' (Fig. 25). The so-called follicular
syphilides consist of pointed, papular lesions related to hair follicles; close
inspection will reveal a hair protruding from the point of the papule. They

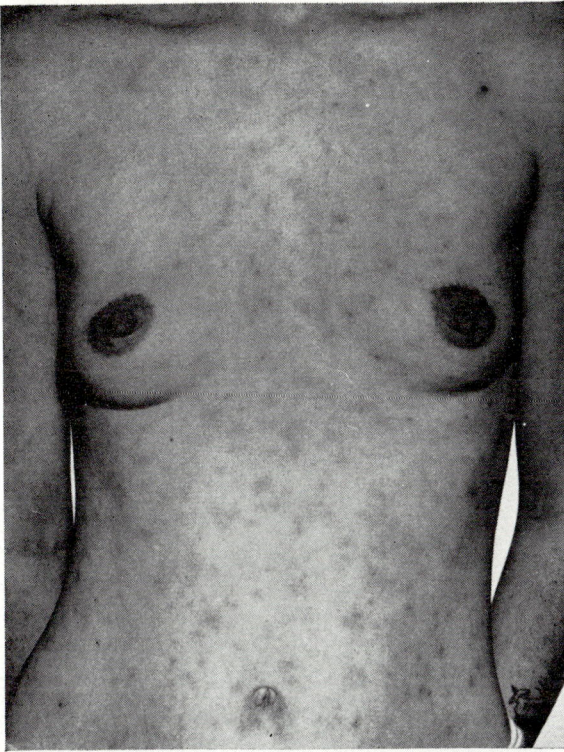

Fig. 19. Secondary stage: papular rash on body.

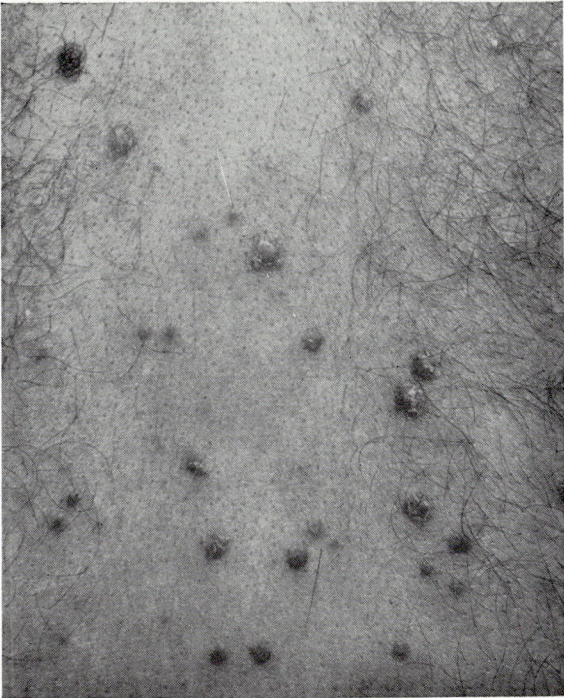

Fig. 20. Secondary stage: close-up view of papulosquamous rash.

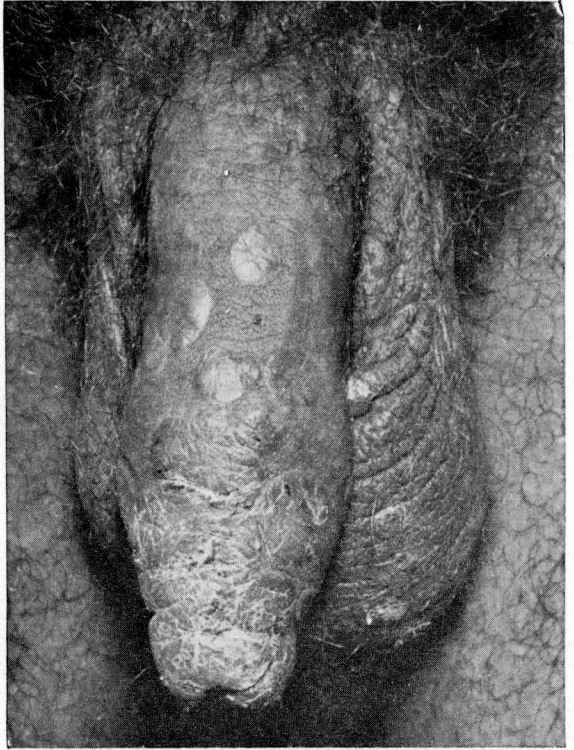

Fig. 21. Secondary stage: psoriasiform rash on the genitals.

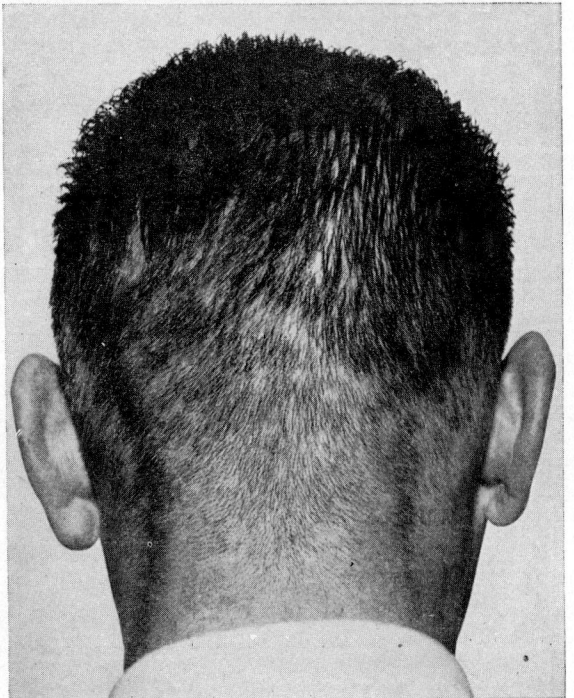

Fig. 22. Secondary stage: follicular rash of scalp with alopecia in a male.

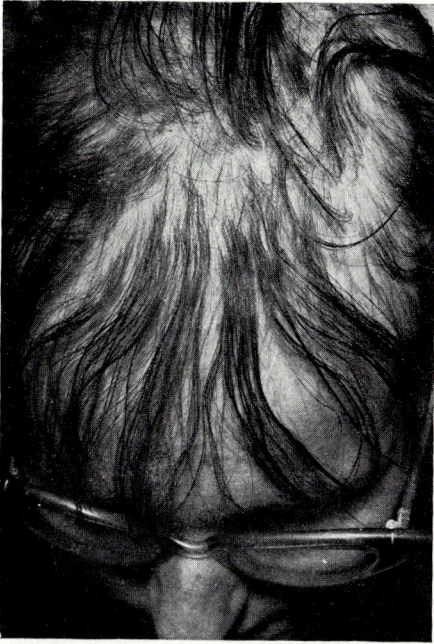

Fig. 23. Secondary stage: follicular rash of scalp with alopecia in a female.

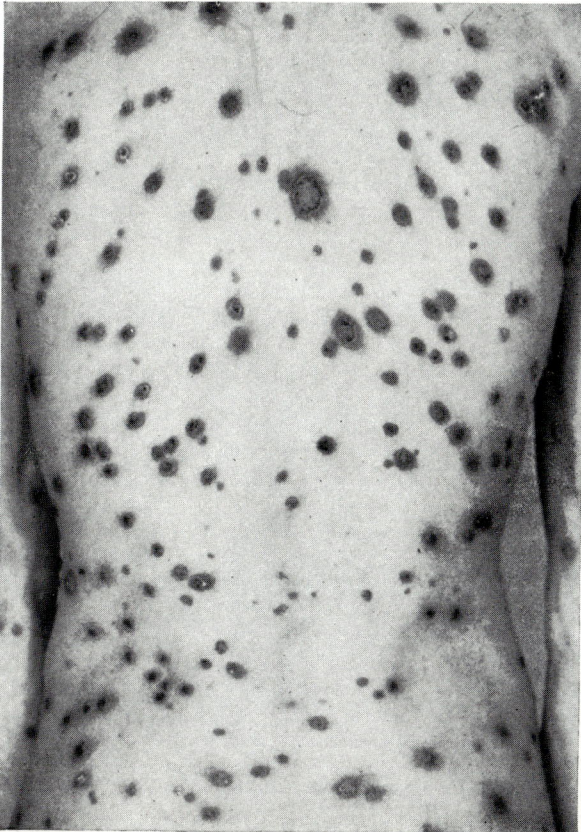

Fig. 24. Secondary stage: 'pustular' rash of body.

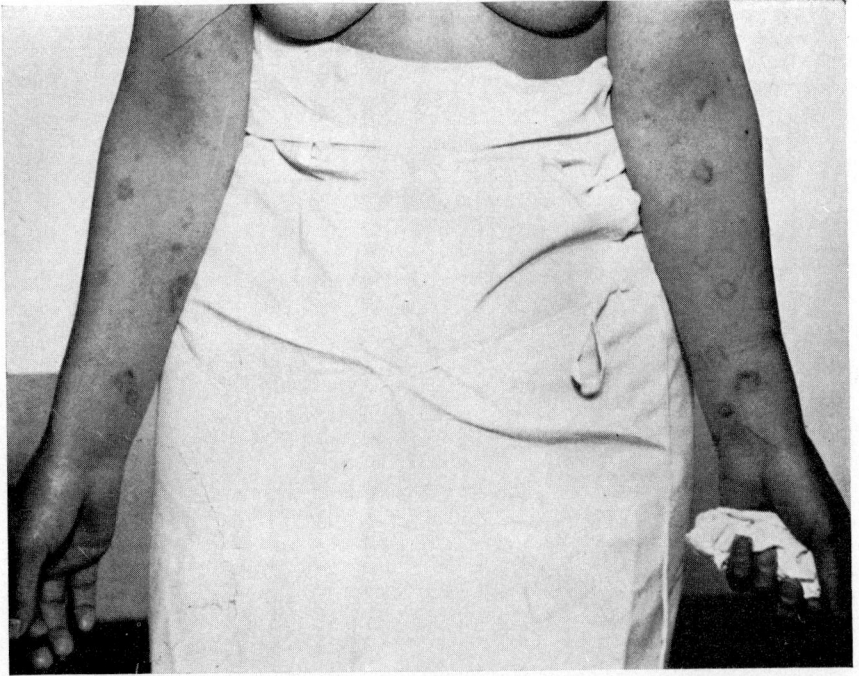

Fig. 25. Secondary stage: annular papular rash on forearms.

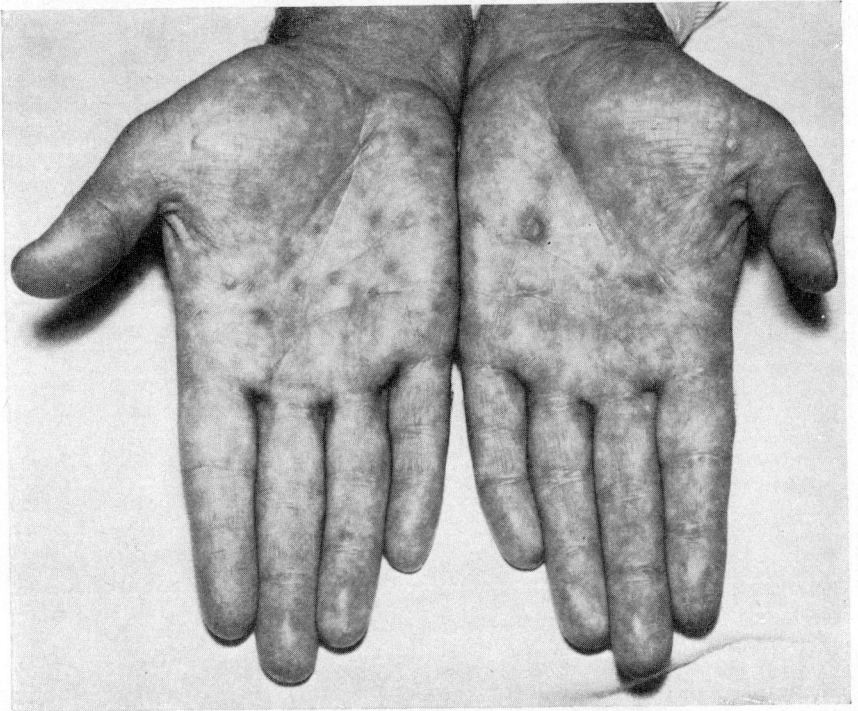

Fig. 26. Secondary stage: palmar syphilide.

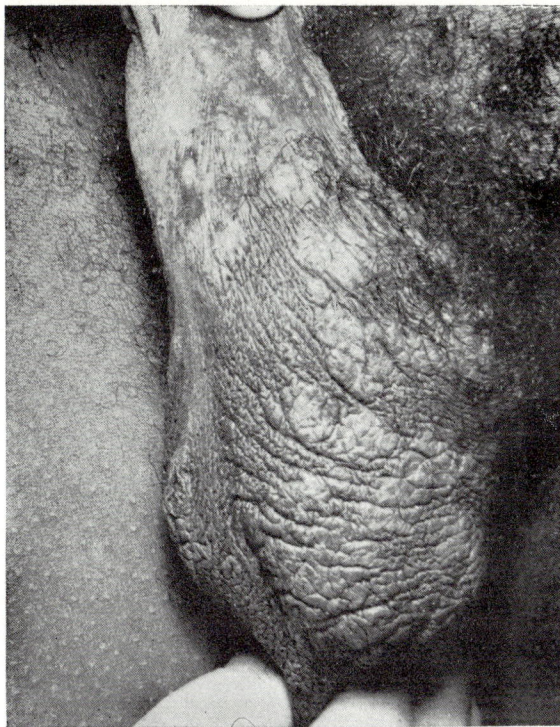

Fig. 27. Secondary
stage: papulo-
squamous rash on
scrotum.

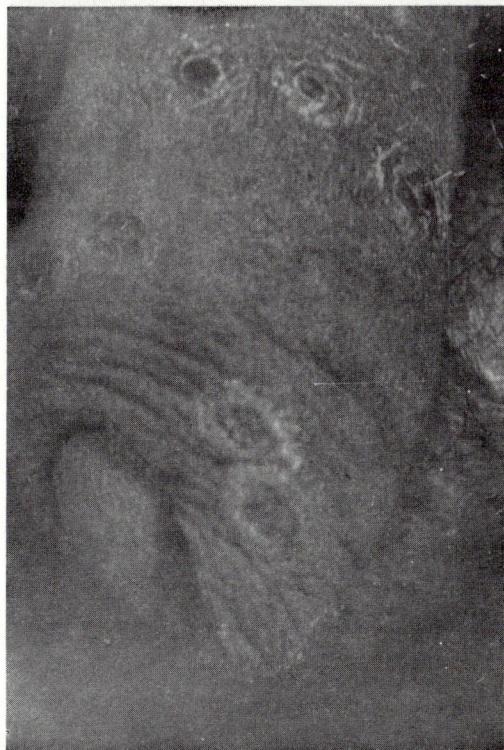

Fig. 28. Secondary
stage: papulosquamous
rash on penis.

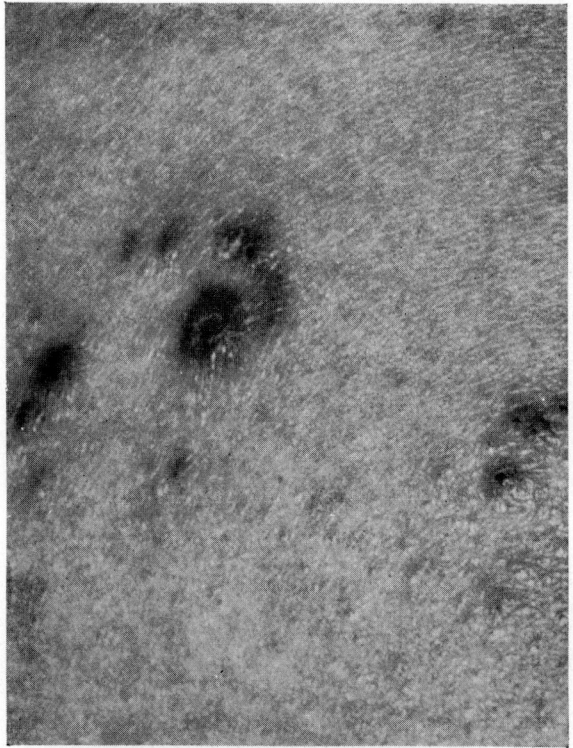

Fig. 29. Secondary stage: corymbose rash.

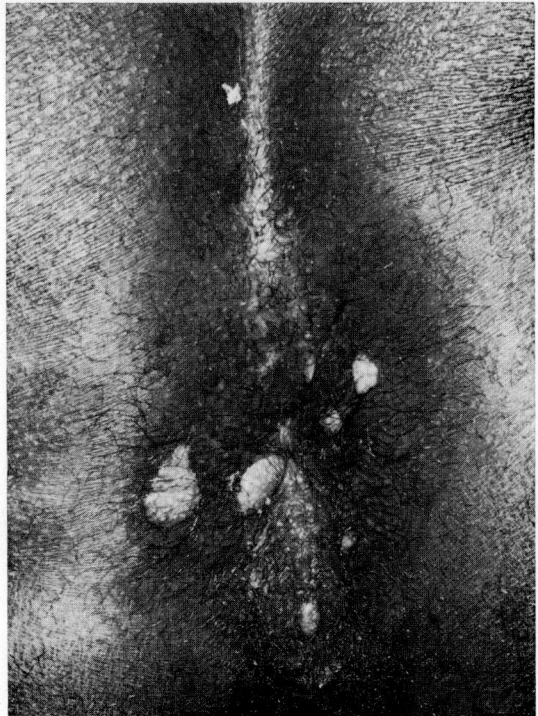

Fig. 30. Secondary stage: perianal condylomata lata in a coloured male.

are common on the scalp where they cause shedding of the hair, with patchy irregular thinning at the sides and back of the head, so-called syphilitic alopecia (Figs. 22 and 23). The eyebrows, eyelashes and beard may also be involved. Follicular lesions occur occasionally on the hairy areas of the trunk, appearing in small clusters of minute dull-red pointed papules. When present they are nearly always on pigmented skins. They may give rise to considerable itching which may mislead the clinician. On the palms and soles, the papular lesions remain flat or only slightly raised because of the tough, horny character of the overlying epithelium. They vary in size from 0·5 to 1 cm in diameter and the surface is apt to show scaling, leaving collars of loosened epithelium surrounding shining papules. In the later secondary stage papular eruptions may recur, but the papules are likely to be fewer in number and asymmetrically disposed. A common form, the 'corymbose syphilide' (Fig. 29), appears as one or a few groups of papules with a large central papule surrounded by smaller satellite papules. It has been likened to the appearance of a large raindrop falling on a pavement and giving rise to secondary splashes around the central patch. The nail beds may be involved, especially in the later secondary stage. The nail becomes brittle and lustreless and is shed; the newly growing nail may be deformed.

The Papulosquamous Syphilide

Scaling of the surfaces of the papules is common, and crusted lesions are usually to be seen among the papules of the papular syphilide. When scaling lesions predominate, the rash is called the papulosquamous syphilide (Plate I iv; Figs. 20, 27 and 28). Sometimes the spots are large and plaque-like with considerable waxy scaling on the surface. These may resemble the crusted lesions of psoriasis and have then been called the 'psoriasiform secondary syphilide' (Fig. 21).

The 'Pustular' Syphilide

As the result of endarteritis obliterans and diminution of blood supply, the lesions (Fig. 24) undergo central necrosis, which extends deep into the papule, and present with a central core of necrotic tissue which may resemble a pustule. Occasional 'pustular' lesions may sometimes be seen among the spots of the papular and papulosquamous syphilide, but multiple lesions with a varioliform distribution are now extremely rare in developed countries. This type of syphilide is believed to occur in under-nourished patients or those with other debilitating disease such as diabetes or chronic nephritis. 'Pustular' lesions may be associated with extensive indolent necrosis of tissue, giving rise to limpet-like crusts which may be discoloured with altered blood. These were called 'rupia' and they were most often seen on the face. A rare form of destructive syphilide, with deeply ulcerating lesions and severe toxaemia which may end in death, is described in the literature[2] under the name of 'malignant syphilis'. It brings to mind descriptions of the first outbreak of syphilis in Europe in the fifteenth century.

Pigmentation and Depigmentation

The surface lesions of secondary syphilis usually heal without evident scarring. As the papules resolve they leave faintly pigmented areas which fade gradually but atrophic macules may persist, especially in dark-skinned races. The condition, known as leucoderma colli or 'collar of Venus', is a residual depigmentation of the skin of the neck (Fig. 35) which is found particularly in dark-haired people, usually women, who have suffered from secondary syphilis. A zone of pigmentation is normally present, extending from the hair margin of the neck to the shoulders. If such a patient has had a well-marked roseolar syphilide, rounded areas of depigmentation, one-half to one centimetre in diameter, may be found in this zone. This depigmentation persists for life and may therefore be found in patients with late syphilis.

Lesions of Mucous Membranes

Mucous membranes, particularly those of the soft palate, the pharynx and the larynx, may show dull-red erythema; but the characteristic lesion is the so-called 'mucous patch' (Plate II iii and Figs. 31–33). These patches appear at the same time as the papular syphilide and may be found on the mucous surfaces of the lips, cheeks, tongue, fauces and palate, the tonsillar beds, the pharynx or the larynx. The lesion is usually a rounded, greyish-white patch edged by a dull-red areola. The greyish-white appearance is due to necrotic tissue. On the pillars of the fauces or elsewhere the lesions may become confluent, presenting as an area with serpiginous outline from which the slough soon separates leaving an erosion which is sometimes called the 'snail-track ulcer'. On the tonsil the mucous patch may ulcerate deeply. If a lesion of this kind appears at the angle of the mouth it becomes fissured. On the dorsum of the tongue the mucous patch appears as a rounded, dull-pink, smooth area where the filiform papillae have been destroyed by the necrotic process. Mucous patches may be found in the nose, on the septum or the floor. In the larynx they occur chiefly on the epiglottis and the aryepiglottidean folds and tend to become eroded and ulcerated. The process is likely to extend to the vocal cords, with redness and oedema, causing the husky voice which may be found in patients suffering from secondary syphilis (syphilitic laryngitis). Mucous patches also occur on the genital mucous membranes, including those of the vulva, the vaginal outlet, the posterior commissure, the cervix, and the glans penis, and on the mucous surface of the prepuce. They are usually eroded and appear sharply defined against the background of normal mucous membrane. They are sometimes

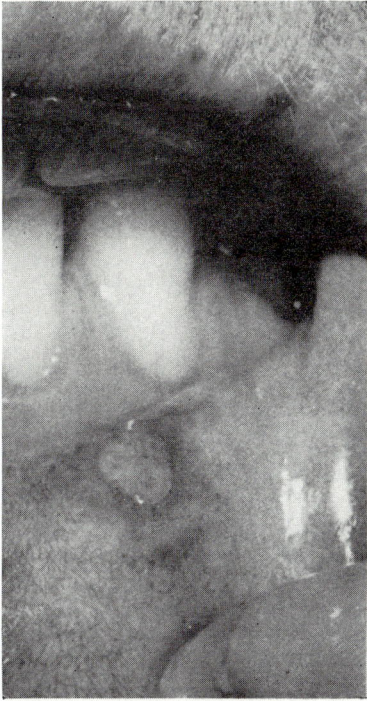

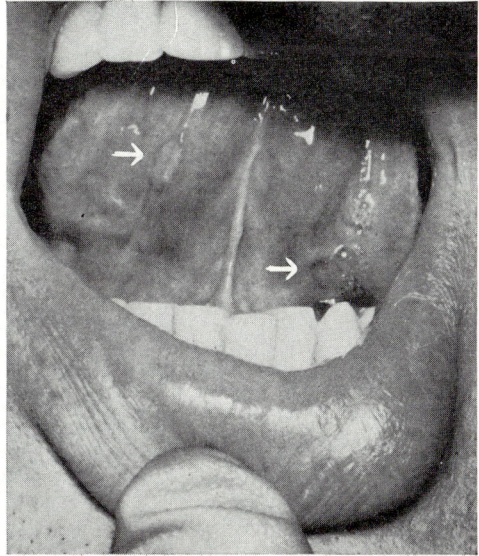

Fig. 32. Secondary stage: mucous patch
under the tongue.

Fig. 31 (*above*). Secondary stage: mucous patch on lower lip.

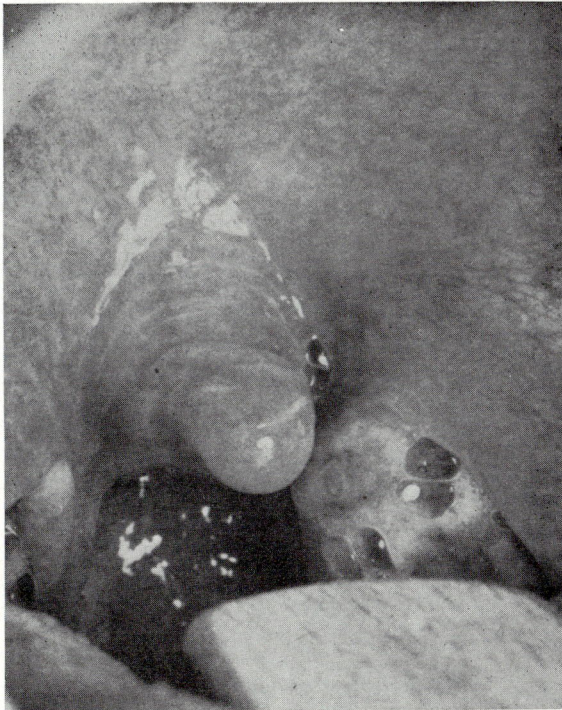

Fig. 33. Secondary stage:
mucous patches on left
tonsil.

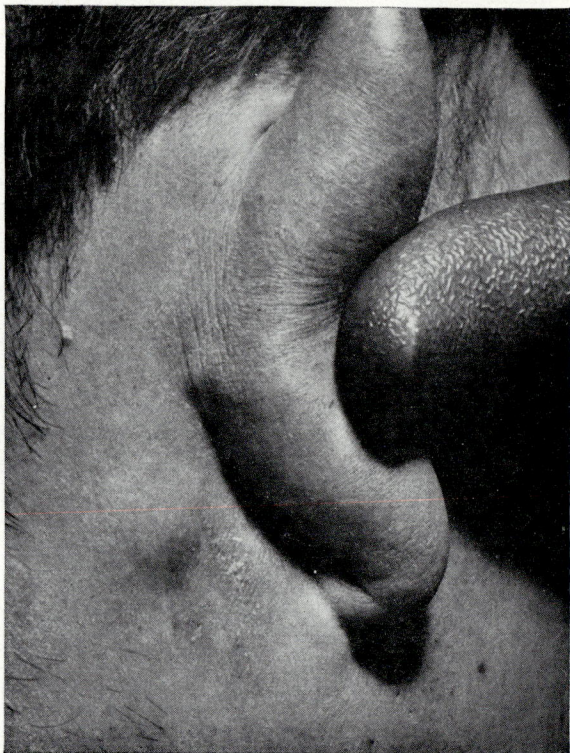

Fig. 34. Secondary stage: enlargement of post-auricular lymphatic node.

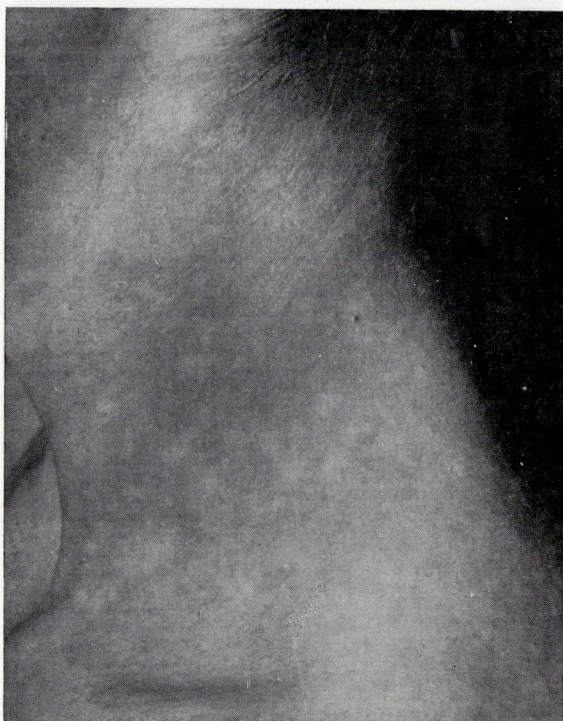

Fig. 35. Secondary stage: residual leucoderma of the neck ('collar of Venus').

called 'mucous erosions'. If other signs of secondary syphilis are absent or inconspicuous, they may be mistaken for syphilitic chancres.

Lesions of mucous membranes are usually painless unless there is super-added pyogenic infection. Patients sometimes complain of persistent 'sore throat', but on questioning it appears that discomfort is experienced and not pain. In the absence of treatment, mucous lesions are likely to persist for weeks, but occasionally they are transitory.

Recently a case has been described[3] of a practising homosexual man who presented with upper abdominal pain, vomiting and loss of weight. On gastroscopy ulcers were found in the distal stomach and motile *Treponema pallidum* were identified in biopsy material. There was no other evidence of secondary syphilis.

Lymphadenitis

Rubbery, discrete, non-tender enlargement of lymphatic nodes is common in the secondary stage of syphilis (Fig. 34). In addition to the inguinal nodes, those of the suboccipital region, the neck, the axilla and the epicondylar region may be found to be involved.

Uveitis and Choroido-retinitis

Anterior uveitis of one or both eyes occasionally occurs late in the course of secondary syphilis, but is more commonly seen during relapse of the early type. It may be differentiated from anterior uveitis due to other causes by the presence of lesions elsewhere and by prompt and satisfactory response to antisyphilitic treatment. Clinically silent anterior uveitis is, in fact, quite common in secondary syphilis.[4]

Acute choroido-retinitis[5] is rare but occasional cases have been reported.

Hepatitis

Hepatitis with jaundice and enlargement of the liver is occasionally found in the course of secondary syphilis. It has been regarded as a rare condition but within the last few years there have been several reports of cases,[6-9] suggesting that it is either becoming more common or more frequently recognized. The clinical picture is that of mild jaundice with moderate tender enlargement of the liver and other signs of secondary syphilis. Laboratory tests show a moderate elevation of serum bilirubin and glutamic oxaloacetic transaminase, with disproportionate elevation of alkaline phosphatase. Liver biopsy demonstrates atypical lesions unlike those attributed to hepatitis due to a virus or drugs or to extrahepatic biliary obstruction. The condition responds promptly to antisyphilitic treatment.

Nephrotic Syndrome

Several cases of nephrotic syndrome have been reported in recent years.[10-13] The renal lesions probably represent an immune deposit disease.

Very rarely haemorrhagic nephritis has occurred.[13] These conditions respond to antisyphilitic treatment.

Arthritis, Bursitis, and Periostitis

Joints and bursae are rarely affected in cases of secondary syphilis, but occasionally effusion occurs. Usually the result is swelling without pain or marked limitation of movement, but very rarely such lesions are painful, especially at night. Tendon sheaths may also be affected. Aching pains in the long bones, the so-called osteocopic pains, may be due to periostitis or to destructive lesions of the cortex. It is rare to find the objective signs of periostitis at this stage of the disease, but X-ray evidence of productive or destructive lesions has occasionally been described.

Neurological and Cardiac Involvement

Examination of the cerebrospinal fluid of patients with secondary syphilis has shown abnormalities in a proportion of the cases which has varied in different series. Cutler et al.[14] found positive reagin tests for syphilis in from 2 to 22·4 per cent of different groups of patients with secondary syphilis. However, it is not routine practice to examine the cerebrospinal fluid at this stage of the disease. The main abnormalities described have been increases in cells and protein; changes in the complement fixation and the colloidal-gold tests have been variable. Clinical signs of involvement are rare at this stage but may be due to acute or subacute meningitis with cell counts as high as 1000 per ml in some cases. The patient may have evidence of raised intracranial pressure with headache, vomiting and papilloedema. Cranial nerve palsies may be associated (see p. 84). Willcox and Goodwin[15] have described three cases of nerve deafness in homosexual men suffering from secondary syphilis. All had abnormalities of the cerebrospinal fluid and all responded well to antisyphilitic treatment.

Various electrocardiographic abnormalities have been described in cases of secondary syphilis and recently a case of the Wenckebach phenomenon occurring in association with secondary syphilis has been reported.[16]

Infectivity

The moist lesions of secondary syphilis are highly contagious; the dry lesions should not be so unless abraded. Condylomata lata and the mucous patches are the most contagious lesions.

Diagnosis

Diagnosis is made with certainty by finding *T. pallidum* by dark-ground examination of serum from a moist papule, a healing primary lesion, a lesion of mucous membrane or a lymph node aspirate. Because of possible confusion with saprophytic *T. microdentium* found in the mouth, immuno-fluorescent staining for treponemes from this site is more reliable. *T.*

pallidum may sometimes be identified in serum obtained after scraping a dry papular lesion.

Reagin tests are nearly always positive in cases of secondary syphilis, although this may not apply to certain African races.[17] The FTA-ABS test is always positive in secondary syphilis and the TPI test almost always.

Differential Diagnosis

The surface lesions of secondary syphilis may simulate many other dermatological conditions. If a patient is seen to have a rash which does not fit into any other well-known clinical syndrome and is chronic and non-irritating, the possibility that it may be due to syphilis should always be considered. The macular rash may be mistaken for measles, rubella, various drug rashes, seborrhoeic dermatitis, or the rose spots of typhoid fever. Glandular fever, in particular, may be closely mimicked because both may present with a rash, enlarged lymph nodes and lesions of the throat. The papular rash may resemble papular urticaria, pityriasis rosea, the papular reaction in variola, lichen planus and, more rarely, pityriasis lichenoides chronica. Other possible sources of error are the nodular lesions of leprosy, papulonecrotic tuberculides and urticaria pigmentosa.

Papulosquamous lesions may resemble psoriasis or seborrhoeic dermatitis. Pustular lesions may be confused with acne vulgaris, ecthyma, pyoderma, acne necrotica, acne scrofulosorum, and eruptions due to bromides or iodides. Annular lesions may be mistaken for fungus infection, erythema multiforme or impetigo; more rarely they may have to be differentiated from the annular type of lichen planus or from granuloma annulare. The rare follicular lesions of the skin must be distinguished from follicular seborrhoeic dermatitis, lichen scrofulosorum, pityriasis rubra pilaris and lichen spinulosus, and on the scalp from alopecia areata, ringworm and the alopecia of lupus erythematosus. Condylomata lata may be mistaken for genital or perianal acuminate warts.

Mucous patches on the throat and tonsil must be differentiated from Vincent's angina, tonsillitis, diphtheria, carcinoma or lesions due to agranulocytosis. Similar lesions in the mouth and on the tongue may resemble aphthous ulcers, erythema multiforme of the Stevens–Johnson type, pemphigus, the oral lesions of Behçet's syndrome, lichen planus, 'geographical tongue' and tuberculous fissures and erosions. Secondary lesions on the genital mucous membranes may resemble herpes simplex, primary lesions, lichen planus, psoriasis and, in the female, the acute vulval ulcers of Behçet's syndrome.

EARLY LATENT SYPHILIS

At this stage, in the absence of clinical evidence and with negative tests of the cerebrospinal fluid, the diagnosis depends on positive blood tests. To confirm the diagnosis it is essential to perform specific tests (e.g. TPI, FTA-ABS or TPHA) as well as routine reagin tests (e.g. CWR, VDRL slide test). The diagnosis should never be made on a single blood examination as there is always the possibility of an error in labelling the specimen in the clinic or of technique in the laboratory. Most clinics test each specimen with one reagin and one specific or group specific test. Recently the combination of the VDRL slide test with the TPHA test has proved very satisfactory. Occasionally attention is drawn to early latent syphilitic infection in a woman as the result of congenital syphilitic infection in her newborn infant.

RELAPSE IN EARLY SYPHILIS

After the early lesions have healed in response to treatment, there is always the possibility of relapse in the first two years of the disease, especially when treatment has been inadequate. As might be expected, the earlier treatment is begun and the more thorough it is, the less chance there is that relapse will occur. Relapse may be clinical, with the appearance of lesions resembling those of secondary syphilis, or it may be indicated by serological tests in which results which had become negative become positive, or by quantitative tests in which titres which had fallen proceed to rise again. So-called serological relapse may occur without clinical signs but clinical relapse is likely to follow.

Relapsing lesions of the secondary type occur in the mouth and throat and on the skin, particularly in the perianal region, but all of them are now rare. On the skin the relapsing lesions may be annular, corymbose or rupial. Sometimes they are 'framboesiform', resembling the early lesions of yaws. Another form of relapse occasionally described is a lesion occurring at the site of the original chancre, which it closely resembles; it is termed a 'monorécidive' or 'chancre redux'.

Other forms of relapse include ocular lesions, lesions of bones and viscera, lesions of the nervous system (so-called neurorecurrence), and the birth of a syphilitic child to an apparently cured female patient.

Relapsing mucocutaneous lesions are highly infectious. It is therefore important to examine patients carefully during the period of surveillance after treatment, in addition to performing the routine serological tests. Special attention should be paid to examination of the throat and of the perianal region.

REFERENCES

1. WAUGH, M. (1972) Br. med. J., 1, 803.
2. DEGOS, R., TOURAINE, R., COLLART, P., DANIEL, F. and AUDEBERT, G. (1970) Bull. Soc. fr. Derm. Syph., 77, 10.

3. SACHER, D. B., KLEIN, R. S., SWERDLOW, F., BOTTONE, E., KHILNANI, M. T., WAYE, J. D. and WISNIEWSKI, M. (1974) *Ann. intern. Med.*, **80,** 512.

4. ZWINK, F. B. and DUNLOP, E. M. C. (1976) *Trans. ophthal. Soc. U.K.*, **96,** 148.

5. MACFAUL, P. A. and CATTERALL, R. D. (1971) *Br. J. vener. Dis.*, **47,** 159.

6. BAKER, A. L., KAPLAN, M. M., WOLFE, M. J. and McGOWAN, J. A. (1971) *New Engl. J. Med.*, **284,** 1422.

7. LEE, R. V., THORNTON, G. F. and CONN, H. O. (1971) *New Engl. J. Med.*, **284,** 1423.

8. PARKER, J. D. J. (1972) *Br. J. vener. Dis.*, **48,** 32.

9. SARKANY, I. (1973) *Proc. R. Soc. Med.*, **66,** 237.

10. BROPHY, E. M., ASHWORTH, C. T., ARIAS, M. and REYNOLDS, I. (1964) *Obstet. Gynec.*, **24,** 930.

11. FALLS, W. F., FORD, K. L., ASHWORTH, C. T. and CARTER, N. W. (1965) *Ann. intern. Med.*, **63,** 1047.

12. BRAUNSTEIN, G. D., LEWIS, E. J., GALVANEK, E. G., HAMILTON, A. and BELL, W. R. (1970) *Am. J. Med.*, **48,** 643.

13. BHORADE, M. S., CARAG, H. B., LEE, H. J., POTTER, E. V. and DUNEA, G. (1971) *J. Am. med. Ass.*, **216,** 1159.

14. CUTLER, J. C., BAUER, T. J. and SCHWIMMER, B. H. (1954) *Am. J. Syph.*, **38,** 447.

15. WILLCOX, R. R. and GOODWIN, P. G. (1971) *Br. J. vener. Dis.*, **47,** 401.

16. INCE, W. E. and MAHABIR, B. J. (1974) *Br. J. vener. Dis.*, **50,** 97.

17. MASAWE, A. E. J., LOMHOLT, G., AHO, K. and LASSUS, A. (1972) *Br. J. vener. Dis.*, **48,** 345.

3

Late Acquired Syphilis

LATE LATENT STAGE

After the second year of the disease, syphilis enters the late phase and is usually non-contagious. The stage commences with a period of latency, in which symptoms and signs are absent, and this may continue for a few or for many years, or even for the rest of life, the patient dying from old age or from causes unrelated to syphilis. Sometimes the fact of infection becomes known because a woman gives birth to an infant with congenital syphilis, but this is less likely than in the early latent stage. The diagnosis can only be made by serological tests and should always be confirmed by at least one of the specific tests (TPI, FTA, and TPHA tests). Infection may come to light because the patient is tested before marriage, as a blood donor, as a prospective immigrant, or during ante-natal investigation. In cases of late latent syphilis, or of late syphilis of any kind, the cerebrospinal fluid should be examined to exclude asymptomatic neurosyphilis, and an X-ray of the aorta taken for evidence of aortitis. It must be emphasized that the diagnosis of latency can only be established when careful examination and accessory tests give no evidence of active disease in any system. The scar of a primary lesion may sometimes be seen on the genital organs and occasionally 'leuco-derma' of the neck gives evidence of an earlier secondary stage. Another occasional residual finding is 'macular atrophy', presenting as small atrophic macules over the body surface at points where the original secondary papules were present (see Chapter 2).

TERTIARY STAGE

The first lesions of the tertiary stage of syphilis are usually seen from three to ten years after the primary stage, but they may appear much later. Many patients give no history of the primary and secondary stages. The tissues most likely to be involved are:

1. The covering structures of the body, that is, skin, mucous membrane, subcutaneous and submucous tissues.

2. The supporting structures, that is, bones, joints, muscles and ligaments.

Because these lesions usually carry no major threat to life or ultimate health, this phase of the disease is sometimes known as 'benign tertiary syphilis'.

PATHOLOGY. The characteristic lesion is known as the gumma. Gummata are usually localized lesions; they may be single or multiple and vary in size from a pin-head to a mass several centimetres in diameter. Diffuse gumma-tous infiltration also occurs. The most typical feature of the localized lesion is the central area of tissue necrosis, which is usually granular but may resemble caseous material. This is surrounded by a zone of granulation tissue which, on macroscopic section, is seen to be dull red in colour. Outside it, is a narrow zone of tough, fibrous tissue (Fig. 36). Microscopic-ally the zone of granulation tissue shows cellular infiltration with small lymphocytes and plasma cells (Fig. 37), particularly concentrated round small blood vessels and giving the appearance of 'perivascular cuffing'. The intima of the blood vessels shows cellular hypertrophy due to endarteritis, resulting in complete blockage of some of these vessels (so-called endar-teritis obliterans) which is responsible for the necrosis of tissue which follows. Epithelioid cells and a few giant cells are also present. Fibroblasts can be seen, particularly at the periphery of the lesion. Search for *T. pallidum* is nearly always unsuccessful. It cannot be found by the dark-ground method and is hardly ever to be seen in stained sections. It can only be demonstrated by inoculation of gummatous material into susceptible animals. The reason for the destructive character of tertiary lesions in the absence of large numbers of demonstrable treponemes remains a mystery. It may be due to some form of local tissue allergy in the host. Sometimes trauma seems to play a part in determining the site of this reaction, but this is not always the case.

The gummatous lesion is not necessarily self-limiting, and it is common to find that, as the initial lesions heal by scar tissue, other lesions appear at the periphery.

In some organs involved in the tertiary stage, the diffuse gummatous reaction is more common than the localized lesion. This is particularly true of the tongue and probably of the testis. The end result of this reaction is a diffuse interstitial fibrosis.

Covering Structures of the Body

In contrast to the secondary stage, when the lesions are symmetrical, late lesions occur singly, or in isolated groups; they are not symmetrically arranged.

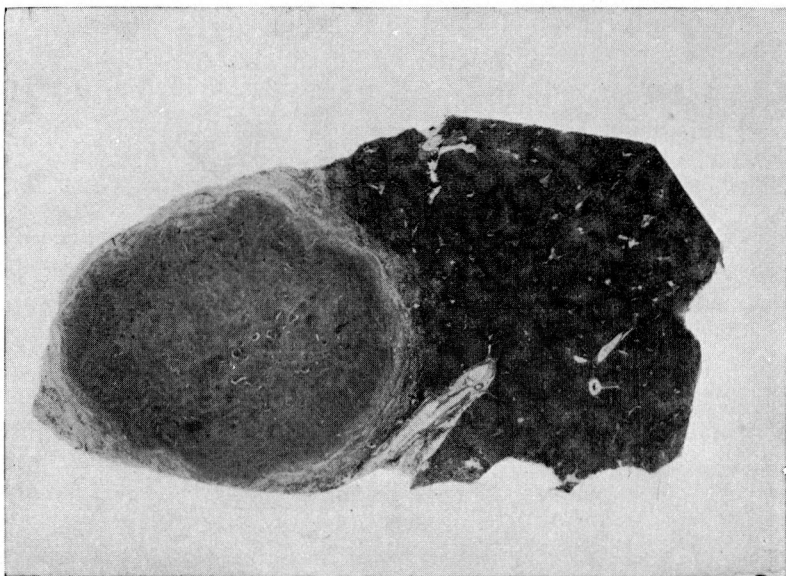

Fig. 36. Gumma of the liver: central necrosis with surrounding fibrosis.
(*Autopsy specimen.*)

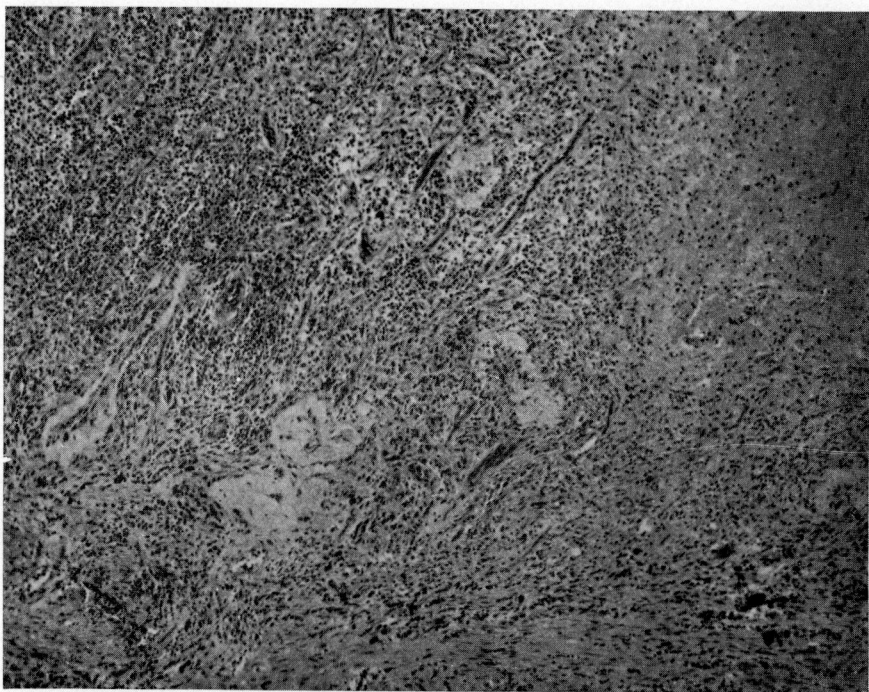

Fig. 37. Gumma of testis with necrosis at upper right corner and surrounding
round-cell infiltration. (*Magnification* × 80.)

Cutaneous Lesions

Gummata involving the skin may be divided into three groups: nodular, squamous or psoriasiform, and subcutaneous.

NODULAR LESIONS. These consist of rounded, dull-red lesions, which vary in size from a pinhead to a pea (Plate III i and Fig. 38). They may occur on any part of the skin surface. They are painless, and develop and regress very slowly. They tend to be arranged in groups, the multiple lesions having a rounded or polycyclic outline. On palpation they are moveable swellings which involve the whole thickness of the skin. The nodules may remain discrete or may coalesce to form a continuous zone. Occasionally they ulcerate, forming small, punched-out ulcers extending into the substance of the nodule, but ulceration is not the rule. Some of them may show scaling on the surface but usually the surface of the nodule is clean and smooth. The regional lymphatic nodes are not involved. In the course of months the nodules heal, but new nodules are likely to appear at the periphery with gradual widening of the area involved which, in untreated cases, may be extensive. When healing has occurred, pigmentation may remain or the skin may show scars of the 'tissue paper' type or adherent crusts. Frequently, however, the skin may look normal after healing. The process may continue for years in neglected cases.

SQUAMOUS OR PSORIASIFORM LESIONS. These are really the same lesions but the tissue reaction seems to be rather more intense (Fig. 39). The main difference is the presence of waxy scaling on the surface of the lesion, which may closely resemble psoriasis. If, however, the scales are scraped away there are no capillary bleeding points. The squamous lesions are often rather larger than the nodular lesions and, although there is peripheral spread, the tendency to central healing is less. There is little tendency to ulceration or scarring. Tertiary psoriasiform lesions sometimes affect the palms of the hands or the soles of the feet.

SUBCUTANEOUS GUMMATA. These present as rounded, painless subcutaneous lesions which may be single or multiple (Plate III iii; Figs. 40, 41, 43 and 44). At first the skin over the swelling is not attached and shows no discoloration. The swelling increases in size and this may be accelerated by the fusion of several gummata into a polycyclic mass. The swelling becomes attached to the skin, which then shows dull-red discoloration and soon breaks down to form a punched-out, destructive ulcer with the rounded or polycyclic outline of the original swelling. The walls are vertical and lead down to a clean-looking floor consisting of dull-red granulations. The necrotic tissue may remain attached to the walls and floor for some time in the form of a tough, yellowish-white slough, called the 'wash-leather slough' (Fig. 45). The intact skin at the margin of the ulcer shows dull-red discoloration and adherent crusts. These gummatous ulcers, as they are called, occur most commonly in the lower leg, where, in contradistinction

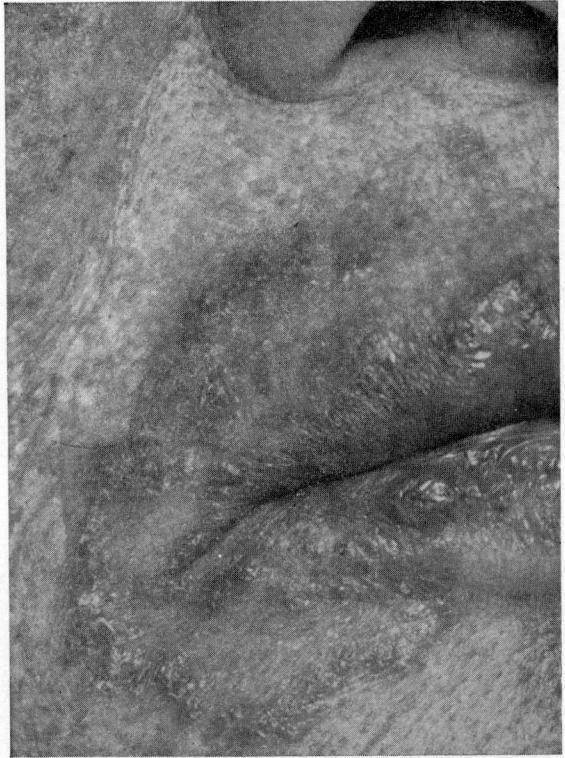

Fig. 38. Tertiary stage:
nodular lesions of the
skin of the face.

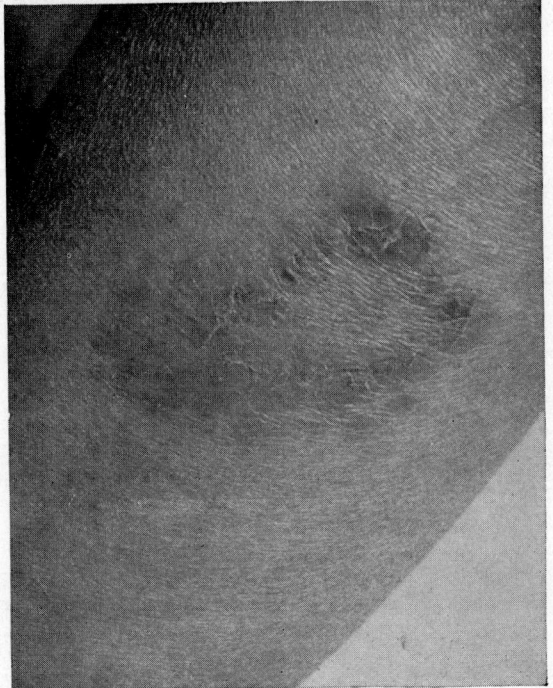

Fig. 39. Tertiary stage:
psoriasiform lesion on
the leg.

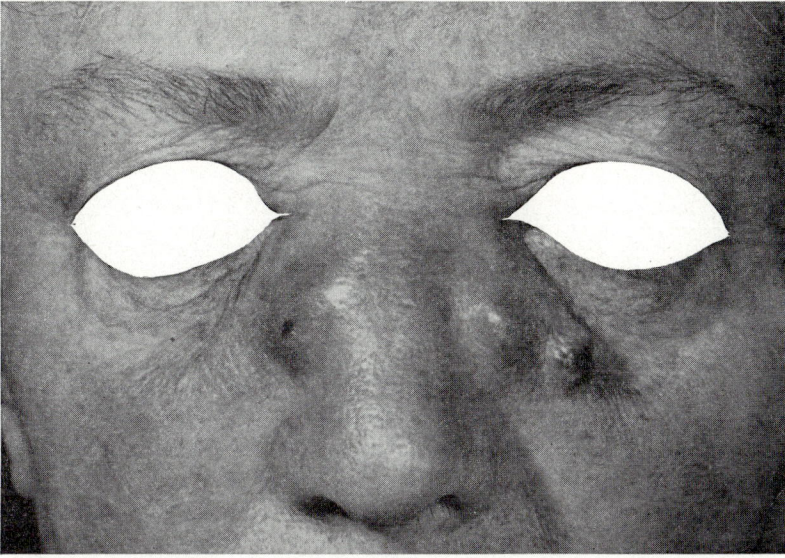

Fig. 40. Subcutaneous gummata of face: commencing ulceration.

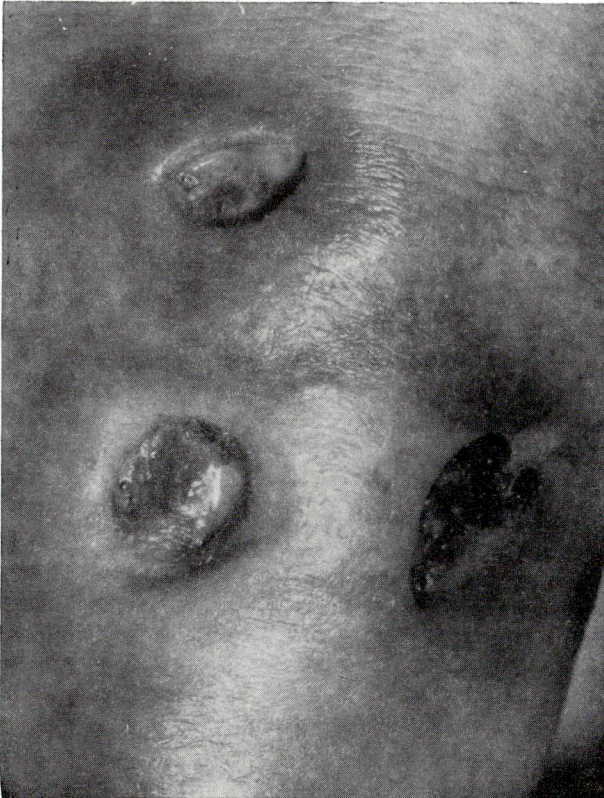

Fig. 41. Gummatous ulcers: the lower lesions are involving the prepatellar bursa.

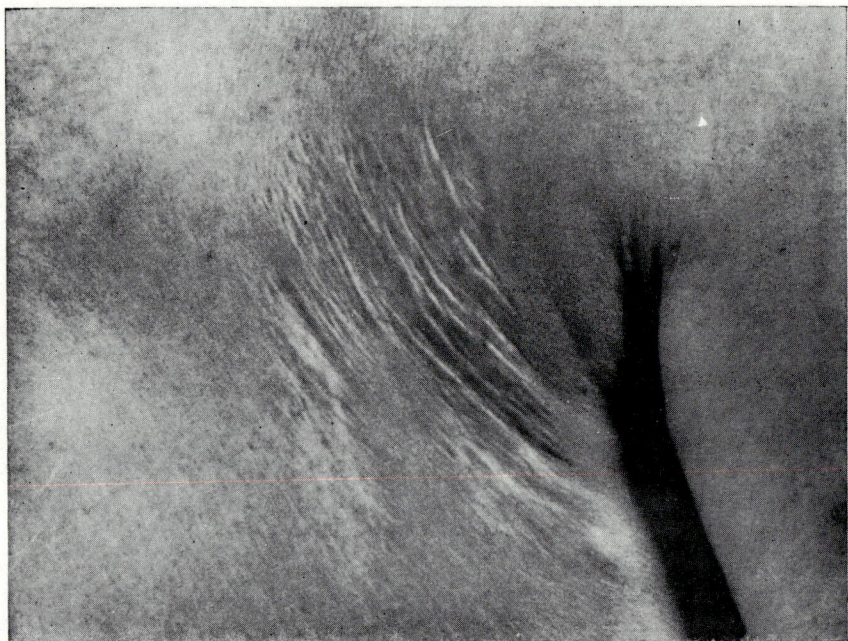

Fig. 42. Tertiary stage: typical 'tissue paper' scarring.

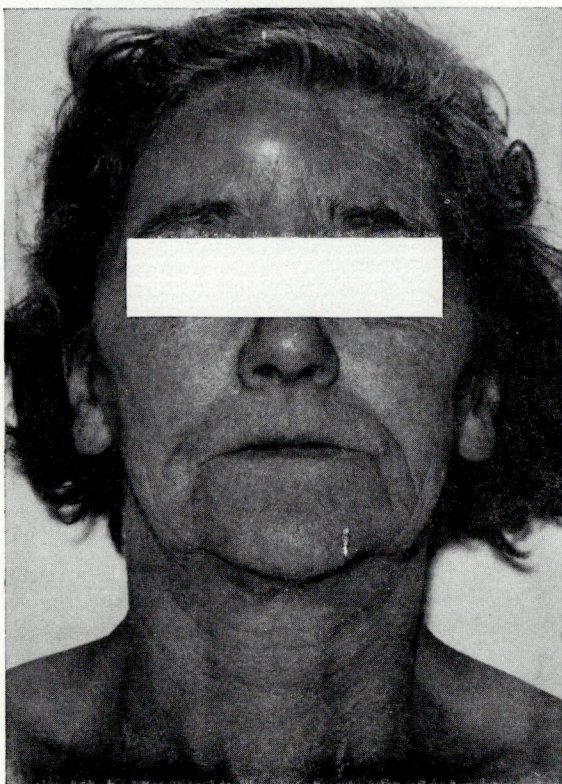

Fig. 43.
Subcutaneous
gumma of forehead.

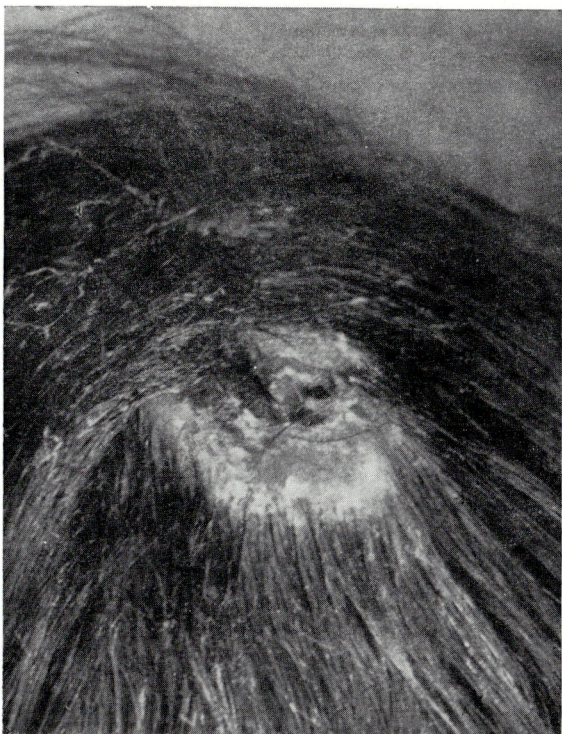

Fig. 44. Subcutaneous gumma of scalp with early ulceration. (From *Roxburgh's Common Skin Diseases*, H. K. Lewis.)

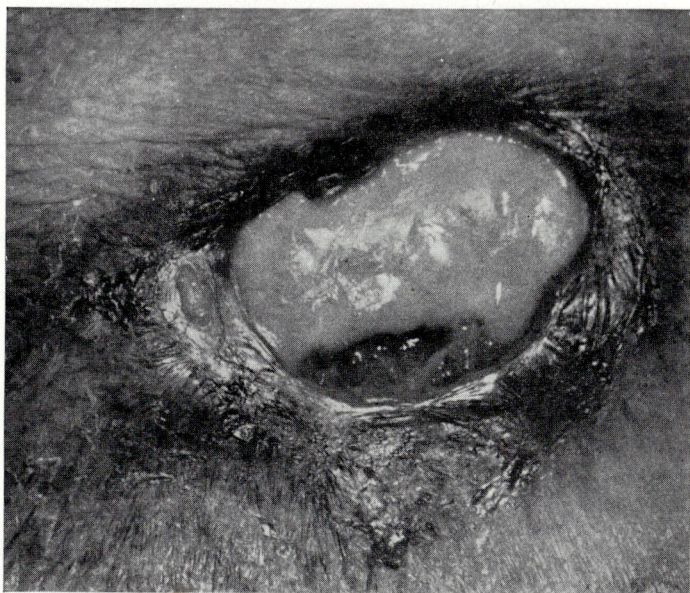

Fig. 45. Gummatous ulcer with 'wash-leather' slough over sternum.

to varicose ulcers, they may affect the upper and outer areas of the skin of the leg (Plate III iii). Other regions commonly affected are the scalp and face, and the skin over the sternum or the sternoclavicular joints and the buttocks. If the subcutaneous gumma has its origin in, or extends to, the periosteum of subcutaneous bone, the floor of the gummatous ulcer may be formed by necrotic bone. Healing of gummatous ulcers is by scar tissue which is thin, papery and non-contractile, often called 'tissue paper scarring' (Fig. 42).

Gummata of Mucous Membranes

Gummatous lesions of mucous membranes may also be localized or diffuse. Localized gummata are most likely to involve the submucous tissue of the mouth and throat, the palate, the pharynx, the larynx or the nasal septum. The condition presents as a painless, localized, rounded swelling, which at first shows no discoloration of the overlying mucous membrane. Soon the latter becomes adherent and shows dull-red discoloration. Then it breaks down to form a characteristic punched-out ulcer with a 'wash-leather' slough. In structures such as the hard palate (see Fig. 51) and nasal septum, the underlying bone is certain to be involved and may be destroyed, with gummatous ulceration on both surfaces and rounded or polycyclic perforation of the organ concerned. Destruction of the cartilage of the nasal septum may lead to collapse of the cartilaginous part of the nose, with obvious external deformity. Lesions of the soft palate lead to destruction or perforation; those of the pharynx and larynx may lead to gross deformity and stenosis. These areas of destruction and deformity in the mouth, nose or throat are always suggestive of gummatous syphilis, especially when the patient's history suggests that the active lesion caused little pain or inconvenience. A nodular type of lesion is sometimes seen on the surface of the larynx and may well be mistaken for a carcinoma, especially when it occurs on the vocal cords. Patients with untreated gummatous lesions of the mouth are very prone to leucoplakia and subsequent malignant changes (see Figs. 49 and 50), and the presence of syphilis should lead to careful consideration of this possibility, which may be suggested by the appearance of the lesion and by its lack of response to antisyphilitic treatment. In the later stages of this change deep infiltration and enlargement of regional lymph nodes will occur. A biopsy should be taken at the earliest opportunity to establish the diagnosis.

THE TONGUE

The commonest change in the mouth due to late syphilis is that which results from diffuse gummatous interstitial infiltration of the tongue (Plate III iv and Figs. 46–48). The syphilitic process follows the vascular supply and infiltrates widely in the muscles of the tongue. The condition is painless and the patient is usually quite unaware of it. Rarely such a patient may disclose that, perhaps two or three years previously, the tongue became swollen and appeared too big for the mouth, and that later it diminished to its former size or smaller. The end result presents some years after and is known by the time-honoured name of 'chronic superficial glossitis'. The name is misleading, because it suggests that pathological changes are limited to the surface of the tongue, whereas the causative process is deep-seated. The condition may present in one of four ways: The patient may begin to have discomfort or pain in the tongue especially provoked by hot, spiced foods or by acids such as vinegar; or there may be no discomfort but the patient notices that his tongue looks odd and seeks advice; or the doctor may notice the condition of the tongue in the course of a routine examination for some other reason; or the patient may present with early carcinoma of the tongue and the characteristic changes of chronic superficial glossitis are noticed.

The signs may be threefold, although not all are present in every case. The surface of the tongue is apt to show deep, irregular fissuring. This is due to the interstitial fibrosis and the fact that some of the sheets of fibrous tissue reach the mucous membrane. Fissuring occurs as the result of sub-sequent contraction. Irregular white patches of so-called leucoplakia are seen on the surface of the tongue. These are patches of keratinized epith-elium attributed to chronic irritation. Apart from syphilis, they have also been described as occurring through friction caused by a carious or broken tooth or by an ill-fitting denture. In the past they are said to have been due to smoking, usually a clay pipe with a clay stem which conducts heat, and to the lavish consumption of spices or spirits. On the syphilitic tongue they probably result from friction with the teeth in eating and talking. The impaired blood supply to the mucous membrane renders the normal process of healing and repair inadequate. The third change is seen on the surface of the tongue at the sides and tip, where the filiform papillae are lost and the surface is smooth and glazed. This effect is probably due to separation of patches of leucoplakia which carry with them the filiform papillae. This change probably causes the sudden onset of discomfort and pain in the tongue in response to certain irritants. The surface heals over and the symptom is relieved spontaneously irrespective of antisyphilitic treatment. Chronic 'superficial' glossitis (Fig. 46) should be regarded as a residual effect which appears after the phase of gummatous activity. It is a pre-cancerous condition, and these patients should be watched carefully for the rest of their lives. Antisyphilitic treatment should be given but there is no evidence that it will make cancerous changes less likely.

Aids to Diagnosis

In cases of late syphilis of the skin and mucous membranes, the reagin blood tests are positive in almost all the cases; negative results do not entirely rule out the possibility of this diagnosis, but they are strong

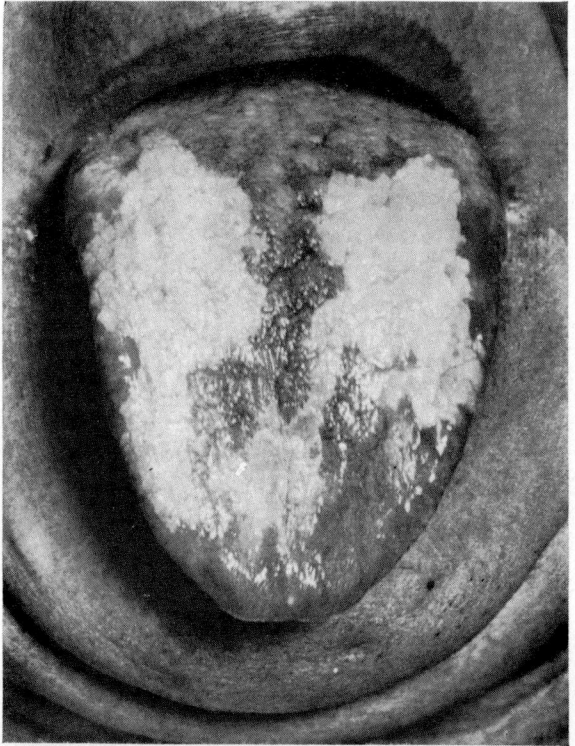

Fig. 46. Tertiary stage:
chronic 'superficial'
glossitis. (From
*Roxburgh's Common Skin
Diseases*, H. K. Lewis.)

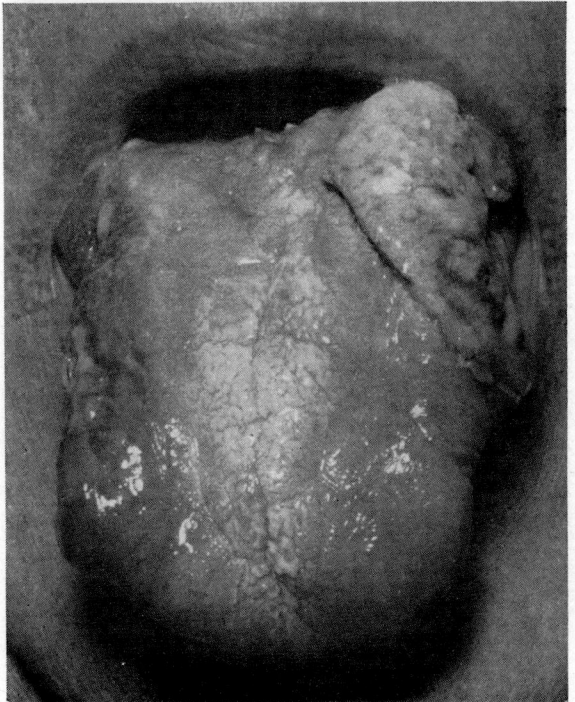

Fig. 47. Tertiary stage:
chronic glossitis with
areas of malignant
change.

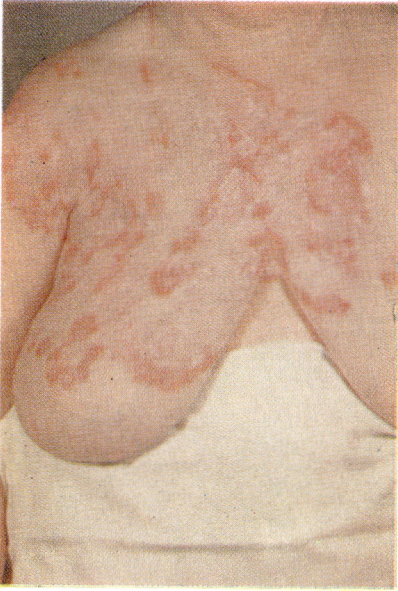

i Tertiary stage: widespread nodular lesions of the skin, with central healing.

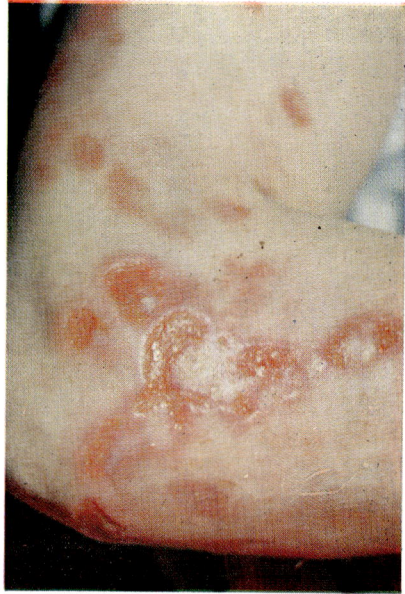

ii Tertiary stage: nodular lesions of skin, with ulceration.

iii Tertiary stage: subcutaneous gummata of lower leg.

iv Tertiary stage: chronic superficial glossitis with leucoplakia, fissuring and loss of papillae at edges of tongue.

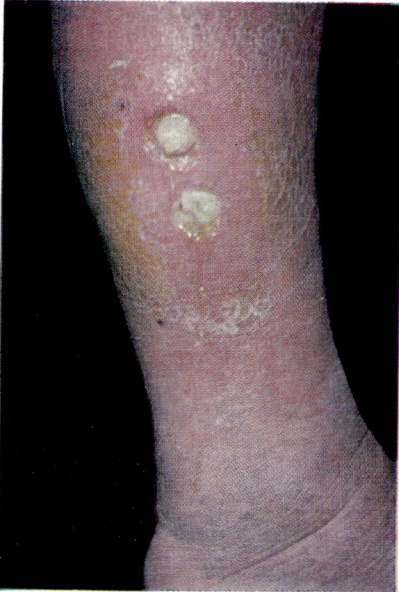

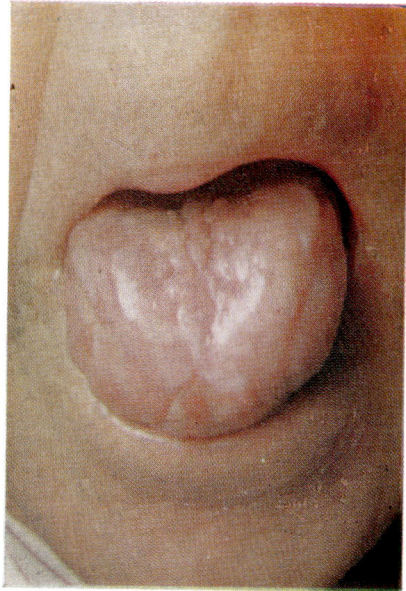

PLATE III: LATE ACQUIRED SYPHILIS

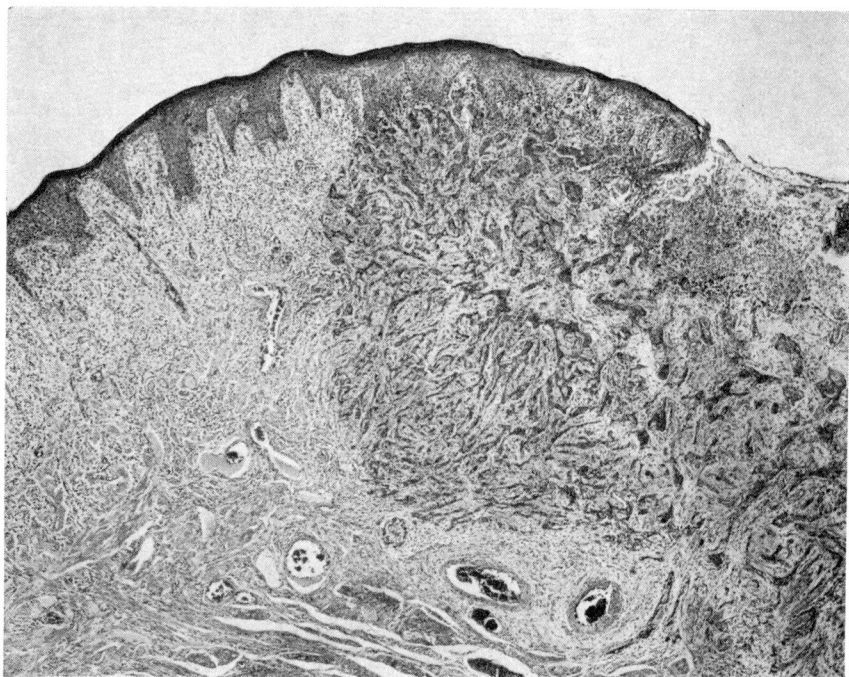

Fig. 48. Tertiary stage: section showing interstitial glossitis with malignant change. (*Magnification* × 60.)

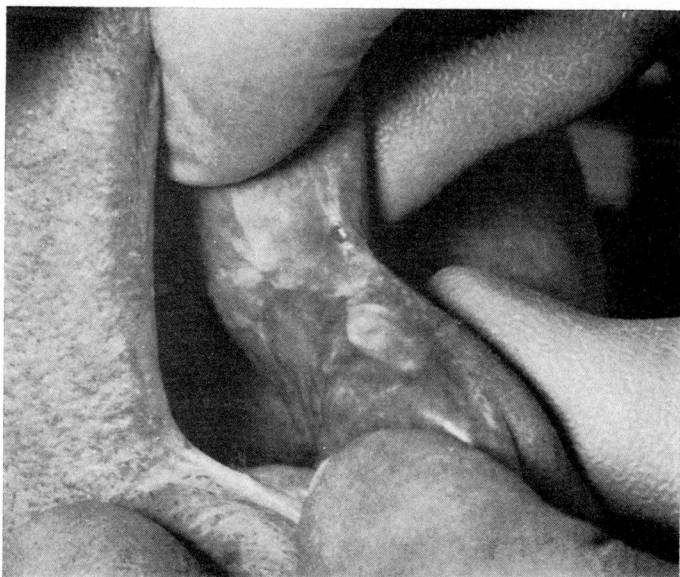

Fig. 49. Tertiary stage: leucoplakia of angle of mouth.

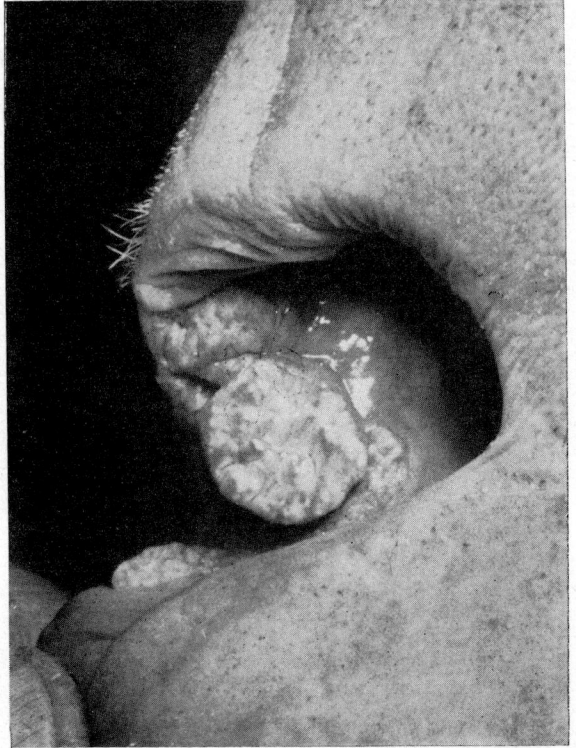

Fig. 50. Tertiary stage: malignant change at angle of mouth.

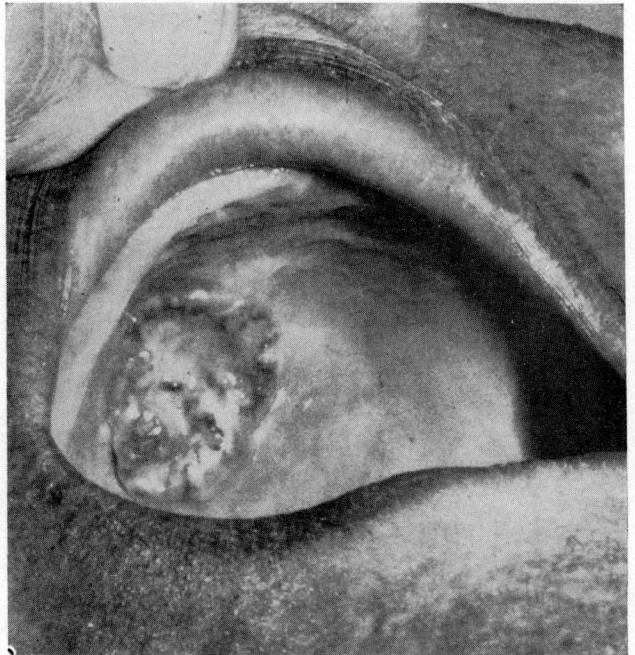

Fig. 51. Gumma of hard palate.

evidence against it. The specific tests should be positive in all cases. The past history of a genital sore or lesions suggestive of the secondary stage, or of early syphilis inadequately treated, may also aid in diagnosis. In addition, there may be clinical evidence of late syphilis of other systems. Examination of the cerebrospinal fluid and X-ray and screening of the aorta should be done in all cases before treatment.

Differential Diagnosis

The skin lesions of late syphilis must be distinguished from those due to other granulomatous conditions, including tuberculosis, sarcoidosis, leprosy, sporotrichosis, and blastomycosis, and from various non-granulomatous lesions, including the plaques of psoriasis and seborrhoeic dermatitis, squamous-cell epithelioma of the skin, various dermatophytoses, lupus erythematosus, erythema nodosum, the surface manifestations of some reticuloses (including mycosis fungoides) and certain types of bromide and iodide eruptions.

The differential diagnosis varies to some extent according to the anatomical site. On the face, lupus vulgaris, sarcoidosis, lupus erythematosus, epithelioma, rodent ulcer, leprosy and rhinophyma must be considered. Palmar lesions may resemble chronic eczema, psoriasis, fungus infection, papulonecrotic tuberculides and possibly granuloma annulare. On the legs, ulcers due to stasis, haemolytic anaemia, erythema induratum and sporotrichosis must be excluded.

Tuberculides spread more slowly than the lesions of late syphilis and they affect younger people. The scars are contractile, unlike the 'tissue paper' scars of healed late syphilis of the skin. Ulcers due to stasis are common and affect the lower part of the leg; they are often associated with varicose veins and an eczematous condition of the adjacent skin with pigmentation round the ankles or with local areas of thrombophlebitis.

Supporting Structures of the Body

Bones (see Figs. 56–58, p. 65)

PATHOLOGY. Lesions usually commence in the fibrous layer of the periosteum and are identical with those occurring in the soft tissue. The cells consist mainly of small lymphocytes and plasma cells with a few epithelioid cells and an occasional giant cell. The infiltration is particularly concentrated round the small blood vessels, which undergo obliterative endarteritis. Fibroblasts appear in large numbers in the area of inflammation. The chronic inflammation in the fibrous layer of the periosteum stimulates activity of the osteoblasts in the adjacent 'osteogenic' layer with new bone formation on the surface of the cortex under the periosteum. The new bone is deposited in irregular fashion, which results ultimately in thickening of the cortex and roughening and irregularity of the surface. The inflammatory process is likely to extend into the cortex of the bone by way of the Haversian systems, causing erosion and destruction of cortical bone, which is promptly replaced by new bone extending from the periosteum. The new bone is more sclerotic than the normal and lacks its usual cortical pattern. It may extend through the cortex and even partly obliterate the medullary cavity. Usually only part of the bone is involved, and the transition from healthy to diseased bone is abrupt. The ultimate effect upon the bone depends upon the degree of osteoblastic activity, which is greater in the long bones than in the flat bones, particularly those which have their origin in membrane. In the great majority of cases long bones are strengthened by the gummatous process, and there is no tendency to bending or to pathological fracture. Occasionally the gummatous process starts in the medullary cavity of a long bone and erodes the cortex from within; this has been called 'syphilitic osteomyelitis'. In the bones of the vault of the skull, the hard palate and the nasal septum, however, destruction outpaces new bone formation and periosteal reaction is slight. There are rounded areas of destruction of bone which may become confluent, and there is little evidence of thickening. In the vault of the skull the process usually starts in the outer table of the bone and may extend to the inner table, involving the dura mater. Extension to the cerebral cortex is unlikely because the dura mater has considerable powers of resistance to chronic infection. Severe degrees of gummatous osteoperiostitis of the skull are often called by the rather fanciful name of 'worm-eaten skull'.

SYMPTOMS AND SIGNS. Tertiary syphilis of bone may be found mostly from five to twenty years after the original infection. It is slightly commoner in men than women. The patient may give a history of trauma. Bones most commonly involved are the tibiae, the cranial bones, shoulder girdle, femur, fibula, humerus and the bones of the forearm; joints are seldom involved. The main symptom is a deep-seated boring pain at the site of involvement. It is usually worse at night and can be very severe. If the skull is involved, the patient may complain of severe continuous headache. Sometimes the pain may be described as 'rheumatic'. Pain is present in about 50 per cent of the cases, and in the remainder there may be no symptoms. If the bone is subcutaneous, the patient may become aware of swelling which may be tender at first. In many cases the diagnosis is made by chance or by routine radiography. Disability is slight and constitutional symptoms are likely to be absent. The process may extend to adjacent subcutaneous tissue and overlying skin, with gummatous ulceration leading down to necrotic bone. There may be evidence of late syphilis in other systems. The results of reagin tests are almost always positive, and these can be confirmed by specific tests.

If a long bone is involved and is near the surface, an irregular bony tumour may be palpable. It may be moderately tender at first. Involvement of the skull is unlikely to give rise to clinical signs. In the mouth, perforation of the hard palate and, in the nose, perforation of the nasal septum may be obvious on examination.

RADIOLOGICAL SIGNS. In the long bones the irregular deposition of new bone on the surface of the cortex is soon evident. The cortex itself may show signs of erosion in the early stages, but the most striking appearance is that of increased opacity of the cortical bone with, in some cases, invasion of the medullary cavity by new bone formation. The new bone formation lacks the normal cortical pattern, and the transition from new bone to normal cortex is abrupt. In the tibia the anterior part of the middle third of the bone may well be the site of the greatest cortical thickening, and this may give the clinical impression of bowing or bending of the bone. The radiographs show that the lines of force are unchanged and that there is no true bending of the bone. In this respect the term 'sabre tibia' or 'sabre-shaped tibia' is apt to give a false impression (see also p. 131).

In the bones of the vault of the skull the appearance is of rounded areas of osteoporosis. In a long-standing case these areas may be seen against a background of increased opacity of the cortical bone, an appearance which is the exact reverse of that found in Paget's disease of the skull, for which syphilitic osteoperiostitis is sometimes mistaken. Following treatment, recalcification of the bone is a relatively slow process occupying some months.

When gummatous lesions of bones are found it is good practice to X-ray other likely bones, where asymptomatic involvement is often found.

DIFFERENTIAL DIAGNOSIS. Syphilis has been aptly described as the great imitator, and late syphilis of bones may resemble many other conditions, some of which are far more common. The following are some of the more likely sources of error: primary and metastatic carcinoma, myeloma, tuberculosis, eosinophilic granuloma, yaws, leprosy, Paget's disease, scurvy, chronic pyogenic osteomyelitis, osteoid osteoma, primary osteogenic sarcoma, and Ewing's tumour.

Cartilage

Perichondritis may occur in cartilage as does periostitis in bone, involving, for example, costal cartilage, the external ear and the cartilaginous nasal septum.

Muscles

Primary gummatous involvement of muscles is rare, but infection may extend to them from subcutaneous tissue or bones. In neglected cases the end result may be contracture with fixation of the related joint.

Joints, Bursae, and Tendon-sheaths

These are rarely the sites of tertiary syphilitic lesions. The parts liable to be affected are those most exposed to stress and strain, such as the knee-joint and the prepatellar bursa (see Fig. 41). The swelling is of soft, rubbery consistency and shows no signs of acute inflammation. It follows the outline of the affected joint, bursa or tendon-sheath. Occasionally, hard fibrous nodules, the so-called juxta-articular nodes, are found along tendon-sheaths or subcutaneously near joints in cases of late syphilis. The histological picture is not characteristic of syphilis, but the nodes disappear with anti-syphilitic treatment.

Viscera

Visceral involvement, other than that of the cardiovascular system, may occur in about four per cent of patients with untreated late syphilis. The pathological changes are those of the gumma in soft tissues. A purely fibrotic reaction is sometimes described, but this is probably due to the fact that healing has occurred before the lesion has been discovered. Clinical manifestations will be described briefly in relation to the following sites: stomach; intestines; liver and spleen; lung; urinary tract; reproductive organs.

Stomach

Gummatous lesions of the stomach are rare. The diagnosis may be suggested in the case of any patient with gastric symptoms and positive serological tests, but even though X-ray examination may confirm the presence of some gastric abnormality, the diagnosis is still a most unlikely one. Even if the patient has late syphilis, the gastric lesion is much more likely to be due to a peptic ulcer or a carcinoma. As described in the literature, the condition is chronic with symptoms of persistent indigestion, or there may be a history suggesting peptic ulceration; there is usually no loss of appetite nor is there marked cachexia. While the disease is active, haematemesis is rare and occult blood is not commonly present in the stools. The emptying time of the stomach is usually not increased and the gastric acidity is normal in the majority of cases. There is not likely to be a palpable tumour. X-ray examination after a barium meal may show a filling defect; there may be distortion of the cardiac end of the stomach with perhaps an hour-glass deformity. The pylorus usually shows no abnormality. Gastroscopy in skilled hands is a possible aid to diagnosis. Obviously gastric syphilis can only be considered in diagnosis when the patient is known to have untreated late syphilis. If there is any question of a gastric neoplasm being present in such a case, exploratory laparotomy should not be delayed. On the other hand, if the findings suggest peptic ulceration, a therapeutic test for syphilis is justified before other medical or surgical treatment is instituted.

Intestines

There are few reports in the literature of syphilitic lesions of the duodenum and small intestine. Gummatous lesions of the large intestine, especially the rectum, have been reported in the past, but the modern view is that all or most of these cases were due to lymphogranuloma venereum with rectal involvement. It is not uncommon for patients with rectal lymphogranuloma venereum to have latent syphilis also, and full investigation (see p. 263) will establish the double diagnosis.

Liver and Spleen

Gummatous involvement of the liver, though now uncommon, is the most frequent type of abdominal syphilis. It has been said to appear either as diffuse interstitial cirrhosis or as a focal gummatous condition progressing to an irregular fibrosis, the so-called hepar lobatum (Figs. 52 and 53). The former is, in fact, portal cirrhosis and has been shown to have a higher incidence at autopsy in untreated syphilitic patients than in non-syphilitic patients;[1] but this could be due to other factors such as alcoholism. The gummatous condition is, of course, a true syphilitic entity with symptoms which vary according to the localization of the gummata. These may involve either the liver capsule or the parenchyma and may press on blood vessels, bile ducts or gall bladder. It must be remembered that amyloid disease may supervene on this chronic condition. Gummatous lesions of the spleen are extremely rare, but slight splenic enlargement accompanying late syphilis of the liver is seen in about 15 per cent of the cases. It is not always possible to prove the diagnosis of late syphilis of the liver by liver biopsy, especially if there is only a single gummatous lesion present, nor is the therapeutic test necessarily effective if diffuse scarring of the organ has already occurred.

Some authors state that involvement of the liver in late syphilis occurs more often in women; others that the incidence is equal between the sexes. Symptoms and signs include loss of weight, jaundice, pain and tenderness in the right hypochondrium, simulating cholecystitis, and remittent or intermittent fever. Other less frequent symptoms and signs are vomiting or haematemesis, due to varicosity of the lower oesophageal plexus of veins, asthenia and anorexia, and vague abdominal tenderness or the awareness of an abdominal mass. The condition is, however, often symptomless.

Hepatic enlargement, the commonest clinical finding, presents as a large firm, irregular mass. The left lobe is apt to be more severely affected than the right. The liver may be tender on palpation, and splenic enlargement may be present but is seldom gross. Ascites may be found in those patients with portal hypertension. Microcytic anaemia is not infrequent. Abnormal liver-function tests indicate damage of the liver parenchyma. It is important to realize that a syphilitic patient may be an alcoholic and that hepatic enlargement, jaundice, or ascites may indicate portal cirrhosis and not syphilitic hepatitis.

In differential diagnosis primary or secondary neoplasm of the liver must

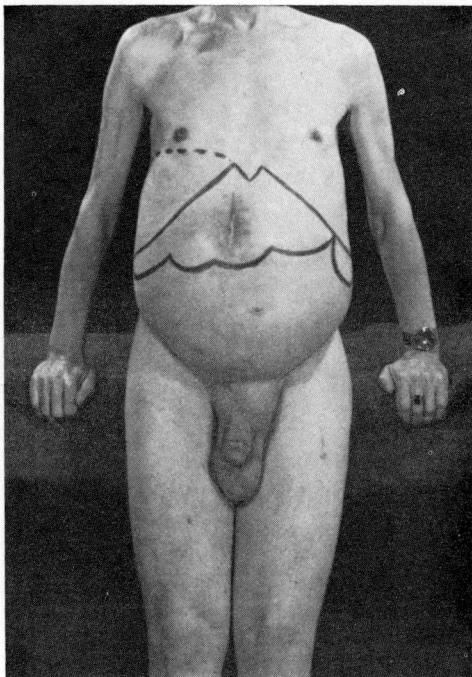

Fig. 52. Gumma of the liver (hepar lobatum) with ascites and splenic enlargement.

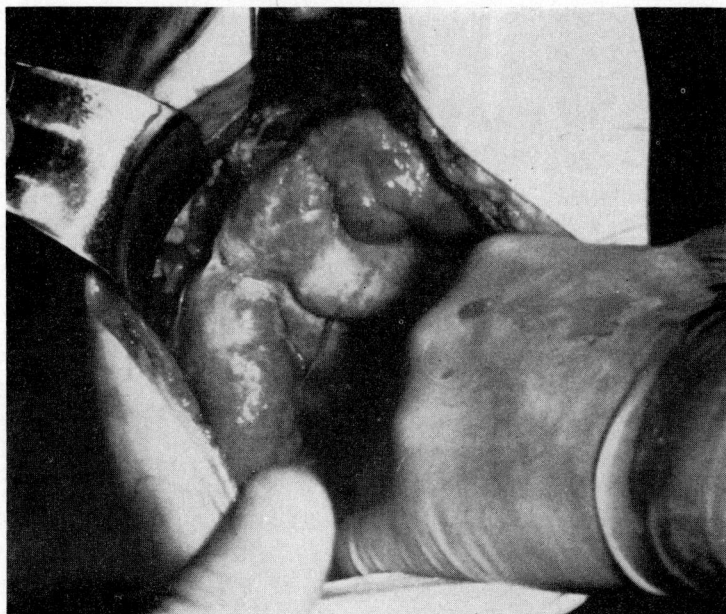

Fig. 53. Tertiary stage: hepar lobatum seen at an operation to relieve portal hypertension. (*Mr. A. Hunt's patient.*)

be excluded by thorough investigation. The possibility of exploratory laparotomy may have to be considered. Other conditions which may enter into the diagnosis include gall stones, cholecystitis, peptic ulcer, appendicitis, tuberculous peritonitis, renal calculi with colic, pleurisy, abdominal angina pectoris and malaria. A past history of syphilis is obtained in less than 50 per cent of patients with hepatic syphilis, but the specific tests are positive and the reagin tests nearly always so. The diagnosis may be aided by finding evidence of old gummatous lesions of skin, mucous membrane or bones, or of cardiovascular syphilis and neurosyphilis. Even if a patient has hepatic syphilis he may also have carcinoma or gall stones or some other serious condition. Sometimes the diagnosis of hepatic syphilis is first suspected at laparotomy by the gross appearance of the liver. In difficult cases the diagnosis can be assisted by a therapeutic test, which may be conclusive if a single large gumma is producing pressure in the portal fissure. It must be emphasized that syphilitic hepatitis is usually a quite benign condition and that some cases are only diagnosed post mortem.

Gummatous lesions of the pancreas are occasionally seen as specimens in pathological museums, but are unlikely to be diagnosed during life. They might simulate malignant neoplasms of this organ if they produced any symptoms or signs.

The Lung

Pulmonary lesions of acquired syphilis are rare. Occasionally a solitary gumma is removed in mistake for a malignant tumour. Multiple gummata may, on healing, result in fibroid lung and bronchiectasis. There are usually no symptoms of the active stage but cough and sputum with, perhaps, low-grade fever and loss of weight may occur. X-rays show localized shadows suggesting tumour formation. The diagnosis is made by exclusion of common diseases of the lung, such as neoplasm and tuberculosis, by positive serological tests, and by a favourable response to antisyphilitic treatment. Such response is, of course, not to be expected with massive fibrosis due to old healed gummata.

Urinary Tract

Gummatous lesions of the kidney, bladder and prostate are rare; but cases are recorded in the literature, and the possibility may be considered in patients with proven untreated late syphilis presenting symptoms referable to the urinary tract.

Reproductive Organs

Gummata of the female genital organs are very rare. On the other hand, gumma of the testis is occasionally seen. It is not so commonly found as might be assumed from the space given to it in textbooks of surgery. The condition may take the form of one or more localized gummata or of

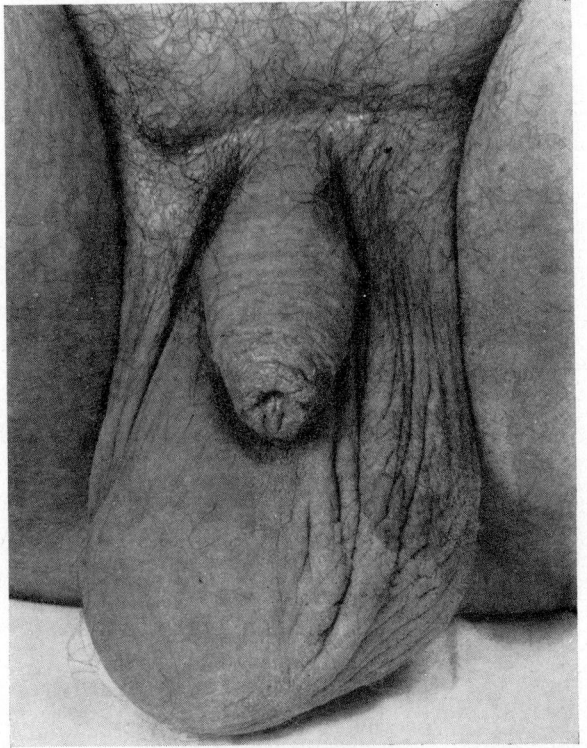

Fig. 54. Gumma of right testis.

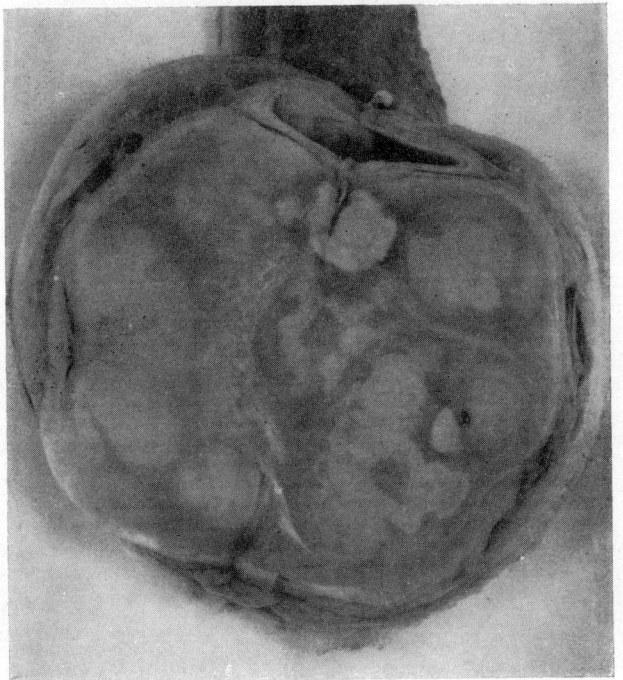

Fig. 55. Gumma of testis: macroscopic section.

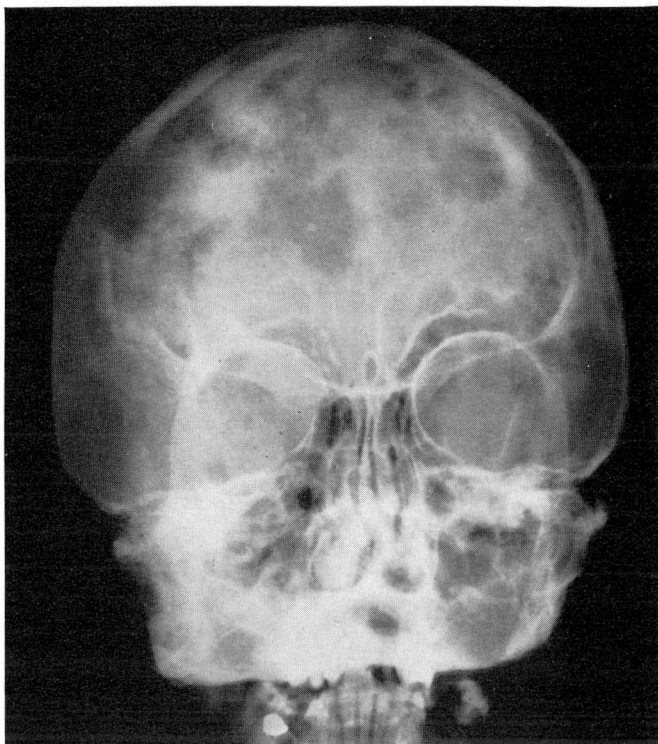

Fig. 56. X-ray showing gummatous osteoperiostitis of frontal bones.

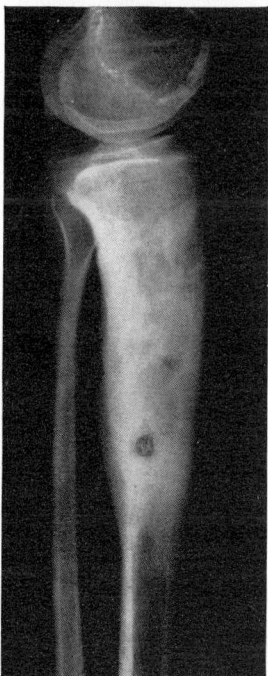

Fig. 57 (*left*). X-ray showing gummatous osteoperiostitis of tibia.

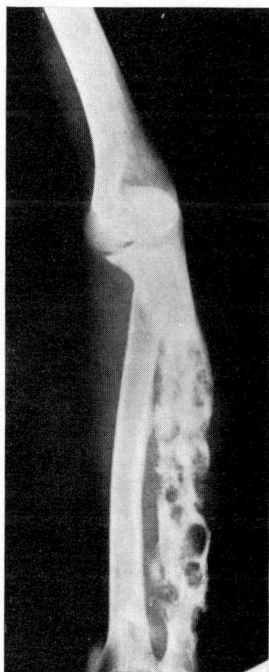

Fig. 58 (*right*). X-ray showing advanced gummatous osteoperiostitis of ulna.

diffuse gummatous infiltration. On healing, the latter causes diffuse inter-stitial fibrosis, and if it is slight in degree clinical signs may not be evident. In most cases the testis slowly enlarges without causing pain. Testicular sensation is lost but the patient is aware of a dragging sensation and altered consistency of the organ. The swelling is usually smooth with a regular surface and feels heavy, presenting as the so-called 'billiard ball' testis. The epididymis is only rarely involved. The process is usually unilateral and there is sometimes a secondary hydrocele. Gummata of the body of the testis do not reach the scrotal subcutaneous tissue and skin and do not ulcerate on the surface (Figs. 54 and 55). Gummata may, however, com-mence in the scrotal subcutaneous tissue and gummatous ulceration follow.

The main differential diagnosis is from neoplasm and from tuberculous epididymitis. The possibility of orchitis of mumps and gonococcal or 'non-specific' epididymitis may also have to be considered.

As with other visceral lesions of late syphilis, biopsy or the application of the therapeutic test may confirm the diagnosis. Serological tests are almost certain to be positive.

Occasionally patients are suspected of having visceral syphilis from the clinical findings, but reagin tests prove to be negative. In these cases, if the condition is syphilitic, the specific tests are positive.

REFERENCE

1.   HAHN, R. D. (1943) *Am. J. Syph.*, **27,** 529.

4

Cardiovascular Syphilis

The indolent chronic inflammatory process of syphilis takes longest to manifest itself in the cardiovascular and nervous systems. The interval from infection to the first signs of this late involvement may take from 10 to 40 years. The chronic inflammatory reaction gradually destroys the affected tissues and serious clinical manifestations may follow.

The incidence of cardiovascular involvement in cases of late, untreated syphilis is probably in the region of 10 per cent[1] but this figure would be higher if it were possible to accept all diagnoses made at autopsy. Pathologists vary in their criteria of diagnosis, which may not be based on the demonstration of treponemes by special staining of sections but may depend on evidence of chronic inflammation. As Rosahn[2] has shown, these changes are not always specific. Cardiovascular syphilis is commoner in negroes than in whites, and commoner in men than in women.

The age of onset depends to some extent on the age of the patient when infected, but may be somewhat earlier in negroes. About 60 per cent of patients with cardiovascular syphilis develop clinical signs of the condition within 20 years. Many patients give no history of the primary or secondary stages. The incidence is higher in those whose occupation has involved heavy physical work. The nervous system is also affected in about 40 per cent of cases of cardiovascular syphilis.[3] At the time of diagnosis reagin tests are positive in about 90 per cent of cases; the specific tests are positive in nearly all cases.

The efficient diagnosis of cardiovascular syphilis during life demands careful clinical examination in every case of syphilis with, in addition, X-rays of the chest (posteroanterior and oblique views) and screening of the heart and aorta by an expert. X-rays should include overpenetrated views for demonstration of calcification. Electrocardiograms, phonocardiograms or angiocardiograms may assist diagnosis in certain cases.

Cases of cardiovascular syphilis may be divided into three main categories: syphilis of the heart, syphilis of the great vessels, and syphilis of the medium-sized arteries.

SYPHILIS OF THE HEART

This is said to take the form of diffuse myocarditis or gumma of the heart. Experience casts doubts on the existence of the former, and the latter is certainly very rare. If such a diagnosis is made at all, it is likely to be made at autopsy. Myocarditis can only be proved to be syphilitic if *Treponema pallidum* can be demonstrated in the cardiac muscle. Gumma of the interventricular septum is occasionally suggested as a diagnosis ante mortem by demonstrating a bundle branch block. A gumma involving the bundle of His is a very rare cause of complete heart block. Gummata involving the myocardium, the various heart valves, the origin of the pulmonary artery, and the pericardium have been reported at autopsy.

SYPHILIS OF THE GREAT VESSELS

Lesions may occur in the aorta, in the pulmonary artery or in the great vessels arising from the aorta (Figs. 59–66). Syphilis of the aorta is by far the most common. Treponemes are presumed to reach the aorta by way of the vasa vasorum during blood-borne dissemination in the early stages of the disease. Inflammatory reaction in the form of exudation of small lymphocytes and plasma cells can be seen about the vessels of the adventitia, and the process appears to extend into the media by way of the perivascular lymphatics of the vasa vasorum. Treponemes have been demonstrated by special staining methods. As the result of endarteritis obliterans, areas of the media supplied by obliterated radicals of the vasa vasorum undergo necrosis, with fragmentation and destruction of the elastic tissue and replacement by white fibrous tissue (see Fig. 59). The areas of intima overlying the patches of mesaortitis undergo thickening due to hyalinization, and subsequently become scarred and thinned. If these changes are extensive they produce gross alterations in the aortic wall. The adventitia is thickened and fibrotic, and stretching of the scarred media produces irregular increase in the transverse diameter of the aortic wall with some lengthening of the section involved. The intimal surface shows longitudinal striation and swollen, greyish, succulent patches, some 5 to 10 mm in diameter, overlying patches of mesaortitis. In other areas, scarring of the intima has occurred leaving the general effect of pitting and irregularity. All these changes are more common and more widespread in the proximal than in the distal thoracic aorta. The damaged intima is often the site of atheromatous changes, which may lead to calcification in the ascending aorta often arranged in a linear fashion. Swollen intimal patches may involve the openings of one or both coronary arteries in the sinuses of Valsalva, and may cause narrowing to as little as one-quarter of the normal lumen. If the patches become fibrotic the narrowing is permanent, producing 'coronary ostial stenosis'.

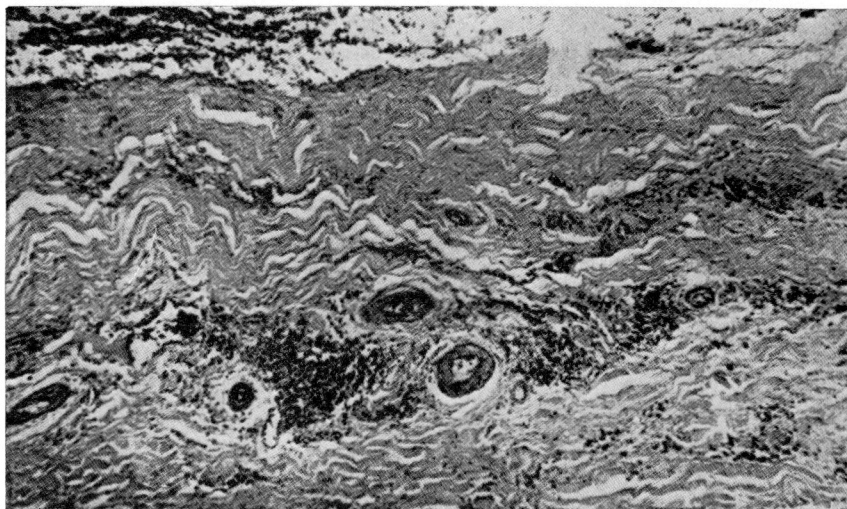

Fig. 59. Cardiovascular syphilis: section of aorta showing degeneration of elastic fibres. (*Magnification* × 80.)

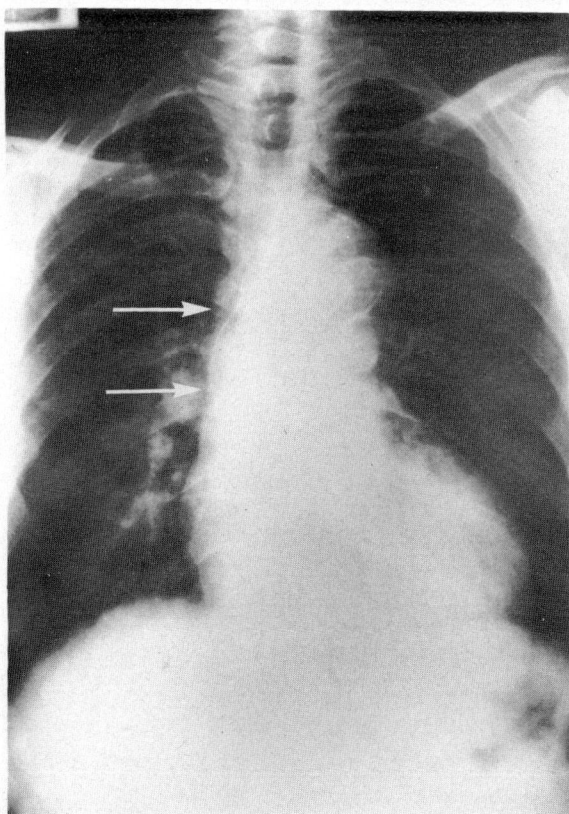

Fig. 60. Cardiovascular syphilis: X-ray of saccular aneurysm of the arch of the aorta with linear calcification in this and the ascending aorta.

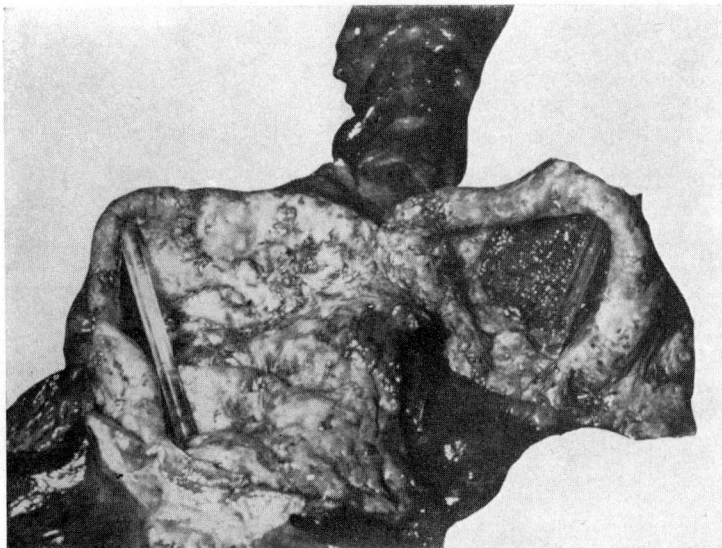

Fig. 61. Cardiovascular syphilis: post-mortem picture of aortitis with clot in small saccular aneurysm.

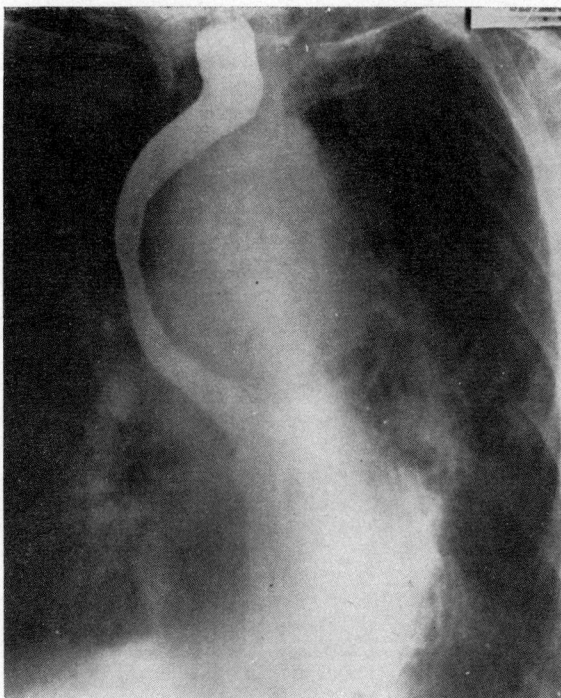

Fig. 62. Cardiovascular syphilis: X-ray of aneurysm of the arch of the aorta shown by a barium swallow.

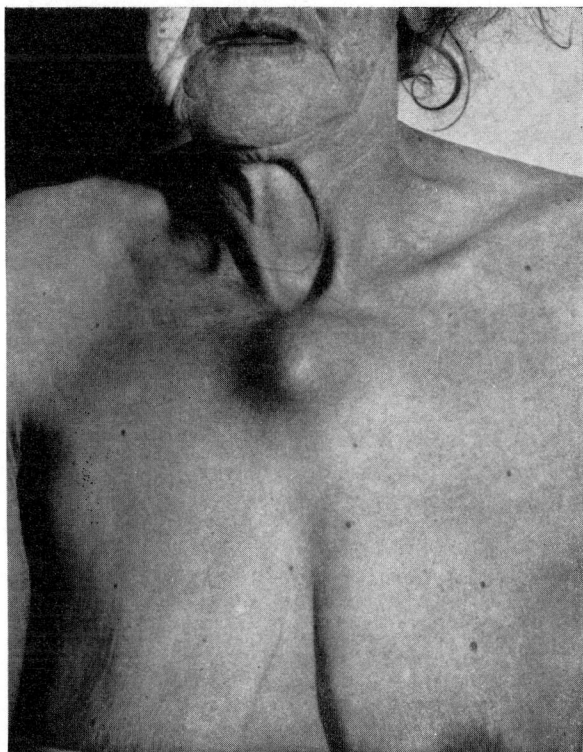

Fig. 63. Cardiovascular syphilis: aneurysm eroding through the upper sternum.

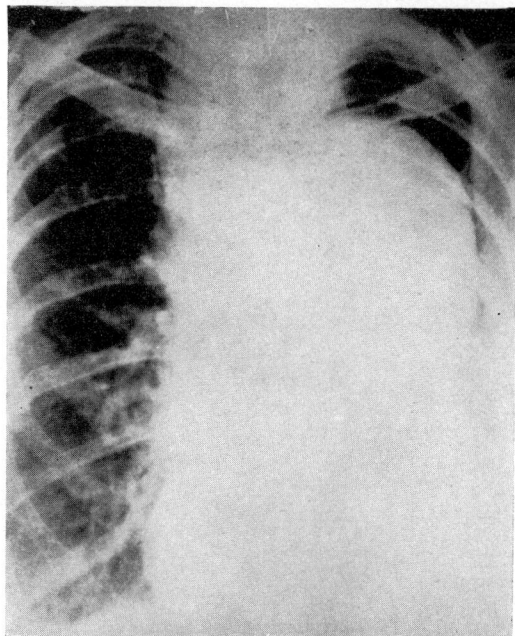

Fig. 64. Cardiovascular syphilis: X-ray of aneurysm of descending part of the arch of the aorta; pressure on the left lower bronchus has caused collapse of the left lower lobe.

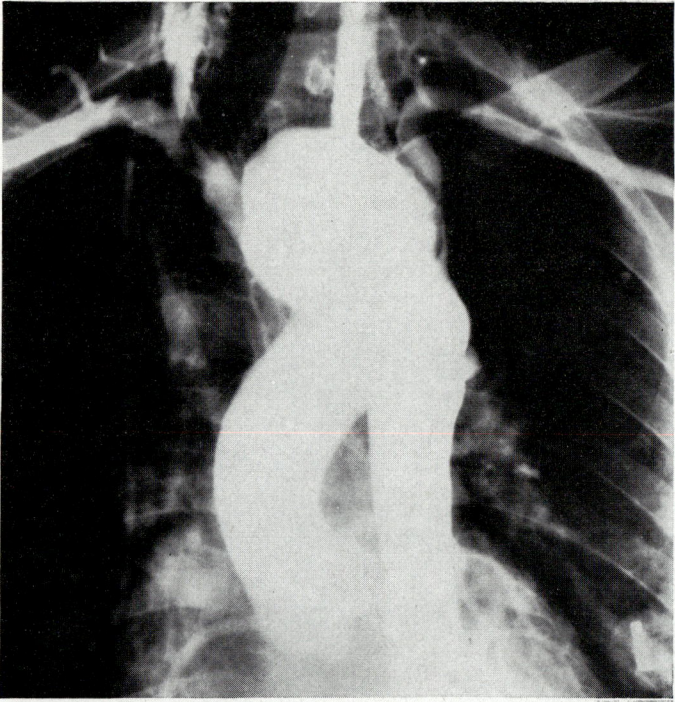

Fig. 65. Cardiovascular syphilis: aortogram of aneurysm of aortic arch pressing on trachea and left subclavian artery.

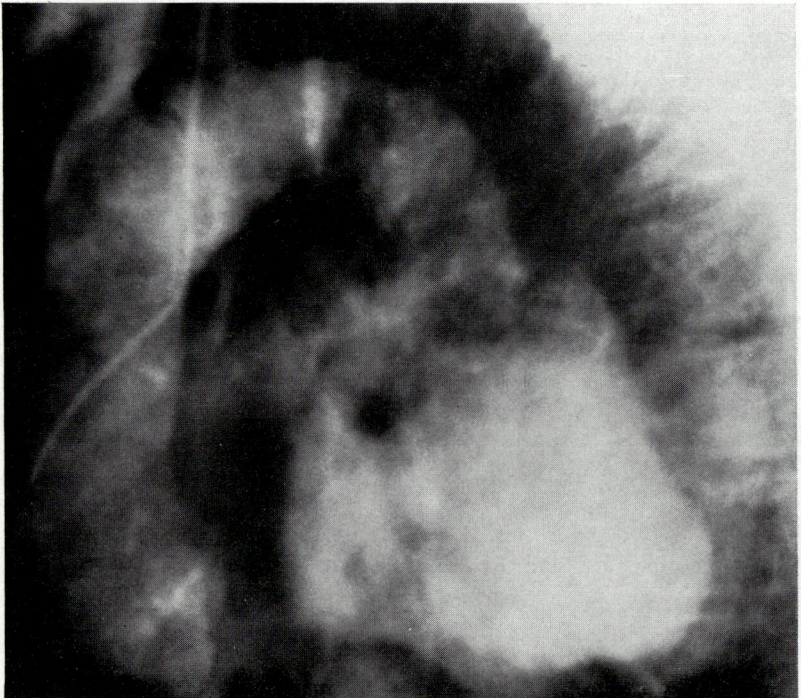

Fig. 66. Cardiovascular syphilis: aortogram of aneurysm of descending aorta pressing on vertebral bodies to cause erosion.

Other clinical results of aortitis are due to the loss of elasticity and fibrosis of the media. If the aortic dilatation is minimal, then the condition is termed 'uncomplicated aortitis'; but if dilatation of the proximal aorta extends to the aortic ring, the valve cusps become separated at their commissures and at their central meeting point and 'aortic regurgitation' (insufficiency) will occur. The intimal process may extend to the valve cusps, causing scarring and deformity, and increasing the insufficiency of the valve. Finally, gross dilatation of the aorta at any point, due to the weakening of the aortic wall and high internal pressure, will cause the condition called 'aortic aneurysm'.

Uncomplicated Aortitis

Ideally it should be possible to make a clinical diagnosis of aortitis which is not complicated by coronary ostial stenosis, aortic regurgitation, or aneurysm. Retrosternal aching pain may occur but symptoms are usually absent and signs are minimal; in fact, it is only when a loud and tambour-like second sound ('bruit de Tabourka') is heard in a patient without hypertension or evidence of atherosclerosis that the clinical diagnosis can be suspected. Nevertheless an aortic ejection sound and soft systolic ejection murmur may arouse suspicion. Radiological diagnosis of the uncomplicated condition may also be difficult, for it is uncommon in these cases for local or diffuse dilatation of slight degree to be demonstrated either in X-ray or by screening. It has been claimed, however, that angiocardiography increases the proportion of cases in which the diagnosis can be made.[4] This technique visualizes the first part of the ascending aorta, which is normally obscured by the heart shadow and is the area most commonly involved. Linear calcification of the ascending aorta is a useful sign of syphilitic aortitis in the absence of significant dilatation. There are no typical electrocardiographic changes in cases of uncomplicated aortitis.

Coronary Ostial Stenosis

The involvement of the ostia of the right or left or both coronary arteries by the syphilitic process may produce narrowing or occlusion. Occlusion is rare but may cause sudden death. In most cases the lumen is still patent, but the narrowing produces coronary insufficiency resulting in myocardial ischaemia. Coronary thrombosis is rare but when it does occur in a patient with syphilis it may be due to coincidental coronary atheroma. Patients with coronary ostial stenosis often have aortic regurgitation and sometimes aneurysm of the ascending aorta as well. The main clinical result of coronary ostial stenosis is angina pectoris; this anginal pain is of the 'referred' type and may radiate up as high as the face and as low as the epigastrium, indicating reflex levels in the cord between C2 and D8. Usually it starts as a sub-sternal ache, which may be gripping in character, and may radiate down the left arm into the hand. A typical attack of angina is precipitated by effort and the patient may collapse. The pain may be agonizing and the patient pale, cold and sweating; but the attack rarely lasts more than 10 to 15 minutes. Sometimes an attack may be precipitated by emotion, such as anger or amusement, or by cold. As the condition progresses, attacks may also occur at rest, particularly at night. Diagnosis can be made from a typical history alone, but in more obscure cases the fact of disappearance of the pain after the administration of nitrites is very suggestive, although these may not be as effective as in coronary atheroma. An electrocardiogram may confirm the diagnosis by showing the typical depression of the ST segment and T-wave inversion. Sometimes these changes can only be demonstrated after exercising the patient to an extent short of producing an anginal attack (see tracings, before exercise and after exercise).

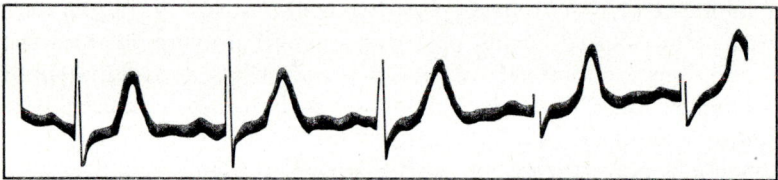

Before exercise

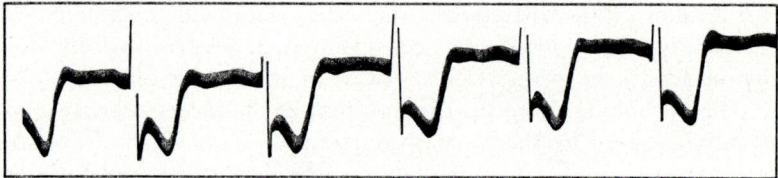

After exercise

Coronary Ostial Stenosis: Exercise Electrocardiogram

Aortic Regurgitation

Insufficiency of the aortic valve is more commonly caused by dilatation of the aortic ring than by primary involvement of the cusps; but, as already described, the cusps themselves may be involved in the intimal fibrotic process, undergoing thickening and distortion, with typical rolled-up edges, resulting in even more severe regurgitation. If coronary ostial stenosis is also present the patient may describe attacks of angina pectoris. It is important to realize that aortic regurgitation is commonly symptomless in the early stages; when symptoms do occur they are most likely to be dyspnoea on exertion and paroxysmal nocturnal dyspnoea due to left-sided heart failure. These patients often state that they sleep with at least two pillows; they may be woken suddenly by a feeling of suffocation, and have to sit on the edge of the bed or in a chair until breathlessness subsides. This symptom is probably due to postural pulmonary oedema occurring when the patient slips off his pillows during sleep. Occasionally, death may result from this pulmonary oedema. Some patients with aortic regurgitation complain of pounding in the head or roaring in the ears or faintness on assuming the upright position. If the condition progresses right heart failure may supervene, with oedema of the lower limbs and over the sacrum, raised jugular venous pressure, marked dyspnoea and enlarged tender liver, sometimes associated with ascites.

Signs of the disease may be obvious, but are sometimes minimal and then may be easily missed. The heart is often enlarged, as indicated by a forceful apex beat which is displaced downwards into the sixth space and outwards towards the axilla. There is a 'blowing' aortic diastolic murmur, usually high-pitched but not musical, and better heard with a diaphragm stethoscope. Its onset is immediately after the aortic second sound which may be loud. It is often widely transmitted over the precordium and may be maximal at the aortic area or down the left of the sternum, particularly in the third or fourth space. It may also be well heard down the right of the sternum and at the apex. The diastolic murmur is accentuated if the patient is made to lean forward and to hold his breath in full expiration and also when the heart rate is slowing after exertion. It is decrescendo in type and lasts through most of diastole. An associated aortic systolic murmur due to the dilatation of the ascending aorta and the increased stroke output is so common that the systolic and diastolic murmurs are sometimes described as 'to and fro' in type. Occasionally the aortic second sound may be absent, which probably indicates involvement of the aortic valve cusps rather than dilatation of the aortic ring alone. A diastolic murmur which is difficult to hear may be more apparent when the ear is applied direct to the chest wall. There seems to be little correlation between the intensity of the murmur and the severity of the regurgitation.

The typical pulse of aortic regurgitation, first described by Corrigan, is collapsing in type; that is, it is forceful with a rapid rise but recedes at once. It can best be felt by grasping with an encircling hand the wrist or forearm and holding it above the level of the patient's heart. The pulse pressure is considerably increased, but it must be remembered that raised pulse pressure may be associated with an inelastic aorta due to arteriosclerosis and be present in other diseases, such as hypertension and high output states such as thyrotoxicosis. In cases of aortic incompetence, estimations of the blood pressure show high systolic and low diastolic levels. The raised pulse pressure with relaxed peripheral vessels results in capillary pulsation, which may be seen in the skin or fundus oculi, or by pressing a glass slide against the everted lip, or by examination of the nail bed of a finger. A 'pistol shot' sound may be heard over the femoral arteries due to the high pressure during systole and collapse of the arterial walls during diastole. An apical mid-diastolic or presystolic 'rumble' is heard in some cases of severe aortic regurgitation (Austin Flint murmur).

This is said to be caused by blood regurgitating into the left ventricle during diastole, impeding the opening of the anterior cusp of the mitral valve and so causing functional obstruction. However, studies employing echocardiography[5] suggest that this may not be the correct explanation. Occasionally a patient is found to have a loud musical or 'dovecote' diastolic murmur which may be audible to the examiner even without application of a stethoscope; it is usually due to rupture, perforation or retroversion of an aortic valve cusp.

X-ray findings may be of additional help in diagnosis when the shadow of linear calcification is present in the ascending aorta (see Fig. 60). The calcification is due to atheromatous change which is very uncommon in the ascending aorta of non-syphilitic patients. Most, but not all, of these patients show enlargement of the left ventricle. The electrocardiogram is likely to show left axis deviation, and changes in the ST segment and T-waves may also be found. They are probably due to left ventricular strain or sometimes ischaemia from coronary ostial stenosis.

DIFFERENTIAL DIAGNOSIS. When a patient is found to have aortic regurgitation, conditions other than syphilis have to be considered; these include old rheumatic carditis, bacterial endocarditis, atherosclerotic aortic valve disease and severe hypertension. The condition is also found occasionally as a congenital abnormality, as a complication of Marfan's disease and it may supervene on a bicuspid aortic valve. It has been described in association with Reiter's disease and with ankylosing spondylitis. These diseases may be present singly or in any combination. Aortic disease due to rheumatic carditis usually commences in younger patients, and there may or may not be a definite or suggestive history of rheumatic fever. Stenosis of the aortic valve is more common than incompetence, and there is often a mid-diastolic or presystolic mitral murmur of mitral stenosis. The latter should not be confused with the Austin Flint murmur. Atrial fibrillation, which is uncommon in cases of syphilis, is often found as a sequel to rheumatic carditis. Screening shows no evidence of aortic dilatation or linear calcification in the ascending aorta, and a barium swallow may show a left atrial 'curve' due to enlargement associated with mitral stenosis. Subacute bacterial endocarditis is more likely to complicate a case of rheumatic carditis, although it has been reported in cases of aortic incompetence due to syphilis. With atherosclerosis regurgitation is minimal and peripheral signs of regurgitation are rare. X-ray evidence of calcified plaques in the aortic knuckle and distal aorta is common and there may be calcification of the aortic valve cusps.

Pulmonary diastolic murmurs are nearly always secondary to severe pulmonary hypertension. Attention to the associated signs should help to distinguish pulmonary regurgitation from aortic regurgitation.

Aneurysm

The term 'aneurysm' indicates a marked degree of dilatation of the aorta and the swelling may be fusiform or saccular in shape. Saccular aneurysm is less likely when there is aortic regurgitation.

A saccular aneurysm may be connected to the aorta by a broad or narrow orifice, and subsidiary or 'daughter' pouches may arise from the sac. Ulceration of the endothelial lining of the sac may occur with rupture or subsequent healing by scar tissue. Thrombosis and calcification sometimes occur in a sac or daughter sac with the likelihood of considerable diminution of pulsation. Fusiform aneurysm results from gross dilatation of one segment of the aorta. Saccular aneurysms of the thoracic aorta are usually caused by syphilis. Fusiform aneurysms are now more commonly due to atheroma than to syphilis, particularly those affecting the descending aorta. Other occasional causes include collagen disease, granulomatous arteritis, dissecting aneurysm, idiopathic aortic arch syndrome, Marfan's disease, Behçet's disease and trauma associated with sudden deceleration accidents. In the abdominal aorta, atheroma is the likely cause of any aneurysm. The diagnosis is sometimes made at autopsy (see Fig. 61) for even large aneurysms may present neither symptoms nor signs, and in such cases ante-mortem diagnosis can only be made by radiological examination.

Aneurysm of the Ascending Aorta ('Aneurysm of Signs')

The ascending aorta is the commonest site of aneurysm due to syphilis. It is likely to bulge laterally into the right lung field and anteriorly against the ribs and sternum, so that parasternal dullness on percussion and arterial pulsation in the second and third right interspaces may be the earliest signs of the condition. There may be a loud aortic systolic murmur and systolic thrill, and loud aortic second sound. As the aneurysm increases in size it may, by its pressure, erode the bones of the anterior chest wall (see Fig. 63) producing the symptom of pain in this region. The superior vena cava may be compressed. Sometimes, however, it extends medially and may displace the trachea to the left or press on the pulmonary artery. Occasionally the aneurysm extends postero-medially, producing pressure symptoms or pulsation of the left upper chest and giving clinical signs suggesting aneurysmal dilatation of the arch of the aorta. An aneurysm of the ascending aorta may cause sudden death by rupture. If this occurs into the pericardium, death is due to cardiac tamponade; if into the pleura, there are signs of collapse of the right lung, due to haemothorax, before death; if into the right bronchus or lung, death follows a severe haemoptysis. Death may also occur after rupture through the skin of the anterior chest wall; occasionally rupture into the pulmonary artery will cause death as a result of right heart failure.

Aneurysm of the Arch of the Aorta ('Aneurysm of Symptoms')

Aneurysm of the arch of the aorta usually arises from its convex surface. It may appear as a pulsating mass in the suprasternal notch and may press on the trachea (see Fig. 65) producing stridor and a brassy cough. It may involve the left recurrent laryngeal nerve causing hoarseness, and on laryngoscopy the left vocal cord may be seen to be paralysed. It may press on and displace the oesophagus but dysphagia is rare. Pressure on the left bronchus at each heart beat may produce the sign known as 'tracheal tug'. To elicit this sign, the patient is seated with the neck moderately extended and the observer, standing behind the head, exercises gentle upward traction on the lower border of the cricoid cartilage, with the two fore-fingers in the episternal notch. A downward tug is felt at each heart beat. Pressure on the left bronchus may also simulate the symptoms and signs of carcinoma of the bronchus. Pressure on the cervical sympathetic chain will produce enophthalmos and a small pupil (Horner's syndrome); while pressure on the superior vena cava may produce cyanosis, oedema, and dilatation of the superficial veins of the arms, upper chest and neck. The phrenic nerve is rarely involved with paralysis of the diaphragm. If an aneurysm of the arch presses on the innominate or left common carotid or subclavian arteries, there may be a loud systolic murmur and signs of diminished or absent pulsation in the neck or arms may be present, produc-ing variation in the systolic blood pressure and also, possibly, asynchronism of the pulses, depending on which great vessel is involved. With pressure upon the innominate or left common carotid artery, patients may complain of dizziness due to cerebral anoxia. This may also result from occlusion of the left subclavian artery ('steal syndrome'). Occasionally the aneurysm projects posteriorly and erodes the bodies of the 4th to the 6th thoracic vertebrae. Pressure on nerve roots may cause severe root pain. Death may result from rupture into the trachea or bronchus, as already described, into the oesophagus with severe haematemesis, into the mediastinum, or into the superior vena cava with severe dyspnoea and cyanosis due to cardiac overload.

Diagnosis of aneurysm of the aortic arch may be aided by X-ray combined with a barium swallow, which shows the indentation of the oesophagus by the swelling (see Fig. 62, p. 70).

Aneurysm of the Descending Thoracic Aorta ('Aneurysm of No Signs and No Symptoms')

Aneurysm of the descending thoracic aorta is rare and usually symptomless. It may project to the left and anteriorly or posteriorly. Symptoms of deep-seated and continuous pain in the back, boring in character, may result from pressure on the bodies of the 7th to the 11th thoracic vertebrae, and occasionally severe erosion may cause involvement of the spinal cord (see Fig. 66). Rupture of an aneurysm at this site is rare.

Aneurysm of the Abdominal Aorta

There is some difference of opinion as to how often an abdominal aneurysm is due to syphilis, but it is certainly much less common than in the thorax.

If the aneurysm is below the level of the renal arteries, syphilis is a very unlikely cause. The patient may complain of pain in the abdomen or back, worse at night, but relieved by change of position. Root pain may occur. On examination, a mass may be felt which shows expansile pulsation, and there may be a palpable thrill and an audible murmur. Radiography may show calcium in the wall of the aneurysm and sometimes erosion of the 12th thoracic and 1st and 2nd lumbar vertebrae. Such a patient may also have a thoracic aneurysm.

The diagnosis of aneurysm is often aided by various radiological techniques. Routine posteroanterior and oblique views of the chest should be taken, and further aid may be obtained by screening. Special help may be obtained by angiocardiography for aneurysms at otherwise inaccessible sites, such as the sinuses of Valsalva, which can be outlined. This method also helps to differentiate aneurysms from other mediastinal or intra-abdominal masses. It must be realized, however, that the necessary technique and apparatus are complicated, involving cardiac catheterization by way of the carotid or femoral arteries with serial X-rays or cine-radiography as the contrast medium is injected. Untoward reactions have occurred.

Aneurysms at Other Sites

The innominate, left common carotid and left subclavian arteries may sometimes be involved by the syphilitic process. Aneurysms in these sites are all rare, but the commonest is an innominate aneurysm which may press downwards on to the aortic arch and push the trachea to the left. There may be lowered systolic blood pressure in the right arm and asynchronism of the radial pulses, as with aneurysm of the arch, and, occasionally, right recurrent laryngeal nerve or phrenic nerve palsy. X-ray shows a dense superior mediastinal shadow with an obliquely sloping right edge; the aortic knuckle is pushed downwards and to the left. Sometimes syphilitic aortitis produces narrowing or even occlusion of the openings of these great vessels due to intimal thickening without any evidence of aneurysm, resulting in systolic bruits and changes in blood pressure and pulse as already described. Atheroma can produce similar clinical features.

SYPHILIS OF THE MEDIUM-SIZED ARTERIES

The cerebral and spinal arteries are sometimes affected, and involvement of the carotid, hepatic, mesenteric, renal, iliac or femoral arteries has been described but is certainly rare. Cerebral and spinal vascular syphilis are classified with neurosyphilis because the main symptoms and signs are neurological. There is destruction of the elastic layer of the media by the chronic inflammation, and aneurysmal dilatation may occur. On the other hand, the relatively small lumen of the vessel, which is further narrowed by intimal thickening, may be the site of thrombosis. In sites other than the nervous system, ante-mortem diagnosis is rare, but occasionally thrombosis of the main vessel to a limb, which may cause gangrene, has been correctly diagnosed as due to this cause.

REFERENCES

1. GJESTLAND, T. (1955) *Acta derm.-venereol. (Stockh.)*, **35**, Suppl. 34, 280.
2. ROSAHN, P. D. (1950) *Vener. Dis. Inform.*, Suppl. 21.
3. O'BRIEN, J. F., SMITH, C. A. and FISHERKELLER, M. A. (1955) *Br. J. vener. Dis.*, **31**, 74.
4. RICH, C. and WEBSTER, B. (1952) *Am. Heart J.*, **43**, 321.
5. FORTUIN, N. J. and CRAIGE, E. (1972) *Circulation*, **45**, 558.

5

Neurosyphilis

Treponema pallidum invades the central nervous system during the early stages of syphilitic infection. The fact of invasion is indicated by changes in the cerebrospinal fluid in from 20 to 37 per cent of cases,[1] and in a minority of these cases there may also be clinical evidence of meningeal involvement. In the absence of treatment, approximately a third of those with this early invasion, whether symptomatic or asymptomatic, will develop signs of late neurosyphilis after the lapse of years.

The following chart indicates the possible sequence of events:

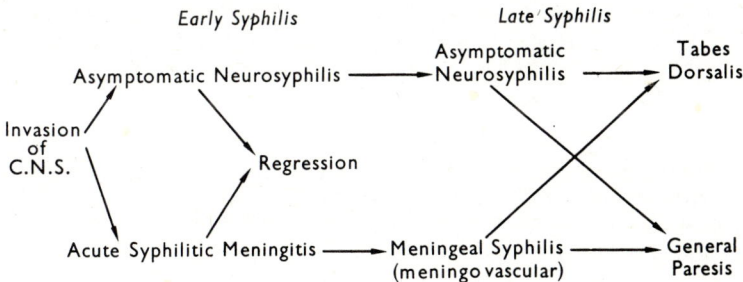

```
        Early Syphilis                    Late Syphilis
                                   Asymptomatic            Tabes
   Asymptomatic Neurosyphilis ───►Neurosyphilis  ───►    Dorsalis
           ↗                ↘                  ╲      ↗
 Invasion                                       ╳
   of               ↘       ↗ Regression      ╱    ╲
  C.N.S.                                                
           ↘       ↗               ↗                  ↘
  Acute Syphilitic Meningitis ───► Meningeal Syphilis ───► General
                                   (meningo vascular)      Paresis
```

Neurosyphilis is less common in women than in men and in negroes and Asians than in whites[2]. There is evidence that patients who develop febrile illness, such as pneumonia, or who become pregnant in the early stages of the disease are less likely to suffer from neurosyphilis. Often there is no history of primary or secondary stages.

CLASSIFICATION of neurosyphilis is a difficult problem because involvement is never confined to the meninges or to the vessels or the parenchyma. Nevertheless the clinical evidence of involvement is usually predominant in one of these tissues. The following is a working classification, but it is subject to the criticism that it depends partly upon clinical and partly upon pathological changes:

Asymptomatic			20 per cent
Meningeal	cerebral ⎱ spinal ⎰		15 per cent
Vascular	cerebral ⎱ spinal ⎰		5 per cent
Parenchymatous	cerebral ⎱ spinal ⎰	15 per cent ⎱ 45 per cent ⎰ 60 per cent	
Gumma	cerebral ⎱ spinal ⎰		Very rare

The presentation can be extremely varied and modified forms occur in which the classical features are absent.

ASYMPTOMATIC NEUROSYPHILIS

The diagnosis of asymptomatic neurosyphilis is established when it is shown that a patient suffering from syphilis has changes in the cerebrospinal fluid, indicating involvement of the central nervous system, but there are no neurological symptoms or physical signs. There may or may not be signs of syphilis in other systems. Cerebrospinal fluid is obtained from the patient by lumbar or cisternal puncture. The former method is routine practice in most countries. The essential investigations are: (a) the cell count, (b) estimation of total protein, (c) one or more tests for reagin, and (d), of more limited importance, Lange's colloidal-gold curve.

CELL COUNT

The fluid normally contains from 0 to 4 cells per mm³. The presence of 5 lymphocytes or more per mm³ may be the first indication of involvement of the central nervous system. The finding suggests a meningeal reaction.

TOTAL PROTEIN

The normal content of protein in the cerebrospinal fluid is usually said to be 20 to 40 mg per 100 ml. An increase in the total protein above 40 mg per cent is commonly considered to be abnormal, but it must be admitted that higher values are sometimes reported from some laboratories without any other evidence to suggest they are of significance.

The level of IgG and IgM in cerebrospinal fluid may be increased in neurosyphilis. Oxelius et al.[3] have suggested that quantitative determination of these immunoglobulins may be of help in assessing the activity of the disease.

REAGIN TEST

Complement-fixation and flocculation tests depending upon the presence of 'reagin' in the cerebrospinal fluid are usually regarded as the only tests which, when positive, give a firm indication of the presence of syphilis of the nervous system. They are not, of course, specific tests, but 'false positive' results are certainly rare in tests of the cerebrospinal fluid. It should be mentioned that a patient suffering from syphilis who has meningitis due to some other cause may show positive tests in the cerebrospinal fluid due to passage of reagin from the blood stream through the choroid plexuses. The specific treponemal tests (TPI, FTA-ABS and TPHA) are nearly always positive in the serum of patients with neurosyphilis, although they may give negative results in cases of very long standing, such as 'burnt-out' tabes. It is extremely rare for these tests to give a positive result on cerebrospinal fluid if it is negative on the patient's serum. The FTA-ABS on the cerebrospinal fluid is generally positive when cells or protein are increased in cases of neurosyphilis.[4]

COLLOIDAL-GOLD TEST

The colloidal-gold test is reported in the form of a graph or by a series of numerals (for full details see the Appendix, p. 393). Notations of o or 1 are considered normal and of 2 to 5 abnormal. Abnormal readings are classified, according to the position of the peak in the graph, into curves affecting the first zone, the mid-zone, or the end-zone. These have also been termed 'paretic', 'luetic', and 'meningitic' curves, but it must be understood that the curves in themselves are *not* diagnostic but reflect changes in the proportions of albumin and globulin in the spinal fluid. These may be produced by other conditions besides syphilis. For instance, a 'paretic' or 'luetic' curve may be found in cases of disseminated sclerosis. Results of the test must be interpreted in the light of other findings in the cerebrospinal fluid and of the whole clinical picture.

If the cerebrospinal fluid is contaminated with blood due to trauma during the lumbar puncture, the results of tests may be invalidated. A rough correction of the white cell count may be made by subtracting one white cell for every 1000 red cells per mm^3. A false positive reagin test due to contamination of the fluid with serum is unlikely to occur unless the cerebrospinal fluid contains sufficient blood to be visible to the naked eye.

Abnormalities of the cell count and protein level are the most sensitive indices of activity of the disease process. They are the first to return to normal values after successful treatment. Tests for reagin or anti-treponemal antibody may remain positive and the colloidal-gold curve abnormal for long periods after the cell count and protein level have become normal.

Classification of Asymptomatic Neurosyphilis

Asymptomatic neurosyphilis can be classified according to variations in these four tests, as follows.

Type I: Minimal changes in cells or protein or both, but negative reagin tests and normal Lange curve.

Type II: Intermediate changes, e.g. raised cells and protein with weakly positive reagin tests and mid-zone Lange curve.

Type III: All four tests abnormal, with strongly positive reagin tests and the colloidal-gold test of the first zone type.

Cerebrospinal fluid of Type III is regarded as specially significant, for it is a warning that, without treatment, the patient is likely to develop general paralysis of the insane. Blood reagin tests are almost always positive when the cerebrospinal fluid shows changes of Type III. It is customary not to examine cerebrospinal fluid before treatment in the primary and secondary stages of the disease, but in all other stages these tests are essential to exclude the diagnosis of asymptomatic neurosyphilis. In cases of pregnancy it is advisable to defer the procedure until at least six weeks after confinement; treatment should not be deferred.

If tests of the cerebrospinal fluid are normal after the secondary stage of the disease, in the absence of clinical signs in the central nervous system, it is the general experience that the patient is very unlikely to develop neurosyphilis, even if no treatment is given.

SYPHILIS OF THE BRAIN

Meningeal Involvement (see Fig. 67, p. 94)

Meningeal involvement can occur in the secondary stage of the disease (see p. 40) or at any time in the later stages; it is sometimes an intercurrent event in the long course of parenchymatous neurosyphilis.

PATHOLOGY

The meninges show perivascular cellular infiltration in which small lymphocytes and plasma cells predominate. This is particularly marked around the vessels in the pia and arachnoid, which show perivascular cuffing, and later there is fibroblastic proliferation. Coincidental with the meningeal reaction there is a general ependymal reaction which results in subependymal gliosis.

In general, the changes produced in the brain may be of four varieties, but any combination of them is possible:

(1) The inflammatory changes affect the meninges over the vertex and spread to the underlying cortex.

(2) The inflammatory changes at the base of the brain involve the infranuclear course of the cranial nerves and the nerves may become compressed by pressure of exudate where they pierce the dura mater.

(3) The circulation of the cerebrospinal fluid is blocked by leptomeningitis which may obliterate the subarachnoid space in the posterior fossa of the brain and produce hydrocephalus.

(4) Subependymal gliosis may interrupt the fibres of the tract that carries the light reflex in the forebrain.

SYMPTOMS AND SIGNS

There may be headache of weeks' or even months' duration. Nausea, vomiting and stiffness of the neck are rare, except with the more acute meningitis of the secondary stage.

The signs are very variable but depend upon the areas affected:

(1) The meninges of the vertex and the underlying cortex are involved. There may be convulsions, aphasia and mental confusion; monoplegia or hemiplegia may occur; papilloedema is common but the pupils are usually normal.

(2) With basal meningitis there may be unilateral or bilateral cranial nerve palsies; there may be papilloedema. The nerves most frequently involved are the 3rd, 6th, 7th, and 8th cranial nerves.

(3) Hydrocephalus is likely to be of the communicating type; there may be marked papilloedema.

(4) The light reflex of the pupils may be lost, and the reflex to accommodation retained. The outline of the pupil may be irregular and the pupils may be unequal in size. If both are grossly constricted ('pin-point') and show the typical changes in reflex response, then the pupils are those described by Argyll Robertson and are called by his name. Changes in the cerebrospinal fluid are usually of Type I or II.

DIFFERENTIAL DIAGNOSIS

Syphilitic meningitis must be differentiated from tuberculous and meningococcal meningitis, from brain tumour or abscess, from osteomyelitis of the skull with extradural abscess, and from other conditions causing papilloedema and signs of raised intracranial pressure. Syphilis should be considered in the causes of epilepsy and mental disease occurring first in adult life, and also in the causes of cranial nerve palsies. Important points in the diagnosis are positive results to serological tests for syphilis, changes in the cerebrospinal fluid, the presence of pupillary abnormalities and, in some cases, the response to treatment.

Vascular Involvement

PATHOLOGY

This is primarily an involvement of blood vessels, but the resulting lesions affect the nervous system because vascular thrombosis results in infarction of nervous tissue. The microscopical changes resemble those of syphilitic aortitis, but in arteries with a much smaller lumen the shrinkage of the intima is the most important factor in pathogenesis because it encourages thrombosis. Aneurysm of cerebral vessels is not caused by syphilis but usually results from developmental defects in the arterial wall.

SYMPTOMS AND SIGNS

There may be prodromal headaches, giddiness, mental disturbances, transient muscular weakness or paraesthesia. The onset of the main attack is sudden; motor paralysis is common. Loss of consciousness is rare, but convulsions or aphasia may occur.

The vessels most frequently involved are branches of the middle cerebral artery, but the anterior and posterior cerebrals, and cerebellar and basilar arteries may undergo thrombosis.

Middle cerebral thrombosis. Branches rather than the main trunk are usually involved, producing contralateral hemiplegia and hemianaesthesia; there may be aphasia.

Anterior cerebral thrombosis. There is mental deterioration with motor aphasia, contralateral hemiplegia and sensory loss of the cortical type, mainly involving the leg.

Posterior cerebral thrombosis. There is contralateral sensory loss, spontaneous pain, hemiathetosis and transient hemiparesis (Déjérine–Roussy syndrome). There may be contralateral homonymous hemianopia.

Cerebellar artery thrombosis. Usually the posterior inferior cerebellar artery is affected. The onset is associated with vertigo and sometimes vomiting. On the side of the lesion there are cerebellar ataxia, Horner's syndrome, loss of sensation to pain and temperature over the face, and dysphagia. There is contralateral loss of pain and temperature sensation over the body (Walkenberg's syndrome).

Basilar artery thrombosis. Thrombosis of the main artery is rare, but sometimes small arteries arising from the upper part of basilar and posterior inferior cerebellar arteries become thrombosed. This results in partial 3rd nerve palsy and crossed hemiplegia of face and leg (Weber's syndrome). Sometimes the red nucleus is also involved (Benedikt's syndrome).

Other vascular syndromes. Sometimes thrombosis of small pontine vessels occurs, producing 6th and 7th nerve palsies with crossed hemiplegia (Millard–Gubler syndrome). There may also be conjugate deviation of the eyes to one side (Forel's syndrome). Thrombosis of small branches of the vertebral arteries may cause 12th nerve palsy, with contralateral hemiplegia or hemianaesthesia.

Changes in the cerebrospinal fluid may be of Type I, but they may be absent in up to 40 per cent of cases. Blood serological tests are positive in almost all the cases.

DIFFERENTIAL DIAGNOSIS

The differential diagnosis is mainly from cerebral thrombosis due to other causes, of which the most common is atheroma. Cerebral thrombosis in younger patients should suggest the diagnosis of syphilitic vascular disease; in older patients atheroma is the more likely cause; but thrombosis due to other conditions may occur in patients who also have latent syphilis, and a distinction is not always possible. Diagnosis must first depend on an awareness of the possibility of syphilis, for without this the specific tests may not be applied.

Meningovascular Involvement

Vascular and meningeal syphilis may occur together in the same patient, resulting in diffuse involvement or in multiple lesions.

Parenchymatous Involvement—General Paralysis (GPI)

PATHOLOGY

Macroscopically, the dura mater is thickened and may be adherent to the vault of the skull. The weight of the brain is diminished due to cortical atrophy, which is more marked anteriorly. Meningeal thickening is variable; the subarachnoid space is dilated and filled with cerebrospinal fluid. The cerebral convolutions are flattened and feel abnormally firm, due to gliosis. The pia mater is firmly adherent to the surface. The ventricular system is dilated and the ependyma has a granular surface with subependymal gliosis, especially in the floor of the fourth ventricle.

Microscopically, there is characteristic inflammatory reaction in the meninges, especially around the blood vessels. Degenerative changes are seen in the parenchyma, involving ganglion cells, axis cylinders, and myelin sheaths; lymphocytes and plasma cells may infiltrate the cortex; glial tissue increases and histiocytes show proliferation and hypertrophy. The latter contain iron in their cytoplasm, a finding which is said to be practically pathognomonic. *Treponema pallidum* may be identified by special staining methods in about half the cases.

SYMPTOMS

The clinical manifestations of GPI do not usually appear until 10 years or more after infection; the patients are often short in stature and of heavy physique.

The symptoms are often slight and indeterminate at first. The patient may well be the last to be aware of them but complaints are made by other members of his family or associates. The patient tends to become irritable and to lose concentration. He tires easily and his memory begins to fail. He reacts too readily to suggestion and may begin to show changes of personality; his behaviour deteriorates and may bring him into conflict with the law. He may suffer from headache and insomnia. As time goes on his judgment becomes very defective and his memory is grossly impaired. He becomes emotionally labile, with gross loss of insight, confused and disorientated, and he suffers from poorly systematized delusions. He may be prone to fainting attacks, to focal or generalized epileptiform convulsions or to 'petit mal'.

SEQUENCE OF MENTAL CHANGES

Period of onset. The onset may be insidious with some of the early symptoms already noted. Relatives and associates may have noticed that the patient has lost drive at his work and is less competent, and he may show less interest in his personal affairs. His condition may suggest a diagnosis of psychoneurosis. On the other hand, the onset may be sudden in the form of a cerebral attack with convulsions, aphasia, confusion and monoplegia or hemiplegia, a so-called congestive attack. Typically these attacks are transient, lasting only for a few hours or days. They may precede obvious mental changes by many months. Sometimes a fully developed psychosis will occur suddenly in the form of a 'brain storm', which may follow a convulsion or a bout of drinking. The psychosis may then improve but will later relapse.

Period of full development. At this stage there has been considerable and irreparable damage to the cortex. The psychosis takes a number of forms. It may be grandiose in type; this is relatively rare, although it conforms to the classical description. The patient is very suggestible and euphoric; he feels 'he has never had it so good'; he may claim that he can run a hundred metres in ten seconds; that he owns a 'Rolls-Royce'; that he won the Grand National last year. The commonest type of psychosis, however, is the deteriorated demented type. Although his mood may be labile, the patient is usually depressed and confused, with defective memory and impairment of judgment. Manic and paranoid types of psychosis may also be seen occasionally.

Period of decline. Mental and physical deterioration become more conspicuous, so that the difference between the various types of psychosis becomes less obvious, with dementia the main feature. Convulsions are common in the terminal stages and there may be 'status epilepticus'. The patient becomes emaciated, bedridden and incontinent, and bedsores develop; death may be due to intercurrent disease, such as pneumonia or renal infection, or may result from respiratory failure associated with convulsions. This period may last for months or years, although most patients who receive no treatment die within five years of developing GPI. Even without treatment clinical remissions may occur occasionally, and, exceptionally, the condition ceases to be progressive.

NEUROLOGICAL SIGNS

In the earlier stages of the disease physical signs may be absent although mental changes are obvious. Pupillary changes are common. Occasionally they are of the Argyll Robertson type, but this suggests that there is an element of tabes present (taboparesis). Sometimes the pupils are large and do not react to light or convergence. There may be dysarthria, with faulty enunciation and slurring of words, which becomes very evident if the patient is tested with a tongue-twisting phrase such as 'West Riding Artillery Brigade' or 'Massachusetts General Hospital'. He may also show impairment of handwriting with illegibility and omission of letters or syllables. In all cases of general paralysis, tests of the mental status should be carried out and a detailed record of both questions and answers should be preserved; this record should include a sample of handwriting. Details of a standard series of tests of mental status are shown in the Appendix (p. 396). It is very important that such tests should be related to the educational and social background of the patient. In addition to their importance in diagnosis, these tests, repeated at intervals after treatment, give a valuable indication of improvement or deterioration. The patient's face has a relaxed, empty expression and there may be tremor of the lips or tongue on protrusion ('trombone tremor'), which can be a very early sign. There is often a mild spastic paraplegia with increased knee and ankle jerks, diminution or loss of abdominal reflexes and extensor plantar responses. Oculomotor palsies or optic atrophy may also be found, and sometimes there are focal signs of hemianopia or hemiparesis. The combination of hemiparesis, convulsions and aphasia has been termed Lissauer's type of GPI. In cases without associated tabes dorsalis, there is no sensory impairment, and when urinary and faecal incontinence occur they are due to mental deterioration.

The cerebrospinal fluid is usually of Type III, but occasionally changes of Types I or II are found. Patients with untreated GPI never have a normal spinal fluid. Blood reagin tests are nearly always positive and the specific tests invariably so.

DIFFERENTIAL DIAGNOSIS

GPI has to be differentiated from meningeal or vascular neurosyphilis. Psychotic manifestations have to be diagnosed from those of cerebral atherosclerosis, manic-depressive psychosis, schizophrenia, central toxic effects of drugs, alcoholism, senility, and the various psychoneuroses. Epilepsy, cerebral tumour or abscess, pernicious anaemia, Huntington's chorea, subdural haematoma, Pick's dementia, Alzheimer's disease, myxoedema, cardiac failure, uraemia, cholaemia, miliary tuberculosis, and carcinomatosis are among the diseases which have to be considered.

Gumma

Gumma of the brain is now a very rare condition. When it occurs it is likely to develop in the meninges, perhaps by extension from bones of the skull, and as it increases in size it may invade and compress the parenchyma of the brain. Gummata may be single or multiple and may occur at the vertex or at the base of the brain. The microscopical changes are those of gummata in other systems. *T. pallidum* is seldom found by staining methods.

SYMPTOMS

The symptoms are those of a space-filling tumour with headache, nausea and vomiting. Convulsions may occur and vision may deteriorate.

SIGNS

There may be signs of increased intracranial pressure such as papilloedema. The localizing signs will vary according to the exact site of the lesion; there may be cranial nerve palsies or hemiplegia. The electroencephalogram (EEG) may show the evidence of a localized 'tumour'. The pressure of the cerebrospinal fluid may be increased and there may be changes of Type I or II. Blood serological tests are positive.

DIFFERENTIAL DIAGNOSIS

The most important diagnosis is from brain tumour, but other types of neurosyphilis, such as meningitis with hydrocephalus, have to be excluded. Because of the rarity of the condition the diagnosis is sometimes made by biopsy following brain surgery. Diagnosis may not be easy, but if anti-syphilitic treatment results in the disappearance of symptoms and signs and the EEG becomes normal, there is a strong presumption that the lesion was syphilitic.

SYPHILIS OF THE SPINAL CORD

Meningeal Involvement—Meningomyelitis

PATHOLOGY

This is similar to that of meningeal syphilis of the brain. It is likely to result in spread to underlying nerve tissue with a tendency to involve the pyramidal and other motor tracts rather than the sensory tracts. Spinal nerves may be affected in the same way as the cranial nerves, producing lower motor-neurone lesions. The meninges may be affected in the cervical or dorso-lumbar regions, separately or together, and this gives rise to three different clinical syndromes, all of which are now uncommon to the point of rarity: (1) dorso-lumbar meningitis mainly involving the pyramidal tracts (Erb's syphilitic spastic paraplegia); (2) cervical meningitis involving spinal nerve roots and spinal tracts (syphilitic hypertrophic cervical pachymeningitis); and (3) a combination of certain features in (1) and (2) (syphilitic amyotrophy).

SYMPTOMS AND SIGNS

Erb's spastic paraplegia. The onset is gradual with progressive stiffness of the legs, so that the patient drags his feet on walking; sensory changes are relatively rare, but bladder involvement is not uncommon and may be an early feature. The patient has an irritable bladder with small capacity, resulting in frequency of micturition. The leg muscles are hypertonic; the reflexes are increased with ankle clonus; and there is bilateral extensor plantar response. The paraplegia is of the extensor type.

Hypertrophic cervical pachymeningitis. The onset is gradual with headaches, bulbar cranial nerve lesions and pains in the neck, shoulders and upper limbs. Horner's syndrome may be present. There are usually lower motor-neurone lesions of the shoulder girdle and arms, with lost reflexes, flaccidity and wasting. Sensory loss from posterior root compression may occur. Progressive spastic paraplegia and sensory loss below the level of the lesion may follow due to compression and ischaemia of the spinal cord.

Syphilitic amyotrophy. The onset is gradual. The signs are of lower motor-neurone lesions affecting the shoulder girdle and arms and the small muscles of the hands or rarely the outer sides of the legs. The affected muscles may be painful at first. Spastic paraplegia may develop but is uncommon.

In these three conditions changes of the cerebrospinal fluid are usually of Type I or II. Blood reagin tests are usually positive and the specific tests virtually always so.

DIFFERENTIAL DIAGNOSIS

Spinal meningeal syphilis has to be differentiated from vascular neuro-syphilis and from gumma of the spinal cord; Erb's spastic paraplegia must be diagnosed from disseminated sclerosis; cervical pachymeningitis from spinal tumour or a cervical disc lesion, and syphilitic amyotrophy from motor-neurone disease. Signs of cerebral syphilis, especially pupillary changes, may be present and help in diagnosis.

Vascular Involvement

PATHOLOGY

As in the brain, vascular thrombosis results in infarction. The spinal cord is supplied by one anterior and two posterior spinal arteries. The former supplies the whole central area of the cord, and when this vessel undergoes thrombosis the clinical onset is sudden and dramatic and not unlike that which results from transection of the cord. The effects vary according to the level at which the artery is thrombosed; it is usually affected in the thoracic or lumbar regions.

SYMPTOMS AND SIGNS

The onset is sudden, with paralysis of the legs associated with urinary and faecal incontinence. There is a sensory level, with loss of sensation of pain and temperature below it. The paralysis is at first of the type called 'spinal shock', with lost reflexes and muscle atonia; this is replaced within two to three weeks by spasticity with increased reflex and extensor plantar responses; the incontinence continues. There are involuntary contractions of the flexor muscles of the legs and abdomen to any pain stimulus (mass reflex), and finally a condition of paraplegia in flexion is established. Trophic ulcers are common. Thrombosis of a lateral branch of the anterior spinal artery produces sudden weakness followed by wasting of muscles supplied by the affected spinal segment. The spino-thalamic tract is often affected leading to loss of sensation to pain and temperature on the opposite side of the body with an upper level a few segments below the site of the lesion. Thrombosis of a posterior spinal artery gives rise to so localized and restricted a lesion that it is unlikely to be diagnosed during life. There may, however, be segmental loss of all forms of sensation with posterior column and pyramidal signs below the level of the lesion on the same side.

Cerebrospinal fluid may be normal but usually there are changes of Type I. Blood reagin tests are positive in more than 90 per cent of cases and the specific tests should be positive in the remainder.

DIFFERENTIAL DIAGNOSIS

The condition must be distinguished from the various types of meningeal spinal syphilis and from gumma of the cord. Transverse myelitis or tumour of the spinal cord may give a similar clinical picture.

Both vascular and meningeal (meningovascular) involvement may occur as in syphilis of the brain (see p. 87).

Parenchymatous Involvement—Tabes Dorsalis (see Figs. 68–76)

PATHOLOGY

Macroscopically, there is shrinkage of the posterior columns of the cord and, on section, they have a grey, translucent appearance. If the optic nerve is involved it is bluish-white in colour. The arachnoid is slightly thickened and opaque.

Microscopically, in early cases, the leptomeninges and the dorsal spinal nerve roots, where they pierce the meninges, are infiltrated with small lymphocytes and plasma cells. Destruction of myelinated nerve fibres is soon apparent. The inflammatory changes become less marked as the condition progresses. In due course, nerve fibres of the posterior nerve roots are destroyed, especially in the lower thoracic and lumbosacral regions; there is an ascending degeneration of the posterior columns of the cord with replacement by glial tissue; the sensory nerve ganglia are involved to a variable extent. There may be similar changes in the retrobulbar parts of the optic nerves leading to primary optic atrophy. There is no firm evidence that *T. pallidum* has ever been found in the nerve tissues in this condition.

SYMPTOMS

The symptoms of tabes dorsalis rarely appear earlier than 10 to 20 years after the onset of the disease, and may appear much later. Usually sensory symptoms, especially pain, precede ataxia by months or years, but ataxia may develop early.

Lightning pains. These pains usually occur in the legs; less often in the back and arms. They may move from one area to another or remain in one place. Attacks may last for only a few moments or for many days; the pain is usually sudden, brief, intermittent and stabbing in character. In other cases it is described as gripping or burning. Hyperalgesia and vasodilatation may occur in the affected area. The pain is not varied by muscular activity. Sometimes attacks seem to be precipitated by changes in barometric pressure, intercurrent infection, or constipation. They may be so severe as to make the patient contemplate suicide. Remissions, during which freedom from pain is absolute, may last for several hours, for days, weeks or months. Usually they tend to grow longer as time passes.

Ataxia. The patient loses his ability to balance when he is not aided by vision. Thus he may first notice unsteadiness in the dark at night, or when he closes his eyes as, for instance, when washing his face in the morning.

Paraesthesiae. Muscle cramps 'like rheumatism' may accompany lightning pains. Other tabetics complain of numbness, tingling or aching sensations of the feet, legs or body. They may describe the feeling that they are walking on cotton wool or on snow. Some feel a 'girdle' sensation like a tight belt round the abdomen, while others experience marked hyperaesthesia of the upper abdomen, flanks and soles of the feet.

Bladder disturbances. These often occur early arising from the fact that because of damage to the posterior roots the patient loses the sensory nerve supply to the bladder and becomes unaware that the bladder is full; there is an interruption of reflex arcs resulting in loss of normal tone and difficulty in expulsion. Chronic overdistension leads to overstretching of the detrusor muscle. There is slowness in starting the act of micturition and an inadequate stream, both of which may be partially overcome by pressing on the suprapubic region. The stream becomes feeble and intermittent, and retention with overflow incontinence may follow. Residual urine leads to urinary-tract infection but symptoms of cystitis may be absent.

Bowel symptoms. The patient may become constipated due to loss of tone of the lower gut and of the musculature of the pelvic floor.

Crises. 'Gastric' or abdominal crises begin suddenly with abdominal pain and vomiting. The pain may be very severe, and persistence of vomiting may cause disturbance of electrolyte balance. The attack often stops equally

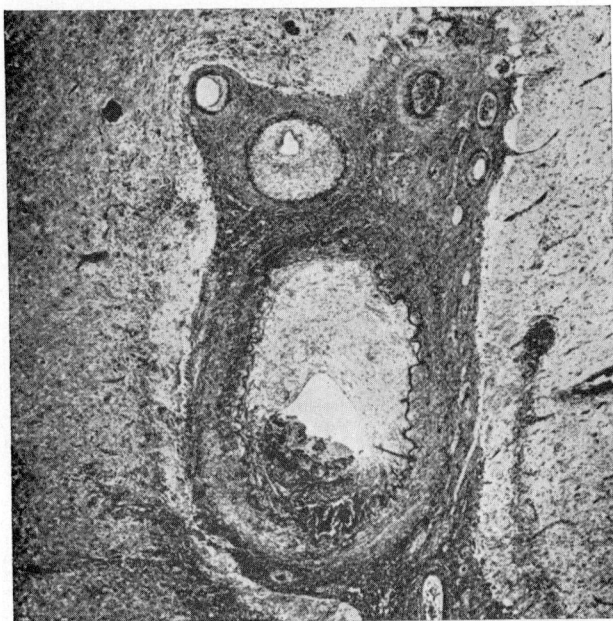

Fig. 67. Neurosyphilis: section across Sylvian fissure showing meningitis. (*Magnification* × 30.)

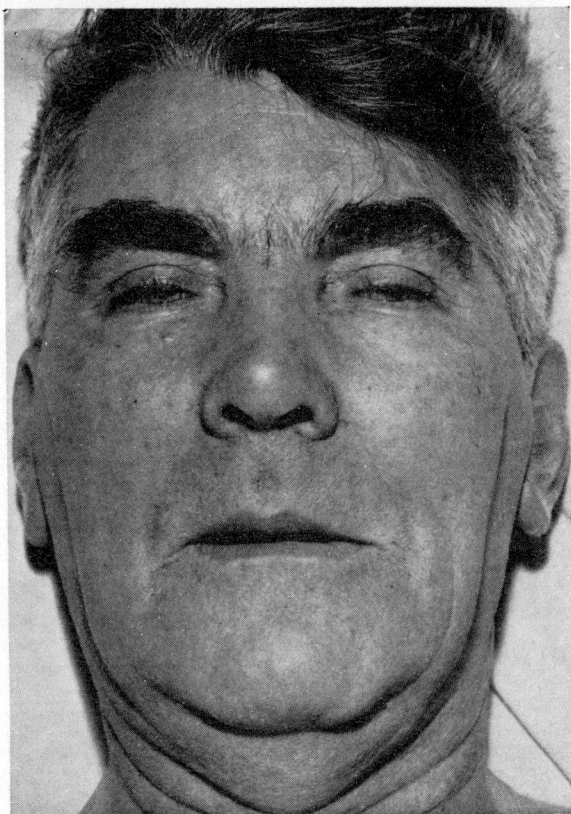

Fig. 68. Neurosyphilis: facies of a taboparetic with dementia and ptosis.

abruptly. Laryngeal crises with stridor, rectal crises with tenesmus, and vesical or renal crises, with urinary symptoms, are rare.

Impotence. Loss of potency may be an early symptom due to involvement of the sacral roots. There may be sexual anaesthesia in the female.

Visual failure. This is due to optic atrophy which may be progressive and lead to blindness.

SIGNS

The tabetic patient is usually thin. Flabby facial muscles together with moderate ptosis and wrinkling of the brow from compensatory overaction of the frontalis muscle result in the so-called 'tabetic facies'. The ptosis is probably due to oculosympathetic paralysis.

Pupillary changes. These eventually occur in over 90 per cent of the cases. They have been ascribed to associated ependymitis with subependymal gliosis involving the light-reflex tracts in the midbrain. Some workers have also reported changes in the iris itself at the neuromuscular junction, which may account for the irregularity of the pupils. The classical Argyll Robertson pupils are small ('pin-point') and often irregular in outline; they do not react to light but react normally to convergence. The smallness of the pupil is probably due to oculosympathetic paralysis. The mydriatic reaction to atropine is rather poor, nor does the pupil dilate with painful skin stimuli. The iris is often pale and atrophic. It must be realized, however, that pupillary abnormalities are not always of this typical pattern. The most usual variants are differences in the size of the pupils, fixation to light and convergence, and the retention of a partial light reflex in one eye.

Areflexia and atonia. These occur mainly in the lower limbs; the atony of the muscles may be so marked that hyperextension of the joints may be demonstrated. Later, loss of power for sustained muscle action occurs due to sensory loss and not to motor paralysis. Tendon reflexes are lost even with reinforcement. This is a more constant finding with the ankle jerks than with the knee jerks. In the early stages there may be asymmetry with only diminished reflexes on one side or the other. The arm reflexes are occasionally lost. The cremasteric reflexes are likely to be absent. The abdominal reflexes may be lost only in the late stages with hypotonia of the abdominal muscles. The plantar reflexes are flexor.

Ataxia. This usually begins in the lower limbs and can be tested by asking the patient to stand with his feet together and then to close his eyes (Romberg's test). If he sways and then loses his balance the result is positive. The ataxic patient walks with his feet somewhat apart and his toes turned out; he lifts the feet unduly high and tends to stamp them on the ground. He has lost proprioception and depends upon vision for standing and walking. He has difficulty in turning and is apt to do so in a series of careful and deliberate movements. He may lose concentration in crowds and become more unsteady. Coordination can also be tested by asking the patient to close his eyes, then to touch his knee with the other heel and to run the heel briskly up and down the leg. If proprioception is lost he is quite unable to do this, and if it is impaired the movements are irregular and incoordinate. Ataxia in the upper limbs can be demonstrated by the finger–nose test.

Sensory changes: (a) *Surface sensation.* Changes in surface sensation are common in cases of tabes dorsalis but vary considerably in extent and degree. Loss or diminution of sensation to pin prick and to light touch may be found over the central area of the face, the nipple area, the ulnar borders of the forearms, the peroneal borders of the legs and the perianal region (Hitzig's zones). Sometimes the loss may be distributed over 'stocking' areas of the lower limbs. On the other hand, hypersensitivity to light touch is sometimes found over the flanks and over the soles of the feet.

(b) *Other sensation.* Deep pain sense, tested by squeezing the Achilles tendons or the calf muscles, is usually diminished or absent. Testicular sensation may also be lost. Vibration sense is usually lost in the lower limbs, but in some cases the earliest evidence of loss of vibration sense is found over the sacrum. Loss of position sense in the toes is a common finding.

Trophic changes: (a) *Charcot's arthropathy* (Figs. 69–74). Loss or impairment of the sensation of pain in joints may lead to severe degenerative effects, especially if the patient sustains trauma to the joint or develops a chronic arthritic condition. One possible sequence of events is that a loose body gets between the joint surfaces, but the patient experiences no pain and continues to use the joint as though it were normal. The cartilage and the subchondral bone are eroded and destroyed, with the formation of more loose bodies. The knee joint is most commonly involved and usually rapid destruction occurs on one side of the joint, causing angulation and deformity. The periosteum reacts with the formation of new bone and osteophytic outgrowths at the margins of the joint surfaces and sometimes in areas more remote. X-rays show, in addition to the destruction and erosion and the osteophytic outgrowths, gross sclerosis of the ends of the bones. Sclerosis may be an early feature and is sometimes the first to be seen. The joint is swollen with fluid, and subluxation, dislocation, fractures and further deposition of new bone may follow, resulting in hypermobility and increasing deformity. These changes may occur slowly over a few years or quickly over a few months. The joint is usually painless but may be painful in the early stages. The amount of pain is never commensurate with the gross derangement of the joint. On examination there is hypermobility due to stretching and destruction of ligaments (flail joint). There is often gross crepitus. Joints most commonly involved are the knee, ankle, hip, foot and spine; more than one joint is involved in some cases. Charcot changes may also occur in syringomyelia, diabetes, and spinal-cord or peripheral nerve injury. In cases of syringomyelia, shoulder, elbow

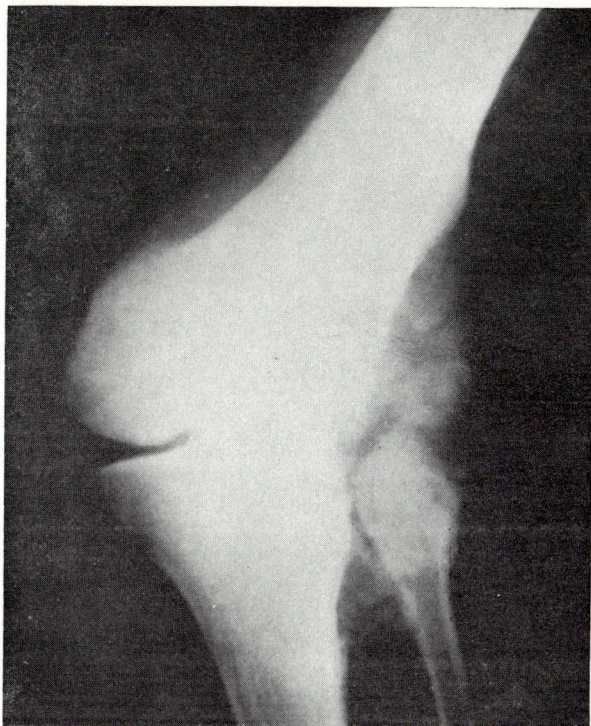

Fig. 69. Neurosyphilis: tabes dorsalis. X-ray showing Charcot knee joint.

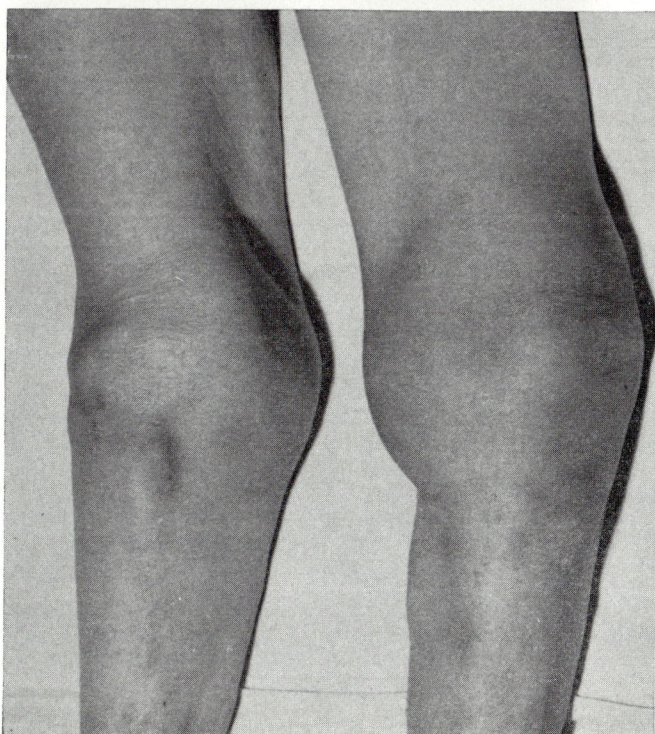

Fig. 70. Neurosyphilis: tabes dorsalis. Charcot knee joints.

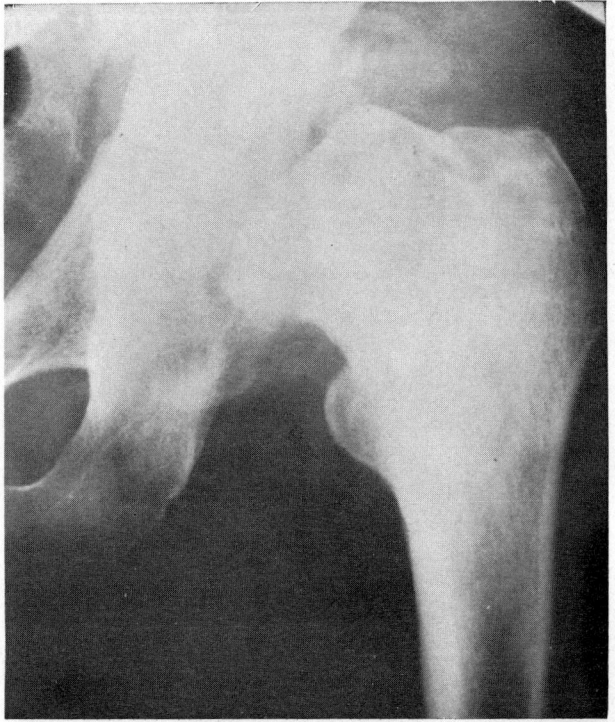

Fig. 71.
Neurosyphilis:
tabes dorsalis.
X-ray showing
Charcot hip joint

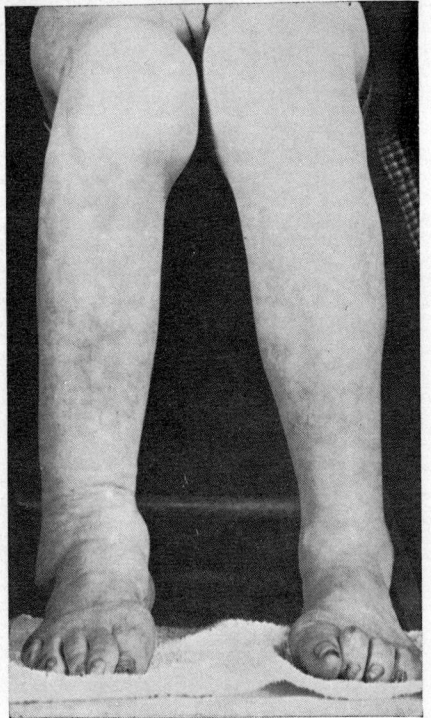

Fig. 72.
Neurosyphilis: tabes dorsalis.
Charcot right ankle joint.

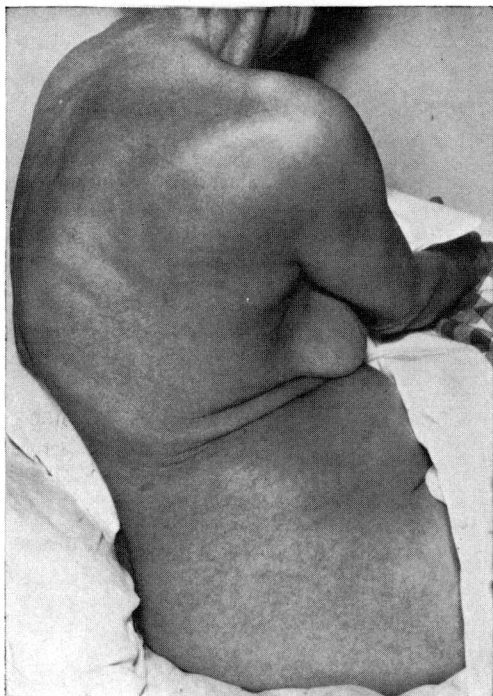

Fig. 73. Neurosyphilis:
tabes dorsalis. Charcot
spine.

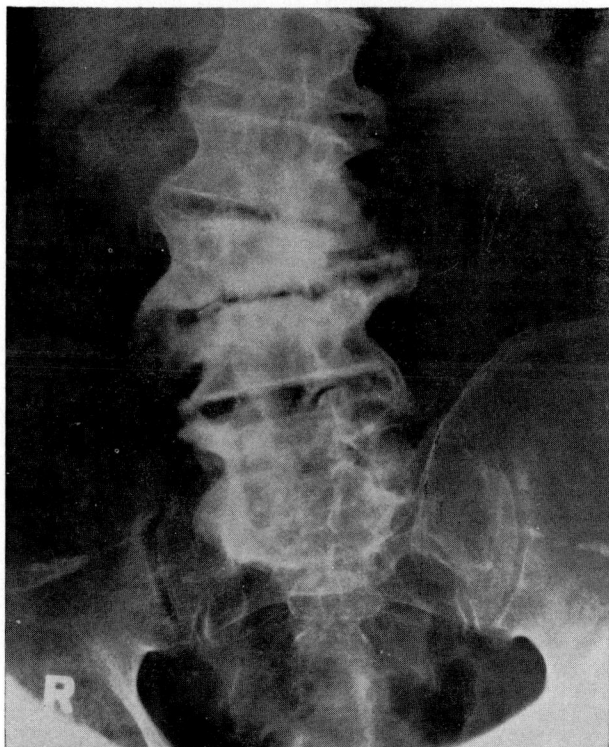

Fig. 74.
Neurosyphilis:
Charcot's
arthropathy
involving lumbar
spine.

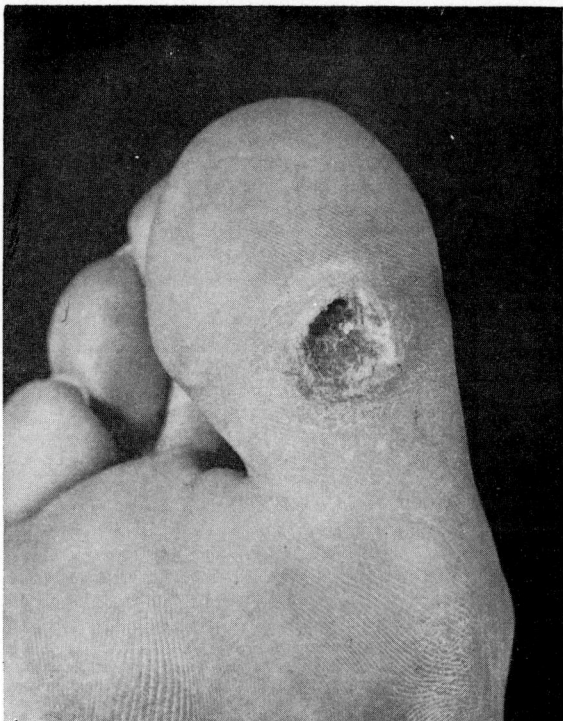

Fig. 75. Neurosyphilis:
tabes dorsalis.
Perforating ulcer of
great toe.

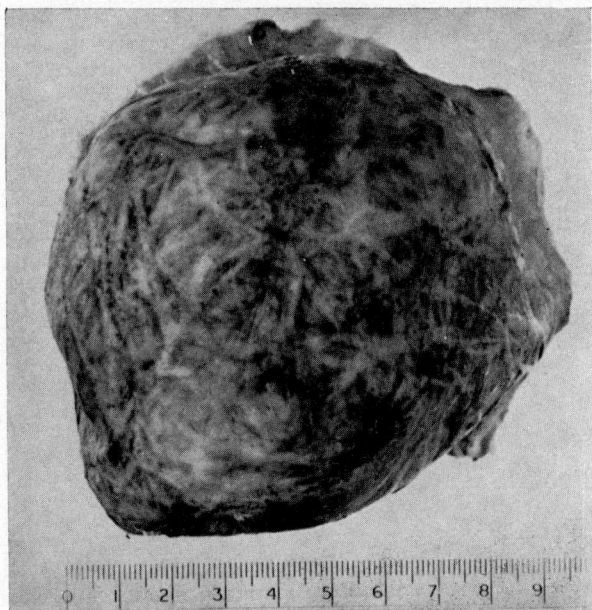

Fig. 76. Neurosyphilis:
tabes dorsalis.
Trabeculated atonic
bladder (post-mortem
specimen). *(Scale in
inches:* 1 in = 2·54 cm)

and wrist are more commonly involved.

(b) *Perforating ulcer* ('mal perforans') (Fig. 75). Loss of deep pain sense and the presence of an enlarging callus at a pressure point or some local trauma to the sole of the foot, such as may result from a nail or other foreign body in the shoe, cause pressure necrosis with the development of an indolent, circular ulcer, often on the under surface of the ball of the great toe. Secondary pyogenic infection may result in osteomyelitis of the underlying bone, or pyogenic destruction of the metatarso-phalangeal joint. These changes in bones and joints can be demonstrated by X-ray.

Primary optic atrophy. This is found in 15 to 20 per cent of tabetics. Gradual diminution of vision often begins in one eye, progresses to a certain point, and then begins in the other eye. In untreated cases, blindness is likely to follow in three to eight years. In some cases, however, the condition is slight and non-progressive. It may be discovered only on routine examination. The earliest sign is generally contraction of the visual fields.

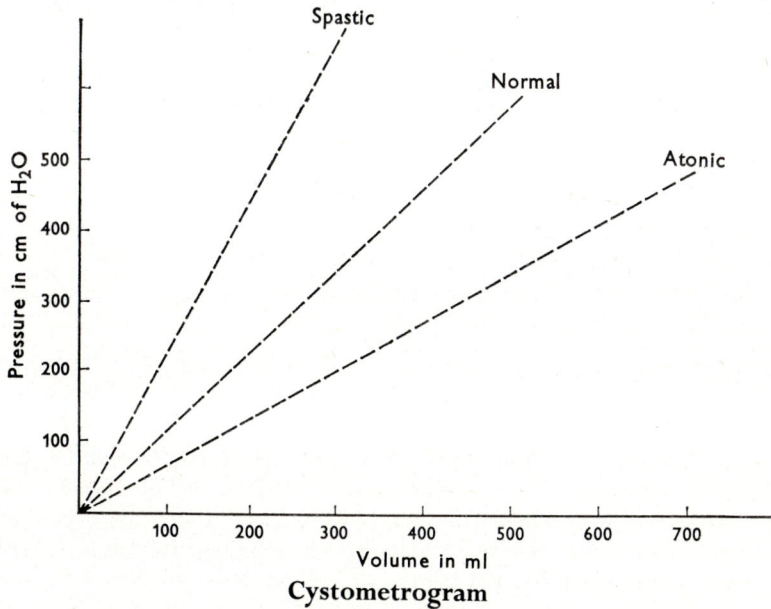

Cystometrogram

There may also be central or peripheral scotomata. Ophthalmoscopy shows that the optic disc has become bluish-white in colour. The disc margin is normal. In the course of time atrophy of the central fibres leaves a funnel-shaped central depression, slaty-blue in colour, which leads back to the lamina cribrosa. The vessels become attenuated and are seen to pass down into and up from this hollow. Loss of central vision may be early or late, depending on when the papillo-macular bundle is affected. Some patients manage to move around independently even when vision is reduced only to the ability to count fingers.

Atonic bladder (Fig. 76). The bladder may be palpable as a central lower abdominal tumour, dull to percussion; it may extend up to the level of the umbilicus. Bladder sensation is lost due to the interruption of the afferent parasympathetic fibres in sacral nerve roots 1 and 2, so that when the bladder fills the usual detrusor reflex is lost. This can be demonstrated by a cystometrogram which measures intravesical pressure with varying vesical content. The graph shows tracings obtained in cases of tabes and Erb's spastic paraplegia (see p. 91) contrasted with a normal tracing.

Cranial nerve palsies. If tabes is associated with cerebral basal meningitis, there may be severe unilateral or bilateral ptosis and perhaps ophthalmoplegia due to involvement of the 3rd, 6th and perhaps 4th nerves. Involvement of the 8th nerve may result in deafness and vertigo; the exact site of the lesion is unknown. Other cranial nerve palsies occur occasionally.

Patients with tabes dorsalis do not necessarily show all the signs described above, and may present initially with almost any variation of the symptoms and signs. Tabes involving the cervical rather than the lumbosacral spinal cord is rare.

Changes in the cerebrospinal fluid are usually of Type II, but in about 11 per cent of cases the fluid shows no abnormality. Blood reagin tests may be negative in almost one-third of the cases. Occasionally all serological tests, including the TPI, FTA-ABS and TPHA, are negative.

Chemoreceptor response. A study by Evans, Benson and Hughes[5] has shown that some patients with autonomic denervation, including tabetics, are unable to adjust their respiratory systems in response to hypoxia.

Postural hypotension. Likewise postural hypotension may occur due to autonomic involvement.

DIFFERENTIAL DIAGNOSIS

Tabes must be differentiated from meningeal and vascular spinal syphilis. Other conditions to be considered are chronic polyneuritis due to vitamin deficiency, alcoholism, lead poisoning, diabetes, diphtheria, infective polyneuritis, peroneal muscular atrophy, Friedreich's ataxia, the lumbar type of syringomyelia, tumour of the cauda equina, subacute combined degeneration and disseminated sclerosis. Adie's syndrome may be confused with the pupillary changes of neurosyphilis. In this condition the pupillary change is usually unilateral, unlike the Argyll Robertson pupil, which is usually present on both sides. The affected pupil is dilated and regular but may be oval in outline. The ordinary light reaction is absent, but slow dilatation occurs in the dark and slow contraction follows on return to the light. Contraction on convergence is slow but very complete. In a number of these cases lower-limb reflexes are absent or diminished. The condition is more common in females than in males but the Argyll Robertson pupil is rather more common in males.

TABOPARESIS. In some cases, parenchymatous involvement of the brain and cord occurs in the same patient, either in the form of GPI with evidence of posterior column involvement but few associated symptoms, or, less commonly, with the onset of psychosis of GPI in a patient with untreated tabes of long standing (see Fig. 68). In all these cases changes in the cerebro-spinal fluid are likely to be of Type III.

Gumma of the Cord

This is a very rare condition. As in the brain, the gumma usually arises from the meninges and enlarges to produce pressure on the spinal cord.

SYMPTOMS AND SIGNS

The onset is gradual and as a result of pressure on the cord there may be a spastic paraplegia, with sensory loss below a well-demonstrated sensory level; trophic ulcers may occur. The cerebrospinal fluid may show changes of Type I or II, and there is a high-protein level due to the loculation syndrome of Froin. Queckenstedt's test will show evidence of spinal block and this may be confirmed by X-ray myelography. Serological tests for syphilis are positive.

DIFFERENTIAL DIAGNOSIS

Gumma has to be differentiated from meningeal and vascular spinal syphilis. It is always difficult to diagnose from a spinal tumour.

REFERENCES

1. STOKES, J. H., BEERMAN, H. and INGRAHAM, N. R. (1945) *Modern Clinical Syphilology.* 3rd ed., p. 609. Philadelphia and London: W. B. Saunders.
2. STOKES *et al.* (*ibid*). p. 608.
3. OXELIUS, V-A., RORSHAN, H. and LAURELL, A-B. (1969) *Br. J. vener. Dis.*, **45,** 121.
4. WILKINSON, A. E. (1973) *Br. J. vener. Dis.*, **49,** 346.
5. EVANS, R. J. C., BENSON, M. K. and HUGHES, D. T. D. (1971) *Br. med. J.*, **1,** 530.

6

Congenital Syphilis

MECHANISM OF TRANSMISSION

The congenital syphilitic acquires infection during fetal life. It is not now considered possible for the father to transmit syphilis to the child without intermediate infection of the mother. The mother of a congenital syphilitic invariably has syphilis, and the evidence indicates that *Treponema pallidum* passes through the placenta into the fetal circulation. This is much more likely to occur when the mother is suffering from early syphilis, particularly in the primary or secondary stages, than when she has late syphilis. Syphilis seems not to cause abortion in the first four months of pregnancy and it has been supposed that the Langhans cell layer provides a barrier against infection of the fetus. Recently, however, treponemes have been demonstrated in nine- and ten-week-old fetuses examined after induced abortion.[1] It has always been believed that syphilis may be transmitted to the third generation. There is no doubt that three generations in a family can have syphilis; superinfection is a possibility (see p. 8), for on very rare occasions it may happen that the individual in the second generation who has congenital syphilis has been superinfected with acquired syphilis. If this occurs, the so-called third generation infection is really ordinary congenital syphilis of the second generation. It remains an open question whether a congenitally syphilitic mother can transmit congenital syphilis to her offspring. It seems impossible to prove the existence of true third generation syphilis in the individual case.

MATERNAL SYPHILIS

There is considerable evidence that pregnancy has a benign effect on syphilis in the mother, although its effect on the fetus may be disastrous. The syphilitic woman who becomes pregnant commonly presents few symptoms or signs of the disease, and after a series of pregnancies, though untreated, she may appear to be cured, with negative tests of blood in approximately 20 per cent of cases.[2] Early in the last century it was observed by Colles that the syphilitic infant did not infect its own mother and his dictum on this subject is called 'Colles's law' (1837). These are his words:

A new-born child affected with congenital syphilis, even though it may have symptoms in the mouth, never causes ulceration of the breast which it sucks, if it be the mother who suckles it, though continuing capable of infecting a strange nurse.

It is now clear that the explanation for this correct observation is that the mother is suffering from latent syphilis and has a degree of immunity to superinfection from her child. It is also true that the longer the duration of untreated syphilis in the mother, the less likely it is that the fetus will die in utero, and the more likely that a live congenital syphilitic infant will be born, or that the fetus will escape entirely. If the mother is suffering from primary or secondary syphilis during her pregnancy, there is probably little chance that the infant will be born normal and healthy unless treatment is given. If, however, she has early latent syphilis there may be a 20 per cent chance, and if she has late syphilis a 70 per cent chance, that the infant will be healthy. It also follows that if a woman with untreated syphilis has a series of pregnancies, the likelihood of infection of the fetus in later pregnancies becomes less. Thus, in successive pregnancies she may have a miscarriage at the fifth month, on the next occasion a stillbirth at the eighth month, next the birth of an infant with congenital syphilis who dies within a few weeks, followed by the birth of two or three infants with congenital syphilis who survive. Finally one or more healthy children may be born. This has been stated as 'Kassowitz's law', but it is far from reliable. This is the disease of exceptions and all kinds of variations are both possible and likely. The possibility that a mother may have given birth to healthy children before she was infected with syphilis must also be borne in mind. From what has been said, it is clear that an obstetric history of repeated miscarriage before the fourth month of pregnancy is not suggestive of syphilis.

PROPHYLAXIS

The prevention of congenital syphilis depends on adequate treatment being given to the infected woman during pregnancy. Details of this treatment will be given in Chapter 8, but the first problem is diagnosis. It is routine procedure to take blood to test for syphilis, as well as for the Rhesus factor, at the first attendance at an antenatal clinic, but not every pregnant woman attends for antenatal care.

There are also certain loopholes in the routine procedure. For instance, the patient may be incubating syphilis, or she may be in the seronegative primary stage, when a hidden syphilitic chancre may easily be missed. Alternatively, she may be infected with syphilis after her antenatal examination. An ideal routine for antenatal clinics would be to examine the patient and take blood for this test as early and as late in pregnancy as possible. It is not usual to perform lumbar puncture on pregnant women with syphilis, and this procedure may be postponed until after the puerperium when the infant is two to three months old.

INCIDENCE

The incidence of congenital syphilis varies considerably in different countries and in different groups of population. It depends upon the prevalence of infectious syphilis in the population concerned, and on the diligence with which cases of syphilis are sought and treated among pregnant women. In Great Britain the incidence is low at the present time. In England and Wales the number of cases of early congenital syphilis treated at clinics for venereal diseases fell from 227 in 1950 to 18 in 1960 and 12 in 1966, since when the figure has remained very low. The number of cases of late congenital syphilis fell from 996 in 1950 to 371 in 1960, 250 in 1966 and 154 (England only) in 1973. In the year ended June 30 1977, the total number of cases of early and late congenital syphilis reported from the clinics in England was 141.[3] In the United States of America the number of reported cases of congenital syphilis in the fiscal year 1972 was 1951, of which 422 (21·6 per cent) were diagnosed in patients under one year of age. The equivalent figures for the fiscal year 1976 were 764 and 170 (22·2 per cent).[4]

PATHOLOGY

Once the treponemes have entered the fetal circulation dissemination to all the tissues occurs at once. These treponemes multiply and, apart from very young fetuses, provoke in many organs the characteristic cellular inflammatory response of small lymphocytes and plasma cells. The fetus may be overwhelmed by the infection and die; it will then be expelled by the uterus, producing either miscarriage or stillbirth according to the stage of the pregnancy. This probably occurs in about 30 per cent of the cases. The syphilitic stillborn fetus may have a macerated appearance with collapse of the skull and protuberant abdomen (see Fig. 78). The skin is of a livid red colour, and on its surface may be seen a number of bullae filled with haemorrhagic fluid. At autopsy the liver and spleen are found to be enlarged, and treponemes can be demonstrated in large numbers in the bullae of the skin and in the viscera (see Fig. 77). Oppenheimer and Hardy[5] have described autopsy findings in a number of cases, including intense pancreatitis and submucosal fibrosis and thickening in the intestinal tract. These changes, combined with alterations in bones, appeared to be patho-

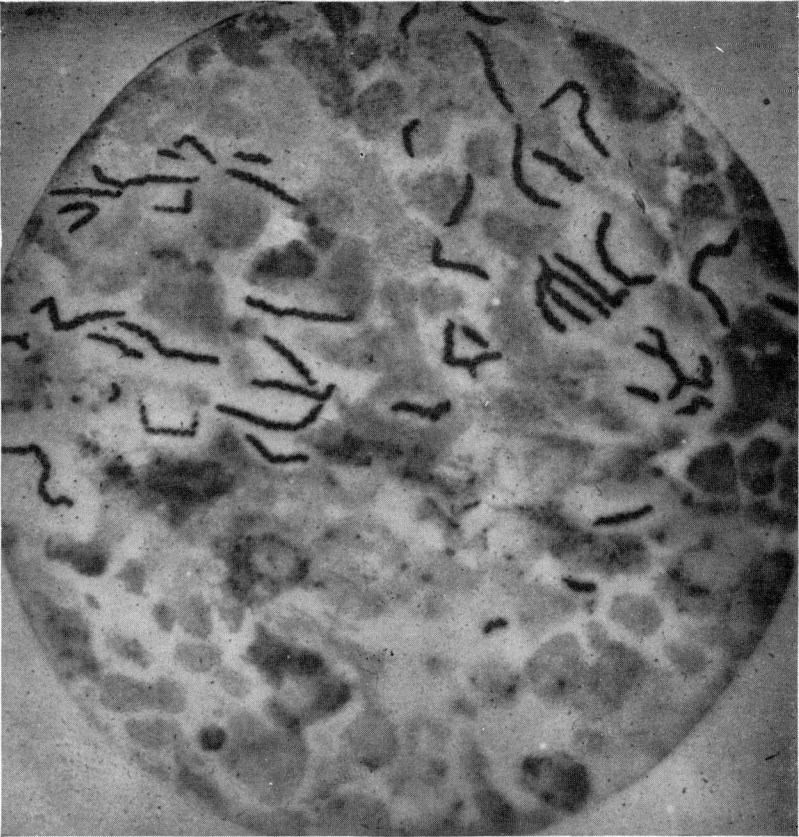

Fig. 77. *T. pallidum* in liver: congenital syphilis (Levaditi staining method). (*Magnification* × 1000.)

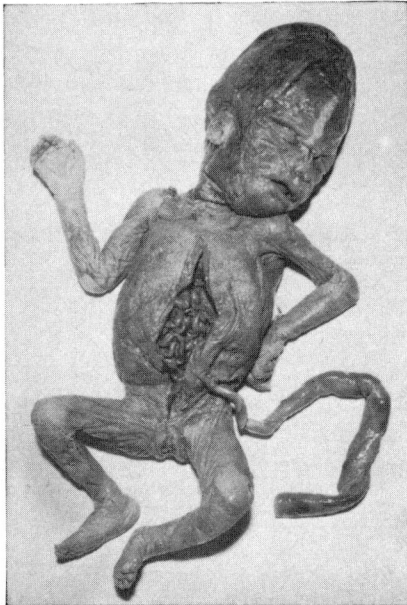

Fig. 78. Congenital syphilis: dead macerated full-term fetus.

gnomonic of the condition, permitting differentiation from erythroblastosis fetalis, congenital virus diseases and toxoplasmosis.

In the past it has been stated that the syphilitic placenta can be recognized by naked-eye appearances and, with more certainty, by microscopic changes in the chorionic villi. This view is now discredited, and it seems clear that examination of the placenta does not help in the diagnosis unless *T. pallidum* can be found, which is seldom possible.

If the treponemal infection does not prove fatal, it may still interfere with normal development at various stages of intrauterine and extrauterine life. Pathological changes in congenital syphilis are, in general, similar to those in acquired syphilis. As the fetal infection is blood-borne there is no stage corresponding to primary syphilis. The early changes are similar to those of the secondary stage of acquired infection, but involvement of bones and viscera is more common. There are also some selective differences in the sites of gummatous lesions; gummata are particularly common in the nasal septum.

There are certain dissimilarities in the later phases of the disease, particularly in the fact that the cardiovascular system is very rarely involved in cases of congenital syphilis. Certain characteristic manifestations, such as interstitial keratitis, perceptive deafness and Clutton's joints, are possibly not direct effects of treponemal activity, and some have believed them to be phenomena of hypersensitivity.

CLINICAL MANIFESTATIONS

These may be divided into early, late, and the stigmata. It is necessary to make an arbitrary division between the early and late stages of the disease and it is customary to place this at the end of the second year of life. Many of the lesions of the first two years of life are infectious and resemble those of secondary syphilis in the acquired form of the disease. Many of the late lesions from the third year onwards are of the gummatous type. They are not infectious. The stigmata are the scars or deformities resulting from early or late lesions which have healed.

Early Congenital Syphilis

As already mentioned, there is no primary stage and signs are similar to those of the secondary stage. If a lesion resembling a primary chancre is seen in an infant, it may be due to acquired syphilis from some chance contact, or transmission may have occurred during birth from a genital lesion of very recent infection in the mother. At birth an infected infant may appear healthy and may not develop signs till it is some weeks old (Profeta's law), but in a few cases signs are present at birth. Blood taken from the umbilical vein ('cord blood') or from the infant may give positive results. But even if these results are confirmed by specific tests they do *not* necessarily indicate infection of the infant with syphilis. The positive results may be due to the presence of reagin and specific antibodies which have passed from the maternal to the fetal circulation (see Chapter 7). It has been suggested[6] that more reliable information can be obtained in these cases from an FTA-ABS test using fluorescein-labelled IgM conjugate in place of an ordinary fluorescein-labelled anti-human globulin. A positive test demonstrates the presence of IgM antibodies to syphilis and these do not pass from maternal to fetal circulations through the placenta. Negative blood tests at birth do not exclude infection. It is not uncommon for an infected infant to have negative tests at birth, but they become positive within a few weeks or a few months. This applies also to the FTA-ABS IgM test,[7] so that, when congenital syphilis is a possibility, follow-up of the infant for at least three months is essential before infection can be excluded. The commonest clinical manifestations in the early stage are various eruptions of the skin and rhinitis.

RASH
RUNNY
NOSE

Lesions of the Skin

The earliest type of eruption is the bullous rash, sometimes called 'syphilitic pemphigus', and this may be present at birth (see Fig. 81). The lesions consist of groups of blebs or bullae distributed symmetrically on the palms and soles, and occasionally on other parts of the body. This is the only bullous or vesicular eruption which occurs in cases of syphilis. The bullae may be as much as 3 cm in diameter; they are circular in outline, and contain serous or seropurulent fluid swarming with treponemes. The floor of the lesion is dull red, rounded and elevated; and when the bulla ruptures, discharging its infectious fluid, it reveals this underlying papule with its dull-red eroded surface covered with scabs or crusts. Infants with this condition are often gravely ill. Other rashes commonly appear some weeks after birth and they are like the rashes of secondary syphilis. The commonest are papular or papulosquamous eruptions with generalized symmetrical distribution. The palms of the hands, the soles of the feet, the buttocks and the genitals are very often affected (Figs. 79 and 80). In moist areas, especially the napkin area, the papules are likely to become eroded and moist. They may be hypertrophic and present as condylomata lata identical with those of the secondary stage in the acquired form of the disease. In moist areas, and where the rash is exposed to friction, the skin between the lesions may become reddened and 'glazed' in appearance. The rash may be very profuse, especially so on the lower part of the face, where it may be confluent. Movement of the lips is apt to produce radiating fissures at the mouth angles which become secondarily infected and leave linear scars. These are common stigmata of congenital syphilis and are called 'rhagades' (see Fig. 96, p. 127). They may also be found about the nares and the anus.

Apart from rashes, the skin may show characteristic changes, especially in severe cases. Loss of weight may produce wrinkling of the skin which is

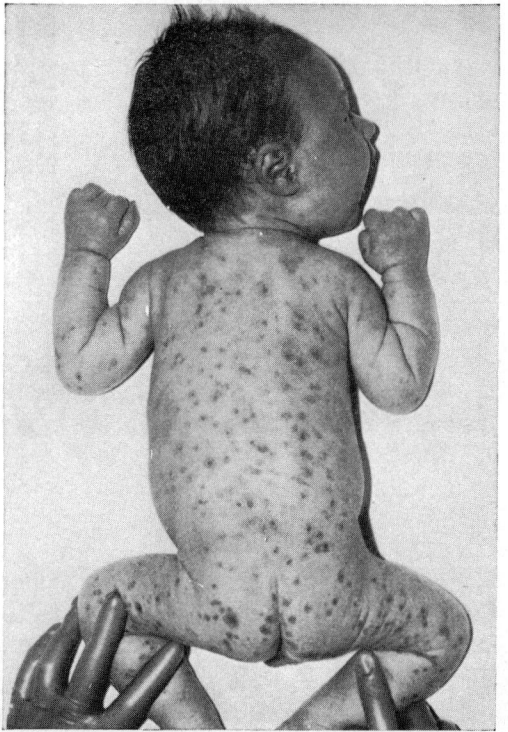

Fig. 79. Congenital
syphilis (early):
generalized rash.

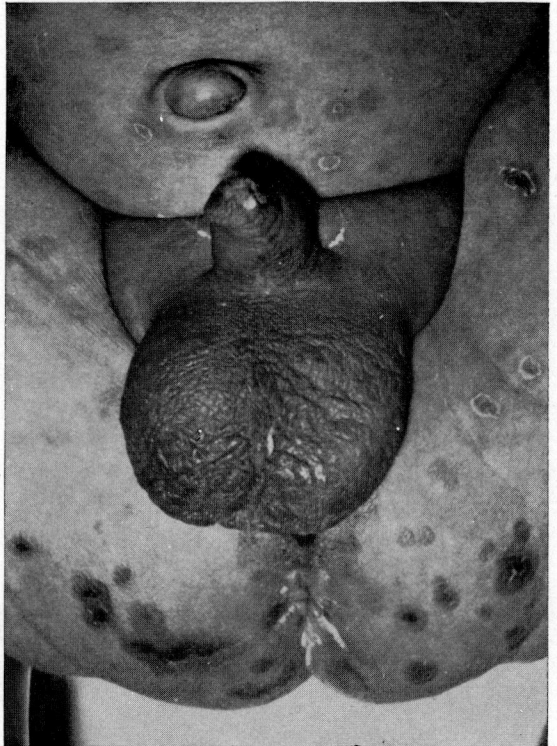

Fig. 80. Congenital syphilis
(early): generalized rash and
early lesions of the buttock
and perianal region. (From
*Roxburgh's   Common   Skin
Diseases*, H. K. Lewis.)

particularly obvious in the face and gives what has been called 'the old-man look'. Sometimes the skin shows a brownish-yellow tint which is called 'the café-au-lait' tint. There may be patchy, irregular loss of hair, especially at the sides and back of the scalp, giving so-called syphilitic alopecia; eye-lashes and eyebrows may also be affected. It has been alleged that, rarely, the syphilitic infant may present with an unusual abundance of rather coarse hair which seems to stop short abruptly at the hair margin, the so-called syphilitic wig. Syphilitic papules may involve the skin at the bases of the nails and extend to the nail beds. The nails may be loosened and shed ('syphilitic onychia'). The newly growing nails may be opaque, irregular and narrowed at the bases, providing another possible but not characteristic stigma of congenital syphilis.

Lesions of Mucous Membranes

Mucous patches identical with those of secondary syphilis may be found on the lips (Fig. 82), in the mouth and in the throat. They may also occur in the larynx, when the infant's cry may be thin or aphonic.

Very similar lesions often occur in the muco-periosteum of the nasal cavity, giving rise to syphilitic rhinitis and the syndrome known as 'syphilitic snuffles'. The effects vary in severity but the characteristic features are nasal obstruction and nasal discharge. Obstruction may be so severe that it interferes with nursing and the infant is unable to take its feeds. This is the likely cause of the rapid loss of weight which occurs in some of these cases. The nasal discharge may be either slight and mucoid, or abundant and mucopurulent or purulent. Sometimes it is bloodstained. It contains large numbers of *T. pallida* and is highly infectious. It may infect the skin of the margin of the nares causing the formation of syphilitic papules.

Mucous patches or moist erosions may also be found on the genital mucosae.

Lymphadenitis

Rubbery, discrete, non-tender enlargement of lymph nodes is frequently present but seldom as well-marked as in the secondary stage of acquired syphilis.

Liver and Spleen

The infant's abdomen may be grossly protuberant owing to enlargement of the liver and, usually, also of the spleen. The cause of the hepatic enlarge-ment can be diagnosed by the presence of other signs of syphilis and is suggested by the fact that the enlargement is usually greater than in other conditions. The liver cells tend to be immature and imperfectly formed. Enlargement of the liver is due to diffuse increase in fibrous tissue and to abnormal persistence of the fetal blood-forming tissues. The fibrosis results from massive invasion by *T. pallidum* and is pericellular in distribution. In

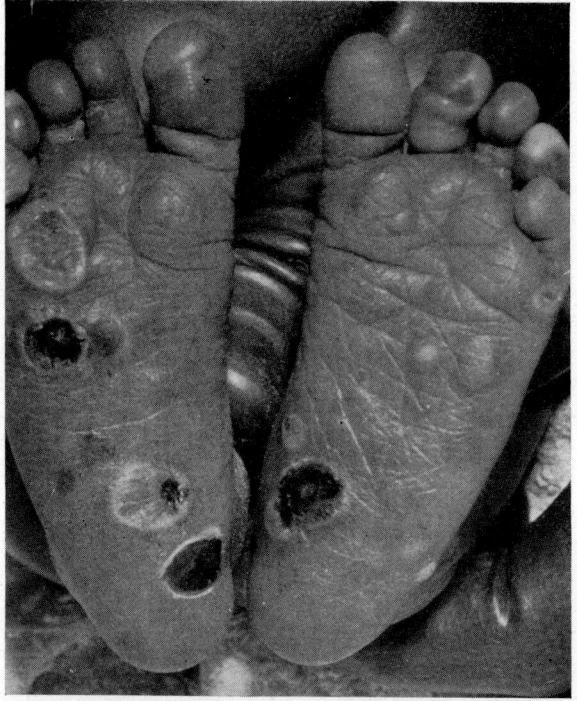

Fig. 81. Congenital
syphilis (early): bullous
syphilide of soles of feet at
birth.

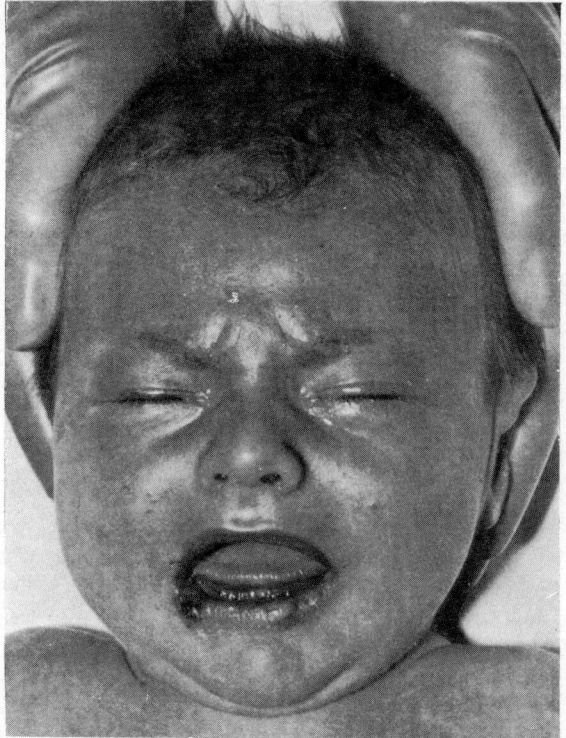

Fig. 82. Congenital
syphilis (early): mucous
patch on lip and snuffles.

these cases hepatic insufficiency is likely to result in failure of protein metabolism and there is marked lowering of the serum protein which may be 4 g per 100 ml or less, together with reversal of the albumin/globulin ratio. Oedema may be present due to this cause. The patient may show a slight icteric tint, but marked jaundice is uncommon.

Kidneys

In some cases the urine shows a little albumin and few or many hyaline and granular casts, but involvement of the kidneys is only of slight degree and not enough to account for the oedema. There have been occasional reports of acute nephrosis ascribed to congenital syphilis; as in acquired syphilis evidence of immune complex deposition has been found.

Lungs

Infants who die of early congenital syphilis are sometimes found to have widespread infiltration of the lungs, so-called white pneumonia.

Testes

Orchitis is described in the older literature as a manifestation of early congenital syphilis, but it must be rare. However Singh, Kaur and Parameswaran[8] have described bilateral orchitis in a newborn infant with congenital syphilis, which responded promptly to antisyphilitic treatment.

Lesions of the Nervous System

Meningeal involvement is not uncommon but the clinical evidence may be slight or absent. There may be convulsions, bulging of the fontanelle, stiffness of the neck, positive Kernig's sign and, occasionally, increasing hydrocephalus. There are changes in the cerebrospinal fluid of Type I or Type II (see p. 84).

Lesions of Bones

The bones may be affected in various ways. In the first six months of life osteochondritis (Figs. 83 and 84) of the long bones is a characteristic finding. Invasion by treponemes is widespread but the most marked changes are seen in the zones of greatest growth near the epiphyses. There is increase in density and irregularity of the zone of provisional calcification where the metaphysis abuts on to the cartilaginous epiphyseal line. Some areas of bony tissue, particularly in the metaphysis, are replaced by granulation tissue, and there is periosteal reaction with deposition of new bone under the periosteum on the surface of the cortex. In severe cases the mother may have noticed loss of movement of the affected limbs, so-called syphilitic pseudoparalysis; or she may complain that the child screams when the limbs are handled, because they are extremely tender. Sometimes there are obviously painful swellings of the epiphyseal ends of the bones. Occasionally a patho-

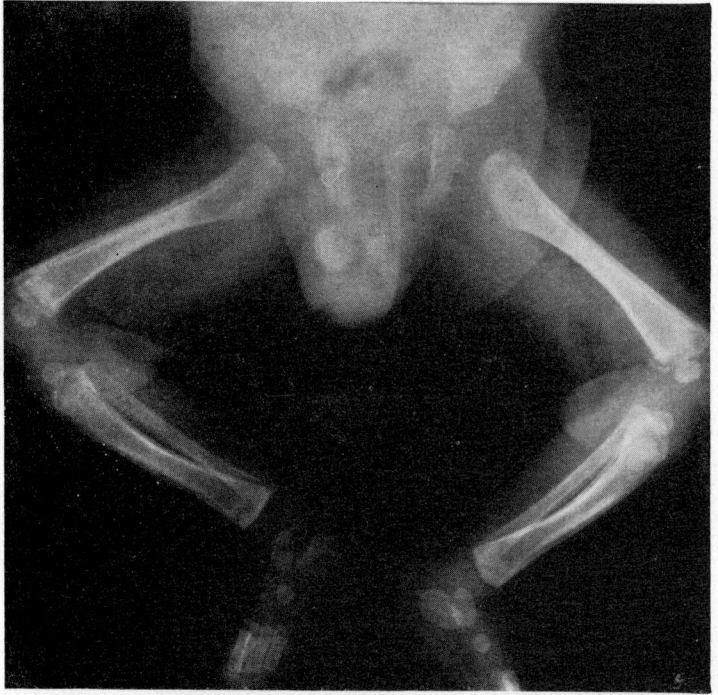
Fig. 83. Congenital syphilis (early): X-ray of legs showing osteochondritis.

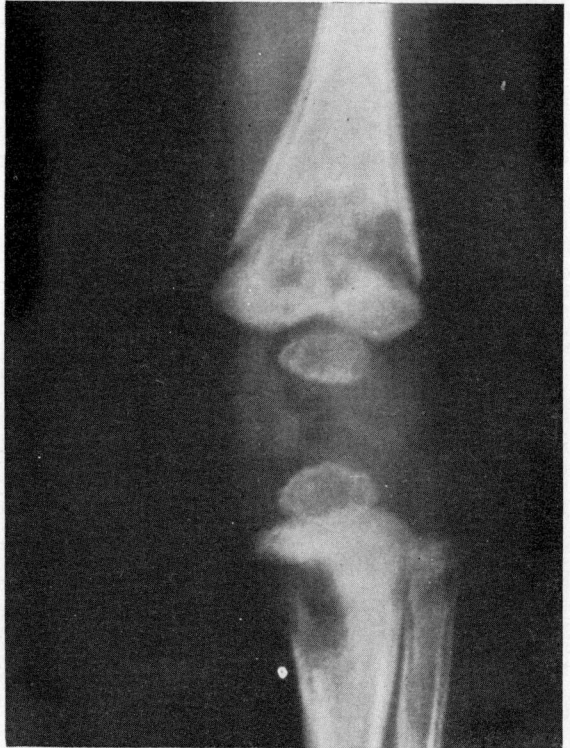
Fig. 84. Congenital syphilis (early): X-ray of femur showing osteochondritis with Wimberger's sign in the tibia.

logical fracture or separation of an epiphysis may occur. Secondary infection and suppuration in the bones may lead to infection of a joint.

In most cases the symptoms and signs are slight or absent, and the condition may only be recognized by radiological examination. It is possible that in all cases the bones may at some time show changes characteristic enough to justify this diagnosis. The earliest X-ray change, which may well be present at birth, is a thin, regular, line of new bone formation on the surface of the cortex. If this is present without other changes it may indicate periostitis due to other causes, but if it is seen in conjunction with other characteristic changes they are together diagnostic. The epiphyses may be enlarged and the epiphyseal line may be broad and irregular. The zone of provisional calcification is abnormally dense and irregular like the teeth of a saw. There are irregular patches of loss of density in the bones, particularly in the metaphyses. The more rapidly growing bones show the most marked changes, particularly the upper end of the tibia and the distal ends of the radius and ulna. There may be evidence of periostitis of the ribs. A very characteristic sign, sometimes called Wimberger's sign, is a loss of density on the medial side of the upper end of the tibia.

The signs of osteochondritis disappear in the second six months of life but periostitis persists and becomes more marked. Successive layers of bone are laid down on the surface of the cortex in regular fashion, giving the radiographic appearance sometimes known as 'onion-peel periosteum'. In the second year of life the characteristic lesion of bones is osteoperiostitis of phalanges, the condition known as 'syphilitic dactylitis'. It is the proximal phalanges which are likely to be affected and the fingers are involved more frequently than the toes. One digit or several may be involved and the condition presents as a painless, fusiform swelling which, unlike the equivalent lesion resulting from tuberculosis, almost never breaks down.

The Eyes

Choroidoretinitis is common in the early months of life but it is likely to be overlooked; residual evidence may be found as a stigma in later life ('pepper and salt' fundus; see p. 130). *Anterior uveitis* is rare.

Infants who are severely affected by early congenital syphilis are very prone to intercurrent infections such as pneumonia or gastroenteritis. Extreme degrees of anaemia are common in early life. In some cases the haemoglobin may be as low as 6 to 8 g per 100 ml. There is a recent report[9] of a three-month-old infant in whose case anaemia was the only presenting manifestation of congenital syphilis. There are no specific features of the anaemia.

Diagnosis of Early Congenital Syphilis

DARK-GROUND EXAMINATION of serum from lesions, especially the moist lesions of skin and mucous membranes, may prove the diagnosis.

SEROLOGICAL TESTS. As already mentioned it is essential to exclude the possibility that positive serological tests are due to antibody from the mother's blood-stream and not to active disease in the infant. Reference has been made to the value of the FTA-ABS IgM test in making this distinction. If blood tests are positive but the significance is uncertain they must be repeated during the first six months of life. In the absence of physical signs, only the presence of a rising titre in quantitative tests or failure of the tests to become negative permits a diagnosis of early latent congenital syphilis.

THE CLINICAL SIGNS. The early bullous rash must be distinguished from the lesions of infantile scabies, which are sometimes bullous, and from bullous impetigo (staphylococcal pemphigus), which does not usually involve the extremities. Lesions of the buttocks may closely resemble a napkin rash, which, however, is more pronounced in the lateral area away from the anus and is absent in folds of the skin.

Periostitis due to syphilis must be differentiated from the periostitis due to other neonatal infections. Similar appearances are sometimes seen in healthy infants.

Late Congenital Syphilis (see Figs. 85–100)

In the majority of the cases found in later years the condition is latent and the diagnosis depends on positive reagin serological tests for syphilis confirmed by specific tests. In adolescents and adults it may be difficult to determine whether the infection was congenital or acquired, and the decision may depend upon the results of examination of other members of the family.

Interstitial Keratitis – hypersensitivity to T.P.

Interstitial keratitis is the commonest late lesion. It may begin at any age between 2 and 30 years, or even later. Most observers have found the condition more common in females. It appears first as circumcorneal vascularization of the sclera, followed by vascular infiltration extending from the sclera into the deep layers of the cornea and cellular exudation into the deep corneal structures. It usually starts in one eye but, irrespective of antisyphilitic treatment, the other eye is likely to be involved after an interval which may vary from a few weeks to many years. The patient complains of photophobia and pain in the affected eye. The first clinical sign is injection of the sclera at the margin of the cornea, but very soon blood vessels extend into the deep layers of the cornea. This vascularization can usually be detected only with the corneal microscope and slit lamp, but if it is very intense it may be clinically obvious as a dull-pink patch at the periphery of the cornea, the so-called salmon patch. At the same time the cellular exudation into the deep layers of the cornea gives a hazy or 'ground-glass' appearance to that normally transparent membrane. The condition is generally associated with iridocyclitis, the signs of which are masked by the severity of the process in the cornea. Antisyphilitic treatment has no effect upon the course of this condition and for that reason, and because *T.*

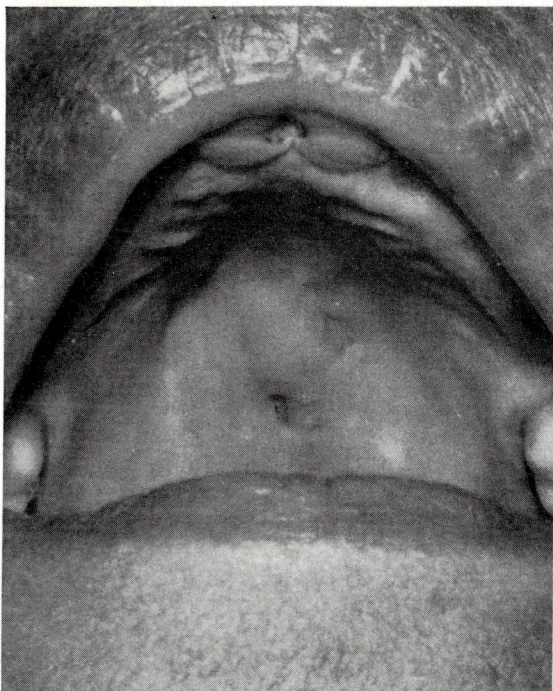
Fig. 85. Congenital syphilis (late): early gummatous destruction of hard palate.

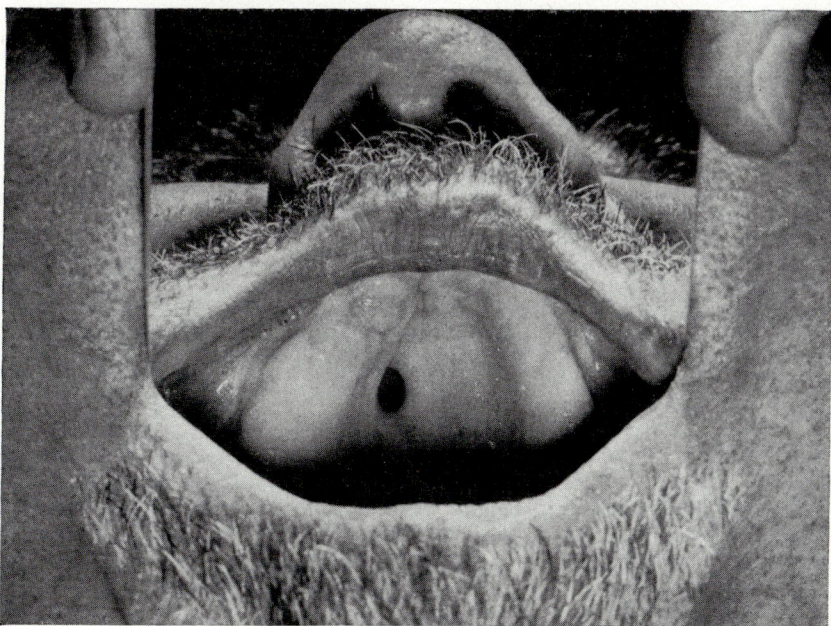
Fig. 86. Congenital syphilis (late): perforation of hard palate seen in a mirror.

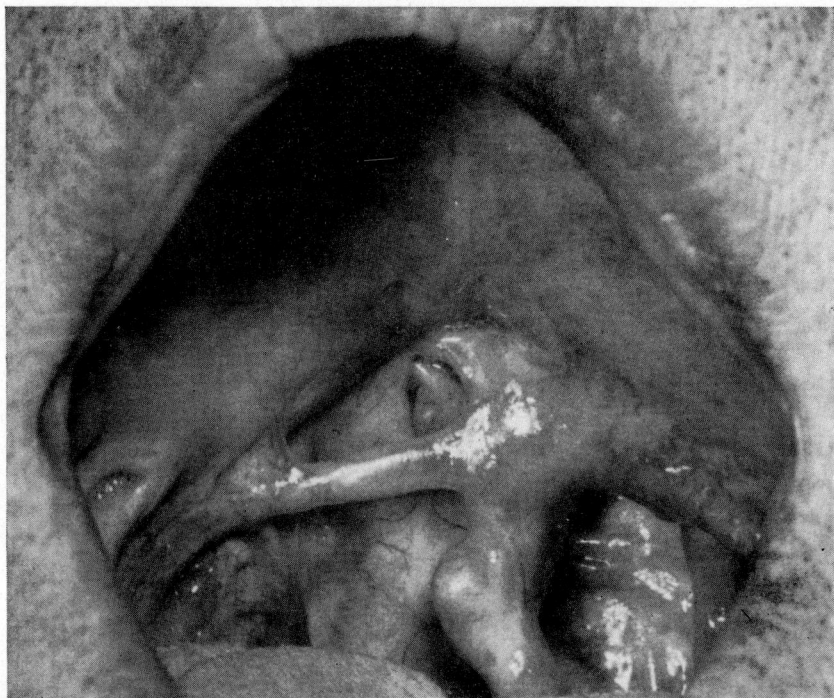

Fig. 87. Congenital syphilis (late): perforation of soft palate.

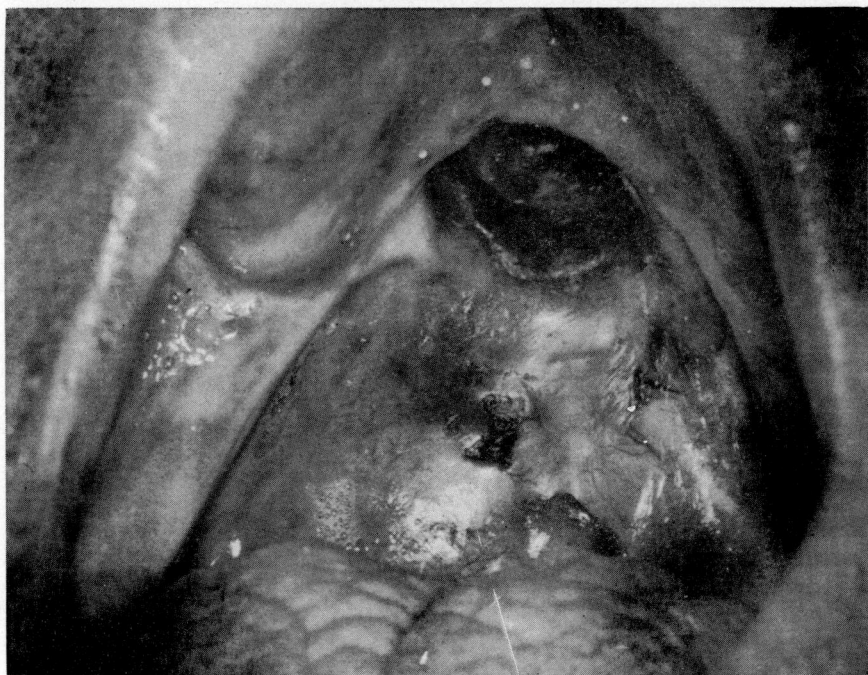

Fig. 88. Congenital syphilis (late): complete destruction of soft palate with scarring of nasopharynx.

pallidum has never been isolated from the cornea in these cases, interstitial keratitis has been thought to be a manifestation of hypersensitivity rather than a direct effect of the activity of the organism. The process in the eye can be suppressed with steroid hormones but if not it may continue for months. In some cases relapses follow in later years. Apart from the effects of steroid hormones, which may well prevent residual damage, the outcome is very variable. Severe lesions are likely to cause corneal scarring, giving rise to opacities. Depending on their size and position, these opacities may cause only slight impairment of vision or may result in complete blindness. Corneal scarring and empty blood vessels, so-called ghost vessels, detectable by slit-lamp microscopy, persist through life as stigmata of the disease.

Late Congenital Neurosyphilis

As in acquired syphilis, treponemes reach the nervous system early in the course of the disease and, as already mentioned, they may give rise to meningitis in the early stage. Other manifestations may follow in later years. The pathological changes in the meninges, blood vessels, and parenchyma are the same as those which occur in acquired syphilis. The following types of involvement may occur: (*a*) asymptomatic neurosyphilis, (*b*) meningeal involvement, (*c*) vascular involvement, and (*d*) parenchymatous involvement.

ASYMPTOMATIC NEUROSYPHILIS

The diagnosis depends on changes in the cerebrospinal fluid, which may be of Type I, II or III.

MENINGEAL INVOLVEMENT

Occasionally convulsions, blindness, hydrocephalus and mental deficiency may be found in older children or adolescents as the late results of early meningitis. The clinical evidence of late meningeal infection is likely to take the form of cranial nerve palsies due to basal meningitis. The cerebrospinal fluid may be under increased pressure and show changes of Type I or II.

VASCULAR INVOLVEMENT

Thrombosis of cerebral or spinal arteries occurs rarely. The results may be fatal, or lead to convulsions, or mental deterioration. There may be sudden onset of monoplegia, hemiplegia, hemianopia or hemianaesthesia. The cerebrospinal fluid may be normal or may show changes of Type I or II.

PARENCHYMATOUS INVOLVEMENT

The changes of juvenile *general paralysis* may appear between the ages of 6 and 21, or sometimes even later. Some of these children have been mentally retarded due to early meningitis but others appear to have developed normally until symptoms and signs of juvenile paresis appear. The earliest changes are in character and intelligence. The child's behaviour becomes eccentric and his capacity at school or work declines rapidly. The type of psychosis is much less developed than in the adult; the main feature is a progressive dementia. He becomes careless, dirty and incapable of concentration. He may show gross changes in character and temperament. Convulsions are common. The physical signs are the same as those found in the acquired form of the disease. It is vitally important to recognize this condition early, for then striking improvement may follow treatment. The results in neglected cases can be appalling. The cerebrospinal fluid always shows changes of Type III.

Juvenile *tabes* is less common. It is frequently asymptomatic and the signs may be detected on routine examination performed for some other reason. These children rarely suffer from lightning pains or severe ataxia. They may present with urinary symptoms or failing vision due to associated optic atrophy. The signs resemble those of tabes due to acquired syphilis, but the course of the disease is likely to be relatively mild. There may be other manifestations of congenital syphilis, such as interstitial keratitis or gummata of bones. Tests of the cerebrospinal fluid may be normal but are likely to show changes of Type II.

Lesions of Bones

Gummatous osteoperiostitis usually occurs between the fifth and twentieth year of life. Most of the lesions result in sclerosis and considerable new bone formation, but destructive lesions occur in the palate and nasal septum. The tibia is the bone most frequently involved, and thickening of the middle third of the bone may give the appearance called 'sabre tibia' or 'sabre-blade tibia' (see Fig. 92). Localized osteoperiostitis of the bones of the vault of the skull may lead to the formation of rounded, bony swellings, called 'Parrot's nodes', which may also occur in early congenital syphilis. These are commonest in the frontal and parietal areas and lead to permanent thickening of the bones. The areas of thickening may give the impression of thinning of the rest of the bones, but it is a false impression and the name 'craniotabes', which is sometimes applied to this condition, is misleading. If gummatous destruction of the nasal septum (see Fig. 90) occurs it is likely to remove the support of the cartilaginous part of the nose, which then collapses, giving the deformity of gross depression of the lower part of the nose and a well-marked ridge between cartilage and bone. The anterior nares may be tilted forward. It should not be confused with 'saddle-nose' (see Fig. 89), which results from failure of proper development of the bones of the nasal cavity, due to 'syphilitic snuffles' early in life, and in which there is flattening of the bony bridge of the nose. Perforations of the nasal septum do not always cause external deformities and therefore all patients with congenital syphilis, indeed, all patients with syphilis, should

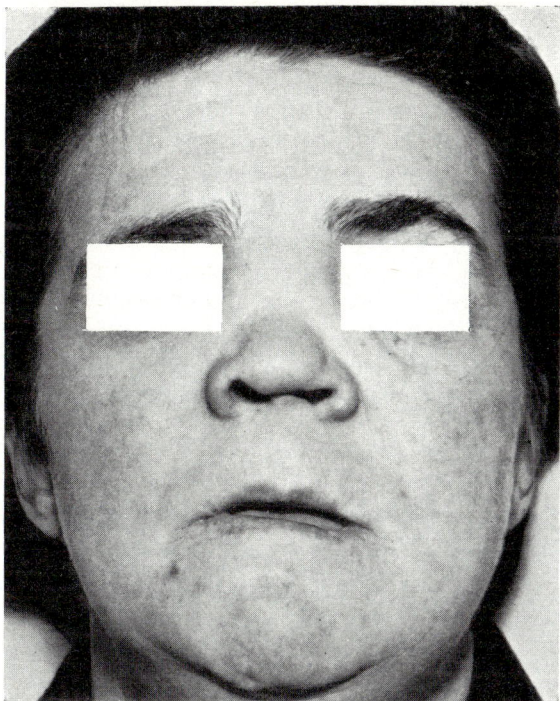

Fig. 89. Congenital syphilis:
saddle-nose.

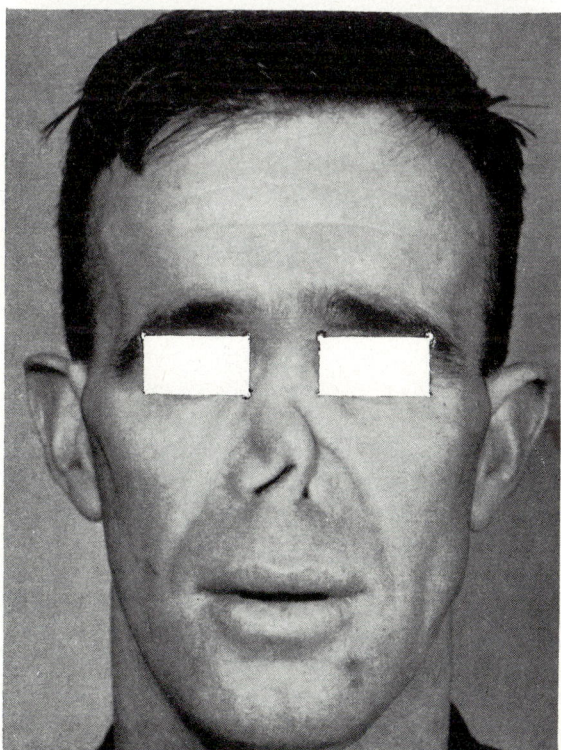

Fig. 90. Congenital syphilis
(late): destruction of
nasal septum with collapse
of 'nose cap'.

be examined by shining a torch into one nostril while observing through the other whether the light shines through to that half of the nasal cavity. Occasionally gummatous ulceration of the nasal septum may spread to the external tissues of the nose, causing partial or complete destruction of the organ. Gummatous lesions may also cause localized or complete destruction of the palate.

Apart from Parrot's nodes, none of these gummatous lesions is peculiar to congenital syphilis, and the decision as to whether the infection is congenital or acquired has to be made on other grounds.

Thickening of the inner end of the clavicle (Higouménakis' sign) and dactylitis are occasionally found in cases of late congenital syphilis.

Lesions of Joints

These patients may suffer from diffuse arthralgia but the characteristic lesion of joints is that described by Clutton and therefore called 'Clutton's joints' (see Fig. 94). The onset is commonly painless and insidious, and the course is chronic. Usually, both knee joints are involved, often simultaneously, but occasionally there may be a lapse of months or even years before the second joint is affected. Rarely, joints other than the knees are involved. Antisyphilitic treatment neither prevents nor cures the condition. The age of onset is likely to be between 10 and 20 years. In most cases the signs are those of a simple effusion without evident inflammatory changes in the joints or peri-articular tissues. There is little impairment of function and what there is seems to be due entirely to the size of the effusion, which is often considerable. X-rays show enlargement of the joint space but no bony changes. *Treponema pallidum* has never been found in the tissues or joint fluid in these cases, and because of this and the fact that the arthropathy does not respond to antisyphilitic treatment, Clutton's joints, like interstitial keratitis, have been thought to be manifestations of hypersensitivity. Recovery is slow, usually taking many months, but full recovery of function is the rule.

The Ear

In the early years of life, infection may spread from the nose and throat to the middle ear, giving rise to low-grade otitis media. The only symptom likely to be present is slight discharge from the ear. The bones of the middle ear may be involved and partial conductive deafness may follow.

The common characteristic lesion is involvement of the terminal fibres of the cochlear portion of the eighth nerve in the labryinth, resulting in perceptive deafness. The onset may be in childhood but it is often much later and may even occur in the middle-aged. It frequently affects patients who have had interstitial keratitis and like the latter it is more common in females. At the onset there may be vertigo and tinnitus but sometimes the only symptom is deafness, which is nearly always bilateral and progressive

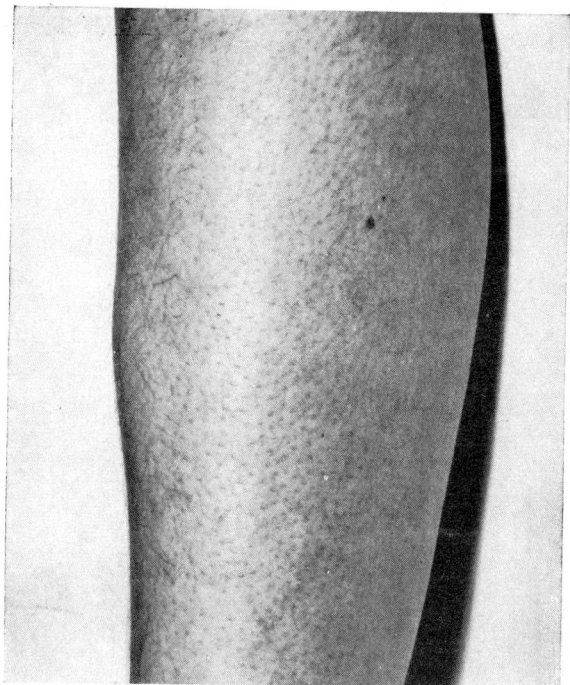

Fig. 91. Congenital syphilis (late): osteoperiostitis of the tibia.

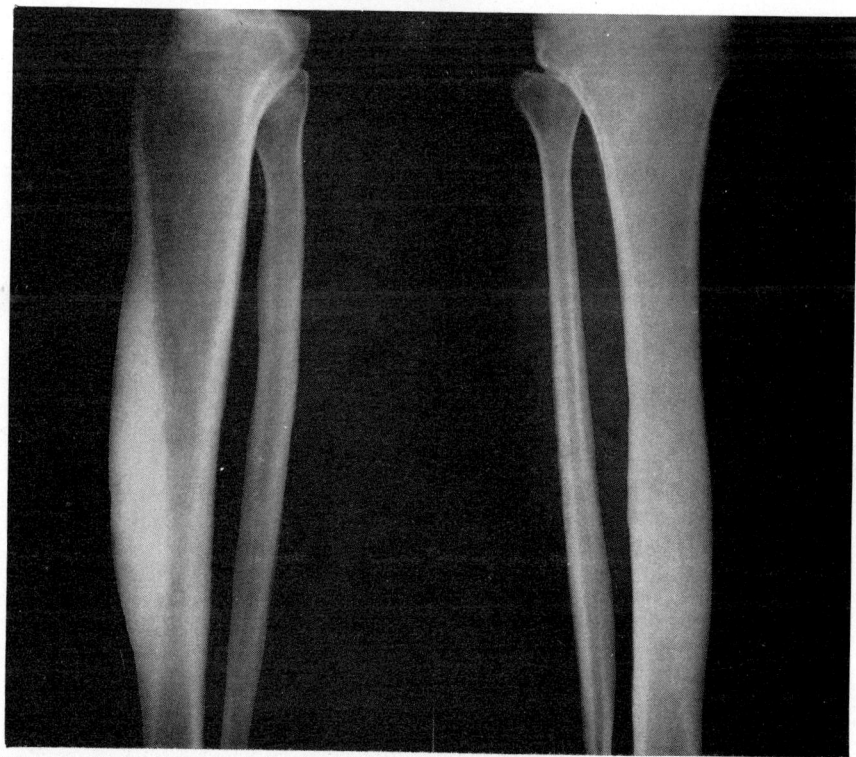

Fig. 92. Congenital syphilis (late): sabre tibia (*left*) lateral; (*right*) anteroposterior.

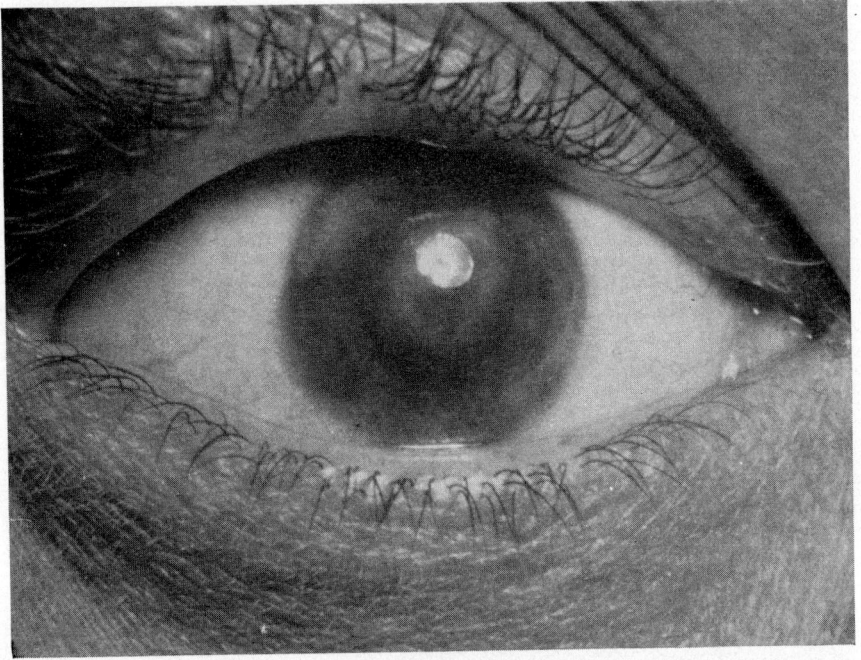

Fig. 93. Congenital syphilis (late): interstitial keratitis (inactive) causing blindness.

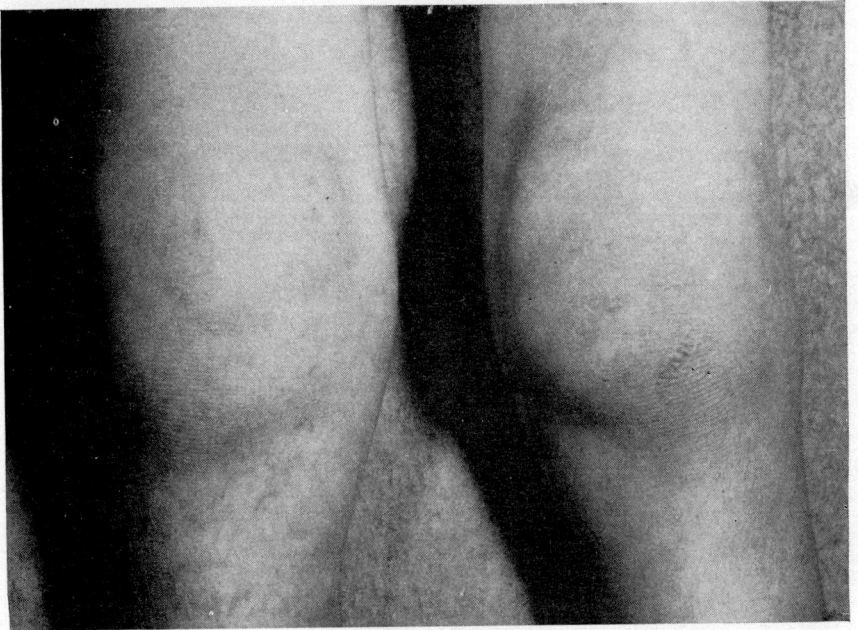

Fig. 94. Congenital syphilis (late): Clutton's knee joints.

and may become absolute. In adults the clinical picture can very closely resemble Menière's disease. On examination the tympanic membrane is normal. Tests for air and bone conduction show that perception of sound conducted by both routes is impaired in contrast with the relative enhancement of bone conduction in middle-ear disease. Sometimes nerve deafness may not be clinically obvious by the usual tests, but an audiogram may indicate loss of hearing; this occurs typically in the high-frequency range but sometimes the curve is flat or the loss for low frequencies greater. Discrimination of speech is particularly affected. Nerve deafness generally takes its course irrespective of antisyphilitic treatment but may be modified by steroid therapy.

The Skin and Mucous Membranes

As in the acquired form of the disease, gummata of soft tissues most commonly begin in subcutaneous or submucous tissues. Gummata may affect any area of skin or mucous membrane but they are particularly common in the soft palate and nasopharynx, and they lead to ulceration and destruction. The pathological processes in these lesions are precisely the same as in those which result from acquired syphilis.

Viscera

Visceral gummata are rare but the liver is occasionally involved. The clinical features are similar to those found in the equivalent condition due to acquired syphilis.

Cardiovascular Syphilis

Clinical cardiovascular syphilis is very rare in congenital syphilis. A few cases of aneurysm and aortic incompetence have been reported.[10] Interstitial myocarditis has been reported as a finding at autopsy.

Paroxysmal Cold Haemoglobinuria

This is a rare manifestation occurring in congenital[11] and also in acquired syphilis. Certain patients if exposed to cold will, within a few minutes, develop chills, malaise, headache, pain in the back and fever. There may also be urticaria. The next specimen of urine passed is dark red or brown. In a day or two the urine returns to normal but the patient may show slight jaundice. The serum of these patients contains a haemolysin which, in the presence of complement, first sensitizes the red cells during the period of chilling, then haemolyses them when the body temperature returns to normal. This type of reaction, the Donath–Landsteiner reaction, can be performed in vitro as a diagnostic test. The test may be positive in long-standing cases of syphilis without the patient having haemoglobinuria. Urine passed during the attack contains haemoglobin, methaemoglobin, occasional red cells and pigment-containing casts. Full treatment with penicillin usually, but not always, alleviates or cures the condition.

The Stigmata

The severe lesions of congenital syphilis have residual effects, such as scars and deformities, which are often characteristic and, of course, remain as permanent evidence of the infection. They are by no means always present and, in the majority of cases of late congenital syphilis, the fact that the infection is inherited is only suggested by the youth of the patient and confirmed by examination of the other members of the family. Stigmata may result from lesions which were active in both early and late stages of the infection.

Stigmata of Early Lesions

FACIES

Facial disfigurement may result from severe and persistent rhinitis in infancy. The infection interferes with growth and development of the nasal septum and other bones of the nasal cavity, with the result that the bridge of the nose may appear grossly depressed, the so-called saddle-nose deformity (see Fig. 89). The maxilla may also fail to develop normally, resulting in a high-arched palate (see Fig. 99). It is then small in comparison with the mandible, which is not involved. The latter therefore looks prominent and overdeveloped by comparison. This is called the 'bulldog jaw' (Fig. 95).

TEETH

One of the most commonly observed of the stigmata is the characteristic lesion of the incisor teeth described by Jonathan Hutchinson, and called 'Hutchinson's teeth' (see Fig. 97). The changes are found only in the permanent teeth. The tooth buds of the permanent incisors are developing in the latter part of pregnancy and in the early weeks of life, when the syphilitic infection is at its most active; the infection may interfere with nutrition of the tooth buds and cause suppression of the middle of the three denticles from which the tooth develops. The lateral denticles expand to fill the gap but succeed only partially. The incisor teeth are smaller than normal and may be widely spaced unless the maxilla is under-developed. The characteristic feature is that the sides of the tooth converge towards the cutting edge like the sides of a peg or the end of a screwdriver. The sides are sometimes, but not always, rounded, and the cutting edge may show a semilunar notch. The notch may be present before eruption or may develop after eruption as the result of erosion of the edge which is deficient in enamel. The upper central incisors are most often affected, but the upper lateral and lower incisors are quite often involved. The deformity is, of course, not apparent until eruption occurs but may sometimes be detected by X-ray examinations within the preceding two years.[12]

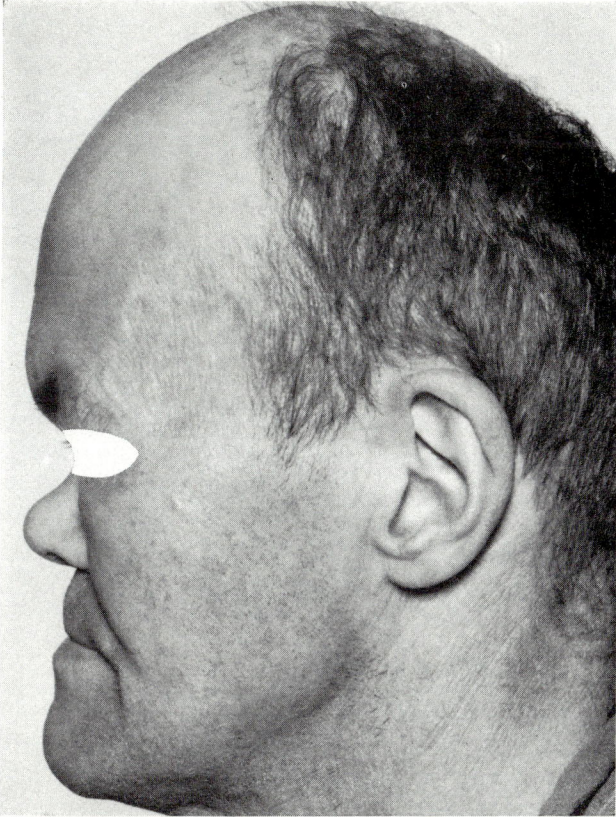

Fig. 95.
Congenital
syphilis (stigma):
bulldog facies.

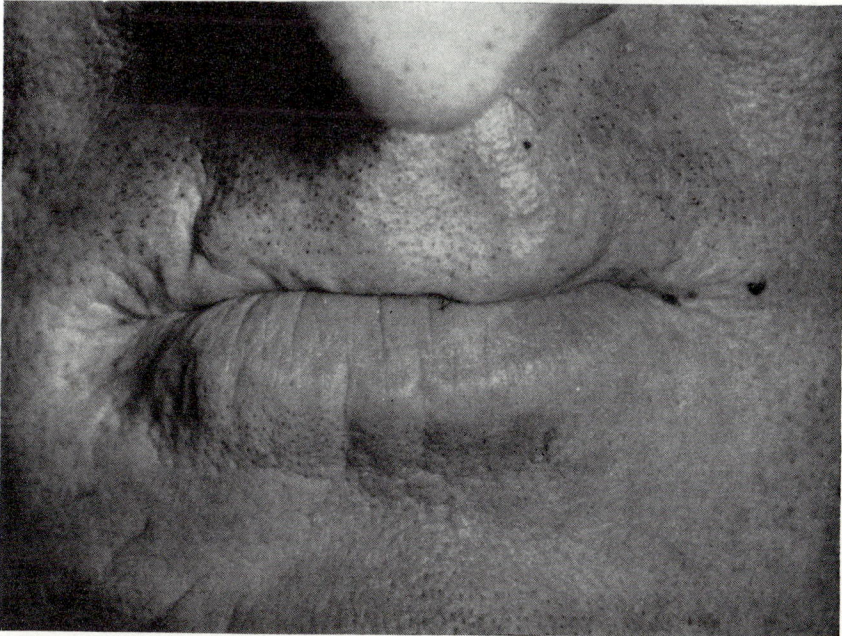

Fig. 96. Congenital syphilis (stigma): rhagades of lips.

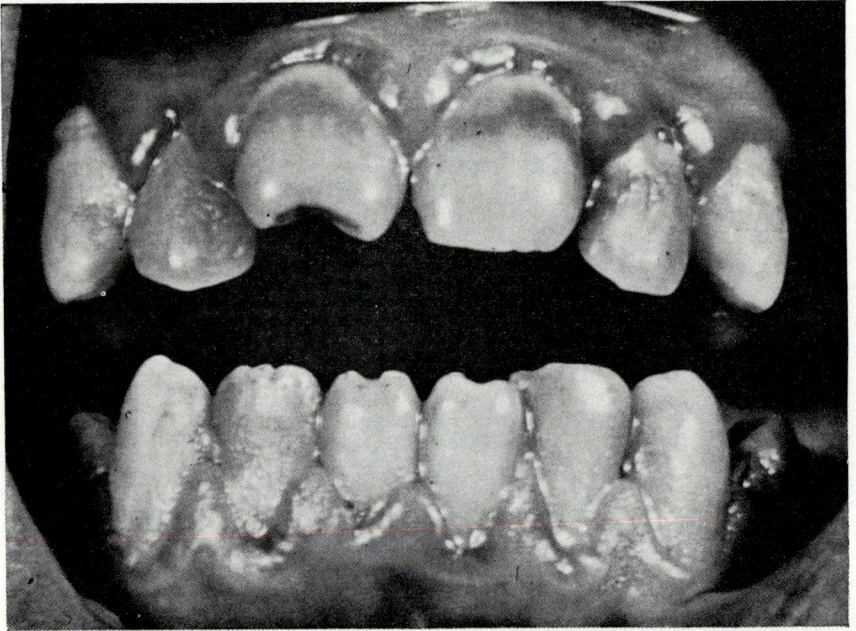

Fig. 97. Congenital syphilis (stigma): Hutchinson's teeth; note 'screwdriver' appearance of upper and lower central incisors.

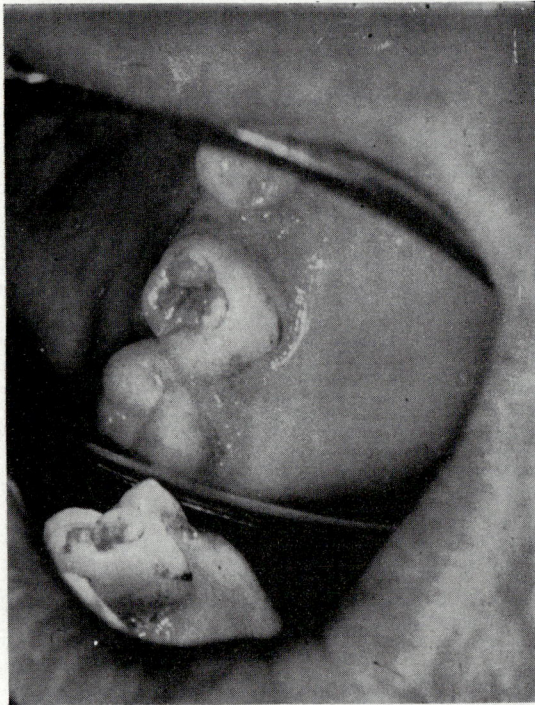

Fig. 98. Congenital syphilis (stigma): Moon's molar.

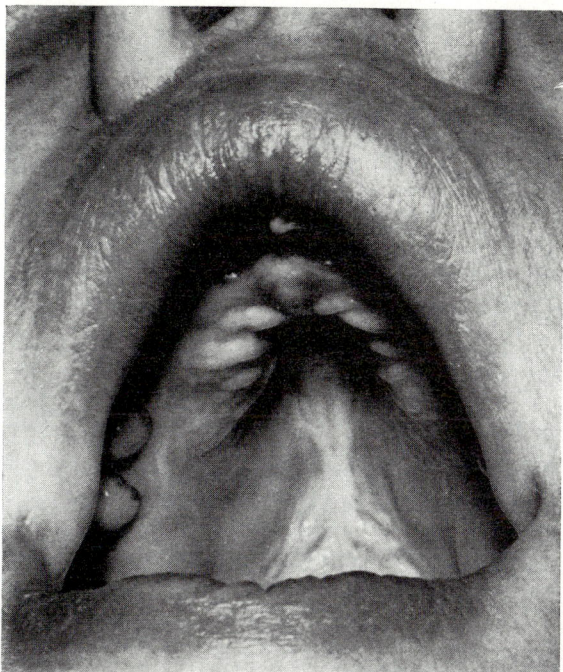

Fig. 99. Congenital syphilis (stigma): high-arched palate.

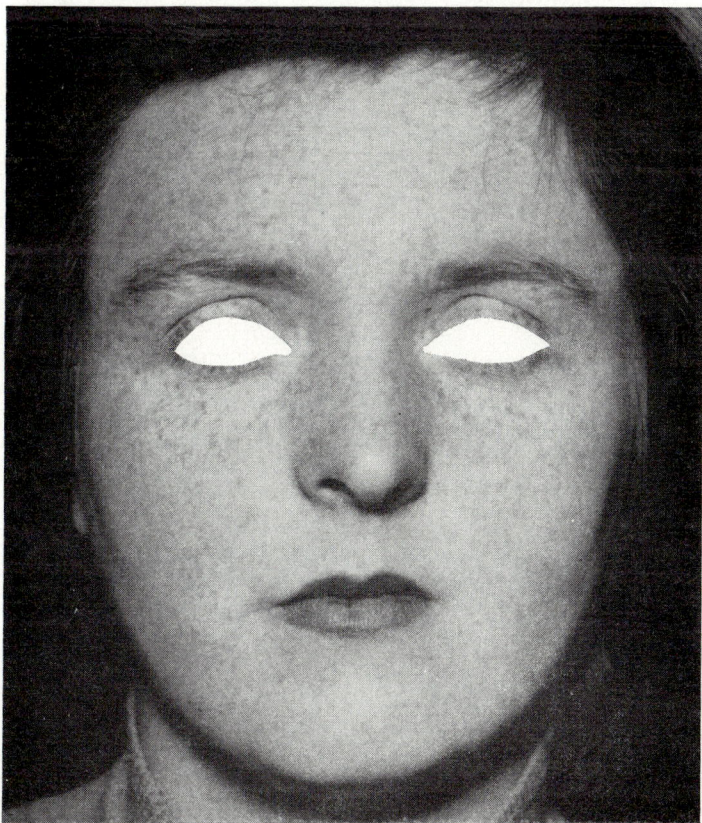

Fig. 100. Congenital syphilis (stigma): Stokes' facies.

The other characteristic dystrophy is that of the first molar teeth. This was described by Moon and the teeth are called 'Moon's' or 'mulberry molars' (see Fig. 98). The first lower molars, which are developing at the same time as the incisor teeth, are most often affected. The cusps are under-developed and poorly enamelled. The biting surface is dome-shaped, with small projections of the ill-developed cusps. This deformity is considerably less common than that of the incisor teeth. The affected molars, unlike the incisors, are very prone to caries and usually they are soon lost.

RHAGADES

These are scars at the angles of the mouth (see Fig. 96). Less often they are seen about the nares and rarely about the anus. They result from the early papular eruption of congenital syphilis which is apt to be profuse and con-fluent on the lower face. Movements of the mouth produce radiating fissures which become secondarily infected, and on healing they leave linear scars which radiate from the mouth angles.

CHOROID SCARRING

Choroidoretinitis occurring in the early stages of congenital syphilis leaves permanent changes visible in the fundus oculi. The scars are rounded, discrete and often widely scattered. They appear either as pale, atrophic areas bordered by pigmentation or as areas of pigmentation only. The appearance is sometimes called the 'pepper and salt' fundus.

THE NAILS

Onychia, in the course of the early eruption, may damage the nail beds and leave permanent change in the nails. These are not characteristic.

Stigmata of Late Lesions

THE CORNEA

Interstitial keratitis (see Fig. 93) may leave opacities in the deep layers of the cornea and so-called ghost vessels, which appear as a network of empty blood vessels extending from the sclerotic into the deep layers of the cornea. They are seen with the corneal microscope and slit lamp.

GUMMATOUS SCARS

Gummatous scars of the skin and mucous membranes may be characteristic in appearance. Scarring and deformity of the throat or perforation of the palate or nasal septum are strongly suggestive of this diagnosis (see Figs. 85–88, pp. 117–18).

BONES

Healed gummatous osteoperiostitis leaves changes which are recognizable clinically or radiologically. The so-called sabre-shin deformity may be present. Healed periosteal nodes are frequently responsible for abnormal prominence and broadness of the frontal region, so-called frontal bossing. The association of this stigma with saddle-nose and bulldog jaw gives rise to the appearance which is usually called 'bulldog facies'. If there is gross frontal and parietal bossing the whole skull is broadened, with intervening and lateral depressions giving the appearance of 'natiform' or 'hot-cross bun' skull.

OPTIC ATROPHY

Involvement of the central nervous system may result in the highly character-istic appearance of primary optic atrophy. Optic atrophy may also result from severe choroidoretinitis.

NERVE DEAFNESS

The presence of nerve deafness for which no other cause can be found suggests the possibility of congenital syphilis.

Other Stigmata

Certain occasional findings have been described as stigmata, but they are not in themselves diagnostic and they sometimes occur in normal people. They include incurvature of the vertebral borders of the scapulae, increased carrying angle of the forearms, ulnar deviation of the middle finger and a very short little finger (Dubois' sign).

Diagnosis

Any of these findings may help to suggest or establish the diagnosis. Hutchinson gave a classical description of three features which are of particular importance in the diagnosis of late congenital syphilis. They are usually called 'Hutchinson's triad', which consists of: the Hutchinsonian teeth, interstitial keratitis, and 8th-nerve deafness.

Stokes has described the facial appearance (sometimes called the 'Stokes facies', see Fig. 100) of many congenital syphilitics who may lack the gross stigmata, in the following words:

The essence of the matter lies in a certain inalertness, a sleepy, tired, fagged, clouded, dreaming or obscured appearance of the upper face; an appearance of veiledness as if a smudge had lightly swept across the brows and eyes and the nasal bridge of a crayon portrait.[13]

The reagin tests follow the same pattern as in acquired syphilis. If they are negative the diagnosis of syphilis can usually be confirmed by the specific tests, but even these tests are occasionally negative in untreated congenital syphilitics diagnosed by the presence of characteristic stigmata.

REFERENCES

1. HARTER, C. A. and BENIRSCHKE, K. (1976) *Am. J. Obstet. Gynec.*, **124,** 705.
2. STOKES, J. H., BEERMAN, H. and INGRAHAM, N. R. (1945) *Modern Clinical Syphilology*, 3rd ed., p. 1083. Philadelphia and London: W. B. Saunders.
3. *A. R. Med. Offr Dept Hlth* (Lond.) (1950–1977) H.M.S.O., 1951–1978.
4. *V.D. Fact Sheet* (1976) U.S. Department of Health, Education and Welfare, Public Health Service, Center for Disease Control, Atlanta, Georgia.
5. OPPENHEIMER, E. H. and HARDY, J. B. (1971) *Johns Hopkins med. J.*, **129,** 63.
6. SCOTTI, A. T. and LOGAN, L. (1968) *J. Pediat.*, **73,** 242.
7. JOHNSTON, N. A. (1972) *Br. J. vener. Dis.*, **48,** 464.
8. SINGH, R., KAUR, D. and PARAMESWARAN, M. (1971) *Br. J. vener. Dis.*, **47,** 206.
9. LASCARI, A. D., DIAMOND, J. and NOLAN, B. E. (1976) *Clin. Pediat.*, **15,** 90.
10. BONUGLI, F. S. (1961) *Br. J. vener. Dis.*, **37,** 257.
11. PARISH, D. J. and MITCHELL, J. R. A. (1960) *J. clin. Path.*, **13,** 237.
12. PUTKONEN, T. and PAATERO, Y. V. (1961) *Br. J. vener. Dis.*, **37,** 190.
13. STOKES, J. H., BEERMAN, H. and INGRAHAM, N. R. (1945) *Modern Clinical Syphilology*, 3rd ed., p. 1134. Philadelphia and London: W. B. Saunders.

7

Serological Tests and their Interpretation

Serological tests for syphilis comprise reagin tests and specific tests.

REAGIN TESTS FOR SYPHILIS

Complement fixation
< flocculation tests

These tests depend upon the fact that in the course of certain diseases, including syphilis, a substance with the properties of an antibody appears in the serum of affected patients. This substance, called 'reagin', has the property of combining with colloidal suspensions of lipoids extracted from animal tissues, which then clump together to form visible masses, a process which is called 'flocculation'. After combining with reagin, the lipoidal particles have the power to fix complement. Thus there are two types of reagin test: complement-fixation tests and flocculation tests.

When Wassermann and his co-workers (1906) first employed the complement-fixation technique previously described by Bordet and Gengou, they used what they thought to be a specific antigen in the form of extracts of liver containing treponemes from infants who had died from early congenital syphilis. It was soon observed, however, that the test also gave positive results in cases of syphilis when aqueous and, later, alcoholic extracts of normal liver tissue were used as antigens. It was not until the Wassermann reaction had been in use for many years that it was realized that reagin could also be demonstrated in the presence of a number of diseases other than treponemal infections. Reagin is part of the gamma-globulin fraction of serum and is probably present in small quantities in all normal sera, although these quantities are insufficient to give positive tests with standard techniques.

Complement-fixation Tests

The Wassermann reaction (WR) is the prototype but there have been many modifications. The presence of reagin is indicated by fixation of complement in the presence of non-specific antigen. The antigen chosen was usually an alcoholic extract of normal animal tissues, such as beef heart, with the addition of cholesterol as a sensitizing agent. The lipoids in the cholesterol-ized alcoholic extract were thrown out of solution by the addition of saline at a pre-determined titre and the resulting colloidal suspension of lipoids and cholesterol in saline was used as the antigen in the test. It was shown by Pangborn in 1941[1] that the active principle of these extracts is a sero-logically active phospholipid called cardiolipin. Although serologically inert by itself, when cardiolipin is combined with lecithin and cholesterol the mixture forms a serologically active antigen for the detection of reagin. The test is applied to blood serum from which the clotted cells have been removed. Human serum contains complement, and this is inactivated by heating the serum at 56°C for 30 minutes. Inactivated serum, antigen and complement obtained from guinea-pig serum are mixed and then incubated at 37°C. The presence or absence of complement fixation is demonstrated by adding an 'indicator system'. This depends upon the fact that sheep's red cells, which have been sensitized by an anti-sheep's red-cell antibody (haemolysin), are lysed by complement. The haemolysin is produced by a process of sensitization in which a rabbit is given repeated injections of sheep's red cells. The mixture of sheep's red cells and haemolysin will only show haemolysis in the presence of free complement. Complement is free in the complement-fixation test only if the patient's serum contains no reagin. Thus haemolysis in the indicator system demonstrates that comple-ment has not been fixed by reagin and the test is therefore negative. If the patient's serum does contain sufficient reagin, it fixes the complement, no haemolysis occurs and the result of the test is positive. If there is only a small amount of reagin present there may be partial haemolysis and the result will be recorded as 'doubtful' or 'weak positive'.

The sensitivity of complement-fixation tests is apt to vary in different laboratories, and results in laboratories with reliable techniques may vary in tests of the same specimen of serum. In the test two tubes are employed, the first as a control from which the antigen is omitted and a second in which all the ingredients are included. The control should show complete haemolysis and then the result can be read from the other tube. Occasion-ally the control shows partial or no haemolysis and the serum tested must then be reported as anticomplementary. This is likely to happen when the serum has become infected or haemolysed and destroys the activity of complement in both tubes of the test. The test must then be repeated with a fresh specimen of serum. Very occasionally, repeated tests give anti-complementary results. Some sera may be inherently anticomplementary in the absence of haemolysis or infection of the serum. Sometimes these sera have an abnormally high level of gamma globulins.

It is important to assess the amount of reagin in a patient's serum; quantitative complement-fixation tests can be done by testing serial dilutions of the patient's serum, whenever a positive result has been obtained with undiluted serum. The titre is expressed as the highest dilution of the serum which gives partial or complete fixation of the test dose of complement.

The crude tissue extract antigens have been superseded by the purer cardiolipin–lecithin–cholesterol antigens. The latter are both more sensitive and specific because they are prepared from chemically defined products. Their level of reactivity can be standardized more easily than was the case with the crude tissue extract antigens.

Flocculation Tests

These tests are technically simpler to perform than complement-fixation tests, and a variety of techniques has been devised. All depend on the ability of serum containing reagin to cause aggregation of a colloidal suspension of lipoid particles into visible clumps.

The Kahn, Meinicke, Kline, Mazzini, Price and other similar tests are all now obsolete and have been superseded by cardiolipin tests. The flocculation test which has found most favour because of its reliability and relative simplicity of technique is the VDRL (*Venereal Disease Research Laboratory*) or *Harris test*. It employs cardiolipin antigen and can be used in either a slide test or a tube test, both of which are well adapted to quantitative estimations. In recent years the VDRL slide test has been widely adopted. In this test a cardiolipin antigen is added to inactivated serum on ringed slides which are rotated mechanically to promote union of antigen and antibody. The slides are then examined microscopically to detect aggregation of the antigen particles, indicating a positive result. Another valuable test is the *rapid plasma reagin test*, in which VDRL antigen is suspended in choline, with finely divided carbon particles as a marker. It is carried out on unheated serum or plasma on disposable cards; a positive result is shown by clumping of the carbon particles visible to the naked eye. The same antigen is used in the *automated reagin test*, designed for use with autoanalyser equipment. Serum is sampled and antigen added automatically, the reaction taking place in a series of mixing coils. The reactants are finally deposited on a moving strip of filter paper. Positive results are shown by clumping of the carbon particles.

False negative results may occur in flocculation tests with some sera containing large amounts of antibody (prozone phenomenon). When such sera are serially diluted in saline and re-examined, positive results are given by the diluted serum. The occurrence of prozone phenomena is an argument for performing both a flocculation and a complement-fixation test, because the latter is not so subject to the prozone phenomenon.

Non-syphilitic Reactions to Reagin Tests[2]

Non-syphilitic reactions, or so-called 'false-positive' results, to the reagin tests for syphilis are of four kinds: 1. technical false-positive reactions,

2. variations in the normal, 3. those due to diseases allied to syphilis, and 4. biological false-positive (BFP) reactions.

TECHNICAL FALSE-POSITIVE REACTIONS

These result from human errors, such as mistakes in the collection and labelling of specimens, the use of faulty materials and reagents in the tests, mistakes in the performance of the tests and mistakes in recording or reporting the final results. They may also occur as the result of testing specimens which are contaminated by bacteria or haemolysed.

The possibility of such errors makes it essential that positive results to these tests which have no confirmation in the clinical findings should always be checked by testing another specimen of serum from the same patient. The use of several tests on the same specimen of serum, which is common practice in many laboratories, is a good precaution against some of these errors.

VARIATIONS IN THE NORMAL

A few normal individuals, for reasons which are uncertain, produce an excess of reagin which may give positive tests; these reactions seem to be more common in the elderly and very occasionally they are familial. The specific tests are negative.

DISEASES ALLIED TO SYPHILIS

These diseases, such as yaws, bejel, and pinta, are caused by treponemata closely related to *T. pallidum* and give positive serological reactions, including those relying on specific antibodies, which are identical with those found in syphilis. These should not be described as 'false-positive' reactions because they give firm evidence of the presence of treponemal disease.

'BIOLOGICAL FALSE-POSITIVE' REACTIONS

These are of two types, transient 'acute' reactions lasting a few weeks or months, and 'chronic' reactions which last for longer than six months and sometimes for many years. The specific tests are negative and there must be no clinical evidence of syphilis. In particular the stigmata of congenital syphilis should be looked for as very occasionally reagin tests are positive and specific tests negative in cases of late congenital syphilis.

The acute type may be associated with infections, especially if these produce fever, for example, bacterial or virus pneumonia or malaria. It may be precipitated by immunization procedures, particularly vaccination against smallpox. Glandular fever has been thought to produce this type of reaction, but this has not been confirmed by recent surveys. Routine serological tests for syphilis during pregnancy may give false-positive reactions but whether or not pregnancy is of itself a cause of such reactions is uncertain.

The only infection known to produce the chronic false-positive reactions is leprosy, more commonly, it is thought, in the lepromatous than the tuberculoid type of this disease. They may be found as but one of the serological abnormalities in autoimmune diseases, especially in disseminated lupus erythematosus, haemolytic anaemia or thyroiditis, and have sometimes been found before the underlying disease is clinically manifest. Investigation may show the presence of other antibodies such as antinuclear or rheumatoid factors, mitochondrial antibodies or cryoglobulins and also abnormal liver function tests and the presence of L-E cells. The chronic false-positive reaction usually appears before the other laboratory abnormalities and is followed by an increase in the erythrocyte sedimentation rate. It may antedate clinical disease by many years. This type of false-positive reaction is found three times as often in women as in men. They have been found in drug addicts, especially in those using the intravenous route of administration. The antibodies responsible for these chronic reactions are usually IgM in nature.

Although false-positive reactions of both types are usually low in titre, the strength of a reaction is no guarantee of its specificity, and high titres are sometimes seen. Individual tests may give discrepant results, one being negative and another strongly positive. The finding of a positive test for reagin, confirmed on a second specimen of serum, in the absence of a definite history or conclusive clinical evidence of syphilis, is an indication for the performance of specific treponemal tests to confirm the diagnosis. Many laboratories in fact now use a specific test as well as a reagin test in routine serological screening.

SPECIFIC SEROLOGICAL TESTS FOR SYPHILIS

Treponema pallidum Immobilization Test

The first specific test for syphilis, and diseases allied to it, was based on the work of Nelson in 1948[3] and developed by Nelson and Mayer in 1949.[4] They showed that the serum of syphilitic patients contains an antibody which, in the presence of complement, inhibits the normal movement of virulent treponemes of syphilis. The organisms are extracted from lesions in experimentally infected rabbits and suspended in a survival medium in which they remain motile and virulent for a limited period but do not multiply. On incubation with syphilitic serum and complement derived from guinea-pigs, the organisms lose their motility and cease to be infectious to rabbits. The antibody is distinct from reagin, and Nelson and Mayer were able to demonstrate immobilization using syphilitic serum from which reagin had been removed. The test is highly specific and positive results are obtained only with serum from syphilitic patients and those with yaws and other diseases closely related to syphilis. The test is called the 'Treponema *pallidum immobilization (TPI)' test.* If 50 per cent or more of the treponemes are immobilized the test is reported *positive.* If 20 per cent or less are immobilized the test is *negative;* but if between 20 and 50 per cent are immobilized the result is regarded as doubtful. It is now accepted that this is a most reliable test, but it can only be done in specially equipped laboratories and the cost is high. There is reason to suppose that there are a number of specific syphilitic antibodies in addition to the antibody demonstrated by the TPI test and called 'immobilizing antibody'.

The test is in no sense a routine procedure replacing the standard serological tests; nor is it a substitute for clinical judgement. It becomes positive later in the course of early syphilis and, like the standard tests, it becomes negative after treatment in cases of early syphilis. However, once the secondary stage is past it is likely to remain positive for the rest of the patient's life, irrespective of treatment. A definite positive result is good evidence of treponemal infection, past or present, but does not give any indication of current activity of the disease. A negative result, while making treponemal infection unlikely, does not rule it out completely because of the relatively late development of immobilizing antibody during the primary stage and its absence in a minority of patients with late syphilis, particularly tabes, and with some congenital infections of long standing. Its particular value is in distinguishing between syphilitic and non-syphilitic reactions to the standard tests, and in the diagnosis of certain cases of late syphilis, particularly those of the cardiovascular system, in which the standard tests may have become negative in the course of time. For the test sterile serum is required and it is important that the patient should not have had recent treatment with treponemicidal drugs, particularly penicillin, as these may render the test invalid.

Reiter Protein Complement-fixation Test

Since 1949 efforts have been made to evolve simpler specific tests which can be used as routine in any laboratory. Tests such as the *Treponema pallidum immune adherence (TPIA) test, treponemal agglutination* and *Treponema pallidum complement-fixation (TPCF)* tests employ killed *T. pallida,* but none of them is entirely satisfactory for routine use, in regard either to simplicity of technique or cost. On the other hand, a test employing a protein fraction derived from the cultivable Reiter treponeme[5] which shares a common group antigen with virulent *T. pallidum* and other treponemes is more satisfactory. The antigen is prepared from an extract of cultures of these organisms and is available commercially. The complement-fixation technique is used, with Reiter protein antigen substituted for non-specific antigen. The test is called the '*Reiter protein complement-fixation (RPCF)' test.* Preliminary incubation overnight of the mixture of antigen, complement and serum at refrigeration temperature before the addition of sensitized sheep cells is said to increase the sensitivity of the test. The cost of the reagents and of the procedure is low. The antibody detected by the RPCF test is, as stated, group specific. It differs from both immobilizing antibody and reagin. False-positive reactions are occasionally found in the RPCF test, and some of these are said to be due to an antibody reacting with a lipopolysaccharide impurity in the protein antigen. The antibody concerned differs from that giving false-positive reactions in reagin tests, so that when the RPCF test is used in conjunction with tests for reagin, the simultaneous occurrence of both 'non-specific' antibodies in the same serum is very unlikely. The RPCF test has proved to be most useful when employed as a screening test in conjunction with a sensitive test for reagin; the combination has a higher detection rate than either test used alone. It is not, however, sufficient on its own to provide full confirmation of the diagnosis of treponemal disease. The test is, in fact, now used much less frequently, many laboratories preferring the TPHA test.

Because specific tests probably depend upon the presence of different specific antibodies, there may not be complete correlation between the results of these tests. However, the TPI and RPCF tests agree in some 90 per cent of the cases.

The Fluorescent Treponemal Antibody Test

The fluorescent treponemal antibody test[6] is an indirect method in which the antigen is a drop of a suspension of dead *Treponema pallidum* (Nichols virulent strain) dried and fixed on a slide. Diluted patient's serum is added; if antibody is present, the treponemes become coated with a layer of antibody globulin. This is detected by the addition of an antiserum prepared against human immunoglobulin labelled with fluorescein isothiocyanate which unites with the film of globulin coating the treponemes. These fluoresce when examined by dark-ground illumination under ultraviolet light. If no antibody is bound in the first stage of the reaction, the treponemes do not fluoresce.

At least two kinds of antibody can be detected by this method. One of these is specific for *T. pallidum* and the allied pathogenic treponemes. The second is a group-reactive antibody which reacts with both pathogenic and commensal treponemes because of antigens shared between them. This group antibody is present at a low titre in many normal sera, probably being produced in response to the normal flora of commensal treponemes, but its titre becomes greatly increased in infection with syphilis in addition to the development of specific antibody. In the *Absorbed fluorescent treponemal antibody (FTA-ABS) test* the effect of the group antibody is blocked by dilution of the serum in a heated culture filtrate of Reiter treponemes (sorbent), thus theoretically leaving only specific antibody free to unite with the treponemal antigen. Although the mode of action and specificity of sorbent is still controversial, the FTA-ABS test has proved extremely sensitive, especially in cases of primary syphilis, and to have a good specificity. However, dilution of syphilitic sera 1 in 5 in sorbent under the conditions of the FTA-ABS test may not remove all group-reactive antibody as is shown by the ability of such absorbed serum to give fluorescence with Reiter treponemes as antigen. This may not be of much importance if the sera are strongly positive with a high titre, but with weakly reactive sera in which the FTA-ABS test is the only test positive and with no clinical evidence to support the diagnosis, it is important to know that fluorescence is due to specific antibody. Wilkinson and Wiseman[7] have suggested that in these circumstances the test should be repeated with an ultrasonicate of Reiter treponemes as the sorbing agent; the absorbed serum should be tested against both *T. pallidum* and Reiter treponemes and results accepted as positive only if there is definite fluorescence with *T. pallidum* and no fluorescence with Reiter treponemes, indicating complete removal of group antibody reactions with the latter antigen. False-positive reactions have been found with sera from patients with balanitis and in cases of lupus erythematosus in which an atypical beaded staining of the treponemes has been observed, although sometimes there is homogeneous staining similar to that given by syphilitic sera. Very occasionally unexplained false-positive FTA-ABS tests occur even after absorption with Reiter treponeme ultrasonicate.

By using monospecific conjugates, the FTA-ABS test can be used to detect the different classes of immunoglobulin antibodies. This has proved of practical use in the differentiation of neonatal syphilis from passive transfer of maternal antibody. IgM antibody does not cross the intact placenta, and the detection of specific IgM antitreponemal antibody in the baby's circulation is suggestive evidence that the child is infected, particularly if the titre rises. There is evidence that after the treatment of acquired or congenital syphilis IgM antibody usually disappears fairly rapidly while IgG antibody persists.[8,9]

Treponema pallidum Haemagglutination (TPHA) Test

In this test the antigen is a suspension of formolized tanned sheep red cells sensitized with an ultrasonicate of virulent *Treponema pallidum*. Serum is added to an absorbing diluent to remove cross-reacting antibodies and the sensitized cells added. Unsensitized cells are added to a second tube as a control and the two left standing. A positive result is shown by the gradual agglutination of the sensitized cells while the unsensitized cells in the control tube form a compact button at the bottom of the tube. The test is very easy to perform, and unlike the TPI or FTA-ABS tests, can readily be done quantitatively. A micromethod is now generally used because of the cost. It has a high specificity and its sensitivity appears to be intermediate between the TPI and FTA-ABS tests; it is less sensitive than the latter in primary syphilis and of comparable sensitivity thereafter. However, when carried out by the original macromethod it appears to be as sensitive as the FTA-ABS test in primary syphilis.[10]

Choice of Tests and Interpretation

Suitable arrangements should be made between clinician and pathologist for the routine of serological investigation. For instance, it may be agreed that one or more tests for reagin and a group specific test such as the RPCF, or a more specific test such as the TPHA, will be done on every specimen of serum. If the tests are positive they are repeated, with the addition of a quantitative estimation, for which the VDRL may be used. In countries such as Great Britain, positive results to the standard and specific tests suggest infection with syphilis in white patients, and syphilis, yaws or other treponemal disease in coloured patients.

If one or more of the screening tests are found positive and there is no conclusive evidence of syphilis, they should be repeated on a second specimen, half of which should be sent to a reference laboratory so that specific confirmatory tests, such as the TPI or FTA-ABS tests, can be carried out. If these are positive, past or present treponemal disease is indicated. There is no serological test which will differentiate syphilis from other treponemal infections, such as yaws. A positive result in these tests does not necessarily mean that the disease process is still active. If the TPI and FTA-ABS tests are both negative, positive tests for reagin are probably non-specific and the cause for this should be sought.

Careful enquiry should be made concerning recent acute disease, vaccination or inoculation. Investigations such as blood counts and a Paul–Bunnell test for mononucleosis, search for malarial parasites and X-ray of the chest for virus pneumonia may be indicated. If the reaction is persistent full investigation for conditions such as autoimmune disease is indicated.

In cases of early syphilis, the FTA-ABS test is generally the first to become positive, the RPCF and reagin tests are usually next, then the TPHA (micromethod) and lastly the TPI test. The FTA-ABS test is particularly useful in the serological diagnosis of early syphilis in the primary stage in cases in which it proves impossible to demonstrate *T. pallidum*.

After adequate treatment of early syphilis, reagin disappears within three to six months in over 90 per cent of cases. Reversal is quicker in primary than in secondary syphilis. The RPCF test may take longer to reverse, as do the TPI and FTA-ABS tests, particularly the latter. These tests may remain positive after many years; such a result indicates the possibility that the patient has received treatment for syphilis in the past, a fact which some patients prefer to conceal or forget. The FTA-ABS IgM test, however, usually becomes negative within a year after successful treatment. When patients are first treated for latent or late infections with syphilis, the serological response is less predictable. In some cases, tests for reagin may show a slow but progressive decline in titre and eventually become negative. In others, the titre may become fixed (the 'Wassermann-fast' cases). The TPI, FTA-ABS and TPHA tests remain positive for many years after treatment for latent or late syphilis; there is some evidence that the TPI test may become negative while the FTA-ABS and TPHA tests remain positive in a small minority of such cases. Because of their persistent positivity, the specific treponemal tests are of little or no value in the assessment of progress after treatment; for this, much more reliance should be placed on quantitatively performed tests for reagin antibody. However, it has been suggested that a persistently positive FTA-ABS IgM test does give an indication of continuing activity of the disease,[8] but the evidence for this is inconclusive.[9,11]

As stated, none of the specific tests is capable of differentiating between syphilis, yaws and the other treponematoses, so that serological interpretation is far more difficult in the cases of some coloured patients. Positive results to the specific tests, with positive, doubtful, or negative results to standard tests, are often shown by the sera of such patients who give the history of yaws in childhood and may have scars on the legs suggestive of this infection. Documentary evidence of earlier infection and treatment cannot usually be obtained. Physical signs may be absent or indefinite, and it may sometimes be in the patient's interest to assume that the infection was syphilitic and to investigate and treat accordingly. A strongly positive VDRL test or strongly positive FTA-ABS IgM test would make syphilis the likely diagnosis. A negative FTA-ABS IgM test does not help differentiate between old yaws and latent syphilis as many patients with apparently untreated latent syphilis, as well as those with old yaws, have negative FTA-ABS IgM tests.[9]

Note: The World Health Organization in its 'Personal Booklet' requests reporting of serological tests as follows:

Non-reactive   (—)
Partially reactive (±)
Reactive   (+)

REFERENCES

1. PANGBORN, M. C. (1941) Proc. Soc. exp. Biol., **48**, 484.
2. KING, A. J. (1964) Recent Advances in Venereology, Chapter 6. London: J. & A. Churchill.
3. NELSON, R. A. (1948) Am. J. Hyg., **48**, 120.
4. NELSON, R. A. and MAYER, M. M. (1949) J. exp. Med., **89**, 369.
5. WALLACE, A. L. and HARRIS, A. (1967) Reiter Treponeme. Bull. Wld Hlth Org., **36**, Suppl. 2.
6. HUNTER, E. F., DEACON, W. E. and MEYER, P. C. (1964) Publ. Hlth Rep. (Wash.), **79**, 5.

7. WILKINSON, A. E. and WISEMAN, C. C. (1971) *Proc. R. Soc. Med.*, **64,** 422.

8. O'NEILL, P. and NICOL, C. S. (1972) *Br. J. vener. Dis.*, **48,** 460.

9. WILKINSON, A. E. and RODIN, P. (1976). *Br. J. vener. Dis.*, **52,** 219.

10. ALESSI, E. and SCIOCCATI, L. (1978) *Br. J. vener. Dis.*, **54,** 151.

11. LUGER, A., SCHMIDT, B. and SPENDLINGWIMMER, I. (1977) *Br. J. vener. Dis.*, **53,** 287.

8

Treatment of Syphilis

The patient must be submitted to full general examination before treatment for syphilis is begun, to assess the extent of damage by the syphilitic process and to detect complicating disease which may modify the patient's reaction to treatment and influence the prognosis. The outcome of treatment depends on a number of factors, including the immunological reactions of the patient, the virulence of the invading organisms, intercurrent infection, allergic reactions, pregnancy, alcoholism and the precise methods of treatment employed. Race and sex are also important factors but mainly in relation to the prognosis of the untreated disease. The mental reaction of the patient to syphilitic infection and its treatment may well be considerable and sympathetic handling of his personal and domestic problems is essential. The patient should be strongly advised not to read medical textbooks.

PAST METHODS OF TREATMENT

The older forms of treatment were potentially highly toxic and their administration to patients was always fraught with some danger.

Mercury

Up to the early years of the twentieth century, mercury was the only drug available for treatment of syphilis which was likely to be at all effective. It was given by mouth, by injection, by inunction or by inhalation. Its toxic effects on skin, mucous membranes and intestines often outweighed its therapeutic value. Its effects were suppressive rather than curative.

Arsenic

Ehrlich's original preparation, arsphenamine (606), was soon replaced by neoarsphenamine (914) and this drug, in combination with intramuscular bismuth, was the remedy of choice in most clinics until the introduction of penicillin. Common practice was to give intravenous injections in amounts of o·3 to o·6 g at weekly intervals for courses lasting 10 weeks, together with weekly intramuscular injections of bismuth, or one of its insoluble salts, in dosage of o·2 to o·4 g. Three to five courses of this treatment were given over periods of from 9 to 15 months, according to the stage of the disease. The results were good when patients attended regularly for treatment and were able to complete it. Unfortunately only 30 per cent of patients received full and regular treatment; the remainder either had to stop treatment through toxic effects or ceased to attend. Neoarsphenamine sometimes produced serious effects, such as exfoliative dermatitis, blood dyscrasias and haemorrhagic encephalitis. Vasomotor disturbance, nausea, vomiting and syncope were fairly common. Accidental extravenous injections produced tissue necrosis. Syringe transmission of the virus of homologous serum jaundice (hepatitis B virus) became a common complication during the Second World War and proved to be due to defective sterilization of syringes and needles. A trivalent arsenical suitable for deep subcutaneous or intramuscular use, sulpharsphenamine, was favoured, mainly by those who were not skilled in intravenous technique, but it was apt to cause painful local reactions, and toxic reactions were common. A more stable and less toxic preparation, oxophenarsine or arsphenoxide (Mapharside) had a considerable vogue before and in the early years of the last war, when it was used for intensive courses of short duration. Intensive treatment with this drug gave a considerable incidence of toxic effects such as gastrointestinal disturbance and encephalitis. A pentavalent arsenical preparation, tryparsamide, was regularly used in the treatment of neurosyphilis, but its value was limited and it was apt to produce toxic amblyopia.

There is now no indication for the use of either mercurial or arsenical drugs in the treatment of syphilis.

PRESENT METHODS OF TREATMENT (PREVENTIVE AND CURATIVE)

Preventive Treatment of Syphilis

A clear distinction must be made between those preventive measures applied before and those after the patient has taken a risk. Consideration of the former would necessitate discussion of the subject of promiscuity and of the social conditions which favour the spread of venereal disease. These are sociological rather than medical problems. They give scope for truly preventive treatment, although the actual nature of the measures to be taken is often a matter of dispute which may involve complex moral issues. Preventive treatment after the risk has been taken is sometimes called 'epidemiological treatment'. Local applications of various antiseptics to the genitalia of those who have taken risks were routine procedures in the Armed Forces of many countries for many years. Opinions have differed as to the value of such methods, but in general they have not been highly regarded. The condom does not provide as complete protection against infection from syphilis as from gonorrhoea because of the possibility of the organism entering through parts not covered by the sheath. There have been advocates of systemic epidemiological treatment and, in their day, mercury, arsenicals and bismuth were all used for the suppressive treatment of syphilis. Within the past 25 years there have been reports of the successful use of penicillin by injection, and also tetracycline, for the prevention of syphilis in individuals whose sexual partners have been known to suffer from infectious syphilis.[1,2] Some of these results appear to be impressive, but the fact is that evidence from these sources indicates only that this treatment diminishes the proportion of those patients who, exposed to infection, develop the early signs of disease. No patients treated in this way have been observed for long enough and with sufficient care to know whether the infection is truly eliminated, or whether the effect of such treatment is merely to suppress the early signs of infection. Treatment of this kind is a violation of a fundamental principle, that is: 'diagnosis before treatment.' Patients who receive it must be observed and tested as though they had truly suffered from syphilis. Anxiety which, with adequate observation and tests, might be limited to three months is prolonged for two years or more. There are restrictions as regards marriage and married life which may destroy happiness and result in the break-up of families. Suppressive treatment should therefore be regarded as an undesirable expedient for which the indications should be carefully and critically examined. It may occasionally be justified as, for instance, in the case of a woman late in pregnancy who has been subjected to a serious risk of syphilitic infection or when infection of a sexual partner is virtually certain but confirmation of infection cannot be established. An opposite view is taken in the United States of America, however, where routine treatment of all sexual contacts of an individual suffering from infectious syphilis is standard practice.

Curative Treatment

The following are the drugs which have been used in the modern treatment of syphilis: penicillin, bismuth, potassium iodide, corticosteroids, anti-biotics other than penicillin (the tetracyclines, chloramphenicol, erythromycin, carbomycin, synnematin B and cephaloridine).

Penicillin

Penicillin was first used for the treatment of syphilis in experimental animals and in man by Mahoney, Arnold and Harris in 1943.[3] It was soon evident that it was both safe and effective. It had very great advantages over the organic arsenicals because it could be given in intensive dosage without toxic effects, and with very considerable shortening of the period of treatment.

The impure, amorphous penicillin of that period was less effective than the pure penicillin which became available later, but good results were obtained with dosage of 2·4 million units given in 60 injections every three hours over seven and a half days. The proportion of failures of treatment was, however, high, being as great as 25 to 35 per cent in some series after two years of observation. On this account, in Britain and other European countries, routine dosage of penicillin was, for a while, combined with one course of an intravenous arsenical together with intramuscular bismuth. In retrospect it seems likely that some of the early failures of treatment, occurring when infectious syphilis was very common, were really due to reinfection of patients who had been cured very quickly and were no longer subjected to the suppressive action of the prolonged treatment of the past. Amorphous penicillin was found to contain a mixture of four different penicillins, called G, F, X, and K. In 1946, in the United States of America, results of treatment with amorphous penicillin began to deteriorate, and this proved to be due to the fact that commercial penicillin contained a progressively greater proportion of penicillin K, which was relatively ineffective against syphilis.[4] The most effective component was penicillin G. Pure crystalline penicillin G was soon produced in quantity and the results of treatment improved greatly. Courses amounting to 2·4 or 4·8 million units were given over periods of a week or more; injections had to be given every two to four hours day and night and this necessitated admission to hospital for the period of treatment. The number of injections was formidable, and attempts were therefore made to produce preparations which acted as depots in the tissues and were slowly absorbed.

The first of these so-called repository preparations was a suspension of calcium penicillin in arachis oil containing 4·8 per cent of beeswax. One millilitre of this preparation contained 300,000 units of penicillin, and a dose of 2 ml given intramuscularly maintained an effective level of the drug in the blood and tissues of a patient for 24 hours, thus making possible the treatment of infectious syphilis in out-patients. Good results were given by eight daily injections of this preparation. However, this mixture was not easy to administer because of its consistency, and there were reactions due to sensitization to its various constituents. The next repository preparation was the chemical combination of procaine and penicillin. Procaine penicillin proved effective when given in watery suspension in daily doses of 600,000 900,000 units for eight to ten days, each injection providing an effective level of penicillin for about 24 hours. A further development was the suspension of procaine penicillin in arachis oil, to which was added 2 per cent of the water-repellent aluminium monostearate (PAM). A standard dose of 300,000 to 600,000 units of this preparation usually maintained an effective level of penicillin in the patient's serum for 72 hours or more, thus dispensing with the necessity for daily injections for patients who could not attend daily, and providing protection for the careless or uncooperative patient who missed odd days of treatment. The daily administration of a standard dose, such as 600,000 units, of this preparation provides a series of depots in the tissues, resulting in a relatively high level of penicillin in the blood at the end of eight to ten days of treatment and a continuing effect which may last for a week or so after the course of treatment is finished. However the main advantage of this preparation is that it need not be given every day but, assuming cooperation of the patient, is given often enough to ensure full supervision during the period of treatment.

High levels of penicillin in the blood are not required for the treatment of syphilis. The experimental work indicated that the minimum level can be as low as 0·03 units per ml; but whatever the concentration it seems essential that the effect should be continuous during the period of treatment. At one stage[5] it appeared that some preparations of PAM which had been put on the market had not conformed to the specifications necessary to ensure slow absorption and prolonged action. In consequence, the World Health Organization laid down definite specifications for preparations of PAM, and these have been embodied in the International Pharmacopoeia. Further prolongation with low levels can be obtained by the use of benza-thine penicillin (dibenzylethylenediamine dipenicillin G). A single dose of 2·4 mega-units of this preparation intramuscularly, of which half is usually injected into each buttock, is likely to give an effective level of penicillin in the patient's blood for about two weeks. It is of great value when patients cannot attend for treatment over a period or when it is clear that they are unlikely to cooperate in treatment. Unfortunately, the preparation is apt to cause pain at the sites of injection.

Penicillin is best given by injection. Although modern oral preparations are likely to be effective, it is so important that treatment should not be interrupted that it is unwise to rely upon patients, who may be careless or uncooperative, to take tablets regularly.

Bismuth

Penicillin is the drug of choice in the treatment of syphilis in all its stages. Increasing experience has served to establish the fact that it is, by itself, highly effective; it is probable that other drugs add nothing to the excellence of results of treatment. Bismuth is still used in some countries for pre-paratory treatment in cases of late syphilis to prevent the Jarisch–Herxheimer reaction (see p. 158), but there is some controversy about the need for this or indeed its efficacy in this regard. Bismuth may also be used as a therapeutic test for patients with lesions which may be due to late syphilis but of which the diagnosis is in doubt.

Insoluble preparations should be used because they are less likely to give toxic effects than soluble bismuth. Suspensions of bismuth metal or of the insoluble salts, such as the oxychloride or salicylate, may be given intra-muscularly in dosage of 0·2 to 0·4 g weekly. Care must be taken to avoid injecting these substances into a vein, because pulmonary embolism may follow. Toxic effects are few. A slaty-blue line commonly appears at the margin of the gums of patients receiving this treatment. It is due to deposits of bismuth sulphide and occurs as the result of pre-existing infection of the gums with pocketing, and then interaction between bismuth in the saliva and H_2S in decomposing food. Care should be taken to ensure that these patients have preliminary dental treatment, but the blue line is not of itself a bar to continuing bismuth therapy. If, however, the gums become spongy, bleed easily or show ulceration, bismuth must be stopped until the mouth has been thoroughly treated, otherwise severe ulcerative stomatitis may follow. Nephrosis is another occasional complication. The urine should always be tested for albumin before treatment; if it is present, the treatment should not be given.

Potassium Iodide

Mixtures containing potassium iodide have been used for many years as an adjuvant treatment for late syphilis. The commencing dose is 0·3 g three times daily, but it may be increased up to 1·3 g or 2 g three times daily, depending upon the tolerance of the patient. It has no treponemicidal action, but is effective in promoting healing of gummatous lesions. It has also been claimed to give relief from the pain of syphilis of bones. Its use is now usually limited to a *therapeutic test*, in which it is often combined with bismuth. These drugs have a much more selective action than penicillin, which should be withheld until the diagnosis is determined.

Corticosteroids

There is evidence that corticosteroids may cause exacerbation of lesions, if given alone and in large dosage, in cases of early syphilis (see p. 8). They are sometimes used as preliminary treatment in cases of late syphilis, in the hope of preventing Jarisch–Herxheimer reactions (see p. 159).

Antibiotics other than Penicillin

No other antibiotic is as effective as penicillin in the treatment of syphilis, but some have anti-treponemal effects and are useful for patients who have been sensitized to penicillin. In choosing an alternative remedy it should be remembered that oral treatment is always less certain than treatment given by injection because of the risk that the patient will not take the treatment correctly. If oral treatment has to be used the patient should be seen frequently during the course to check on this.

THE TETRACYCLINES

Chlortetracycline, oxytetracycline and tetracycline have been used in the treatment of syphilis, and all are effective. They have the disadvantage that they are best given by mouth, and patients who are treated for syphilis with these drugs should be carefully supervised. In general, their toxic effects are not severe, but occasionally they have caused severe and even fatal enteritis through disturbance of the balance of the intestinal flora, by destruction of susceptible organisms and overgrowth of those which are not susceptible. The United States Public Health Service[6] recommends tetracycline hydrochloride 500 mg four times a day (one hour before or two hours after meals) for 15 days in cases of early syphilis and for 30 days for syphilis of more than one year's duration. Doxycycline, a newer derivative of tetracycline, is particularly well absorbed and, unlike ordinary tetracycline, absorption is not significantly decreased by food, including dairy products. Dosages of 200 mg or 300 mg daily, taken after food, for 15 to 30 days are recommended. Experience of this and other substitutes for penicillin in the treatment of syphilis is still inadequate, and careful follow-up is essential in these cases.

CHLORAMPHENICOL

The experimental work indicates that this drug is likely to be less effective than the tetracyclines in the treatment of syphilis. Nevertheless, good results have been reported from dosage similar to that of the tetracyclines. Because other and probably better substitutes are available and because of its dangerous toxic action on the blood-forming organs, *chloramphenicol should not be used* for the treatment of syphilis.

ERYTHROMYCIN

Experimental work suggests that erythromycin may be more effective than the tetracyclines in the treatment of syphilis, but experience with it is less. The United States Public Health Service[6] recommends erythromycin (stearate, ethylsuccinate or base) 500 mg four times a day for 15 days for early syphilis and for 30 days for syphilis of more than one year's duration. Absorption of the drug is said to be best if it is taken at the beginning of a meal or with 250 ml of water on an empty stomach. Exceptionally close observation and follow-up are essential. If this drug is used, it is probably better to avoid use of the estolate salts, from which a number of cases of jaundice have been reported,[7] particularly in pregnant women. There is also doubt about the ability of erythromycin to cross the placental barrier and a dosage of 3 g daily for 12 days was inadequate to prevent a case of congenital syphilis.[8] If it is used in pregnancy it should be given in this dosage for at least 21 days and, even so, it would be a wise precaution to treat the newborn infant with penicillin.

CEPHALORIDINE

Experience with this drug is small but it is known to give good response in cases of early syphilis, and the fact that it is given by injection is a further recommendation. Courses of 2 g daily, preferably as 1 g twice daily, by intramuscular injection for 10 to 14 days are recommended for early infection. It has been shown to cross the placenta readily. Because of the possibility of cross-allergy it should not be used for patients who have had serious reactions to penicillin, although its use may be justified for patients who have had mild delayed reactions if other antibiotics are unsuitable.

CARBOMYCIN AND SYNNEMATIN B

These two antibiotics have been used in the treatment of small numbers of cases of early syphilis, apparently with success. Information about their effects is quite insufficient and at present their use must be regarded as purely experimental.

Fever Therapy

Fever, induced by mechanical means or by inoculation of agents of other diseases, such as malaria, has been used in the past in the treatment of syphilis, either alone or as an adjuvant. Its only present use is as an additional method in certain types of neurosyphilis when penicillin therapy alone has failed to cure. Such treatment is now very rarely required.

Details of Curative Treatment

Early Syphilis

In the treatment of early syphilis the evidence suggests that relatively small doses of penicillin give success in the seronegative primary stage, but that larger amounts are needed in cases of longer duration. It is simpler, however, to establish a routine which is likely to be effective in all stages of early syphilis, because treatment is never prolonged and the dangers of moderate over-dosage are slight. The following methods have proved effective in the treatment of early syphilis:

1. *Aqueous procaine penicillin*, 600,000 units intramuscularly daily for 10 to 12 days, totalling 6 or 7·2 million units.

2. *PAM*, 2·4 million units intramuscularly followed at intervals of three days by three more injections, each of 1·2 million units. Total—6 million units.

3. *Benzathine penicillin*, 2·4 million units in one injection (1·2 million units may be given into each buttock).

These methods may be expected to cure in more than 95 per cent of the cases. Because some of these patients are careless or uncooperative, some venereologists who favour Method 1 prefer to begin with a single, large dose of PAM, such as 2·4 mega-units, in case the patient fails to return for further treatment. With such a dose, infectiousness can be controlled and there is a chance of a cure. As already described, Method 3 has the disadvantage that the injections are apt to be painful. If the patient has been sensitized to penicillin, another antibiotic should be used, as described on pp. 149–51.

There are minor differences in accepted practice in different countries and, indeed, among individuals in the same country. The United States Public Health Service recommends the following schedules[6] for the treatment of early syphilis at the present time:

1. *Benzathine penicillin G*, 2·4 million units by intramuscular injection.

2. *Procaine penicillin G* in oil with aluminium monostearate (PAM), 4·8 million units, usually given as 2·4 million units at the first session and 1·2 million units in each of two subsequent injections three days apart.

3. *Aqueous procaine penicillin G*, 600,000 units daily for eight days to a total of 4·8 million units.

In cases of early syphilis the patient should be instructed to avoid sexual intercourse. Local treatment is not required for surface lesions.

Late Syphilis (Benign Gummatous Type and Late Latent Syphilis)

In the treatment of late syphilis of the benign gummatous type and of late latent syphilis, the same treatment is effective and there seems no need to prolong it unless it has proved impossible to test the cerebrospinal fluid through refusal on the part of the patient or technical difficulties. Whether it is a useful precaution to start with intramuscular injections of bismuth is a matter of some controversy but this method is now seldom used. If penicillin is given at once there is probably slight danger from the Jarisch–Herxheimer reaction (see p. 158). The reaction cannot be prevented by starting with small doses of penicillin, but Jarisch–Herxheimer reactions of any severity are rare in cases of late syphilis, and it must be conceded that many physicians have started treatment with penicillin in late cases of this disease and have seen no ill-effects. If precautionary measures are deemed necessary it is probably better to rely on the preliminary administration of corticosteroids (see p. 159).

The following routine methods of treatment are recommended for these cases.

1. If tests of the cerebrospinal fluid are negative, give treatment as for early syphilis.

2. If tests of the cerebrospinal fluid cannot be done, the following alternatives are suggested:

(a) *Aqueous procaine penicillin*, 600,000 units intramuscularly daily for 20 days, totalling 12 million units.

(b) *PAM*, 2·4 million units followed at intervals of three days by eight injections, each of 1·2 million units, totalling 12 million units.

(c) *Benzathine penicillin*, 3 million units (1·5 million injected in each buttock) weekly for three weeks, totalling 9 million units.

With the residual effects of destructive gummatous lesions the patient's lot may sometimes be improved by various surgical and other procedures. For instance, destructive lesions of the face may be improved by tissue grafts; perforation of the hard palate may be closed by an obturator carried by an upper dental plate, and portal hypertension resulting from gummatous hepatitis may justify a portal-shunt operation.

Cardiovascular Syphilis

In the treatment of cardiovascular syphilis assessment of the value of anti-syphilitic treatment is difficult because of the varied character of the lesions and the uncertainty of prognosis in individual cases. General measures are of great importance and if the patient's occupation is physically strenuous he should be advised to change it. Anti-syphilitic treatment may be expected to bring about healing of the syphilitic lesions and, particularly in early cases, to prevent progression, but damage to the aortic wall is permanent, and complications may result from scarring which follows healing. Jarisch–Herxheimer reactions are rare in cases of cardiovascular syphilis, and many physicians have practised giving penicillin at once without ill-effects. This is common practice in the United States of America. There is possibly some danger in cases with involvement of the coronary ostia, when pre-liminary steroid therapy may be indicated (see p. 159). Injections of a standard preparation of procaine penicillin may be given daily in dosage of 600,000 units for 15 to 20 days, with total dosage of 9 to 12 mega-units. Usually no further antisyphilitic treatment is required; but there is a school of thought which believes that a series of courses of treatment should be given in these cases, a view which appears to be based on opinion rather than sound evidence. Benzathine penicillin has also been given in doses of 3 million units at intervals of seven days, to a total of 6 to 9 million units.

Depending upon the severity of the condition, patients suffering from cardiovascular syphilis may need to modify their ways of life. A patient with uncomplicated aortitis without evidence of coronary ostial involvement should be able to lead a normal life, provided that the heaviest type of work is avoided; whereas a patient with aortic insufficiency who has passed through a phase of congestive failure, or a patient with severe angina of effort, or with a large pulsatile aneurysm, should be limited to a sedentary occupation. Such a patient should be instructed to walk and to mount stairs slowly, to avoid excitement, and to avoid sexual intercourse. An attack of congestive failure may be precipitated by an upper respiratory-tract infection and patients should be protected from this hazard as far as possible. When congestive failure occurs the patient should be admitted to hospital. He should be digitalized and given diuretics; he should also be given light sedation and, if he is obese, the diet should be of low caloric value. Apart from the obvious benefits of bed rest, close supervision of treatment and relief from anxiety, a period in hospital gives an opportunity for accustoming the patient to those parts of the treatment regimen which will have to be continued when he leaves hospital. The patient's common sense should be taken into account especially when choosing a diuretic. If his condition permits a choice, an unreliable patient is probably best treated with injections of diuretics such as mersalyl or mercaptomerin. Patients may become confused about their tablets and prolonged accidental over-dosage with chlorothiazide or frusemide may produce serious effects from sodium and potassium depletion; the effect of digitalis may be potentiated by potassium loss. Once it has been decided to give digitalis, dosage must be maintained at a level which is effective and it must be made clear to the patient that tablets cannot be discontinued because he is feeling better. The anxious patient with angina should be assured that trinitrin tablets (tab. glyc. trinit. 0·2 mg) may be taken frequently with safety. There must be a restriction of physical activity but patients should not be allowed to sink into unnecessary invalidism. If a change of occupation is required, it is reasonable, if the patient agrees, that prospective employers should be told that heart trouble is the cause of the disability. The syphilitic origin of the condition must not be divulged; at this stage it is in any case irrelevant.

There are various techniques for the treatment of saccular aneurysms which are increasing in size, causing pressure symptoms or threatening to rupture. If a major operation is justified, aneurysms which cannot be removed may be strengthened by the application of polythene membrane which causes periarterial fibrosis; however, the results are often disappointing. If the aneurysm can be removed, it can be replaced by an Orlon tube or by an aortic graft. In these days even elderly patients may be good risks for these operations if their health is satisfactory in other respects. Removal of fusiform aneurysm of the aortic arch carries a high mortality and will seldom be justified.

Operations have also been devised for the relief of aortic incompetence, of which cardiovascular syphilis is one of the commoner causes. The insertion of ball-valve prostheses, plication operations, prosthetic reconstruction of the valve and other procedures have been used with varying success. All have their hazards and they are justified only in carefully selected cases. With severe coronary ostial stenosis improvement has followed operative removal of obstructing intimal proliferation. Some highly successful results have been described in a few cases.

Neurosyphilis

For neurosyphilis penicillin is the treatment of choice. There is no evidence that additional fever therapy improves the ultimate results and it is, of course, a potentially dangerous treatment. No amount of antisyphilitic treatment of any kind can influence the damage to the nervous system which remains after adequate treponemicidal remedies have been given. Preliminary bismuth has been used, but it is not helpful in preventing Jarisch–

Herxheimer reactions in cases of general paralysis. In all types of syphilis of the nervous system daily injections of 600,000 units of procaine penicillin should be given for at least 15 days and preferably for 20 days, totalling 9 to 12 mega-units. If for some reason injections are given every other day, PAM should be used, and the period of treatment should be extended so that the total amount of the remedy is not less than would have been given by daily injections. Benzathine penicillin has been recommended in these cases in doses of 3 million units weekly for three weeks, but there are reservations because of the inability to produce measurable levels of penicillin in the cerebrospinal fluid by this means.[9] Additional courses of treatment are seldom required but may be necessary in some cases of general paralysis and occasionally other types of neurosyphilis. In such cases it might be advisable to give doses that will produce higher levels of penicillin in the cerebrospinal fluid. One method is to give crystalline penicillin 500,000 units intramuscularly every six hours together with probenecid 0·5 g by mouth every six hours, both for 15 to 20 days. Dunlop et al.[10] have shown that this produces treponemicidal levels of penicillin in the cerebrospinal fluid. Physicians in the United States of America seem to favour the intravenous route for this purpose, giving 12 to 24 million units of crystalline penicillin daily (2 to 4 million units every four hours) for 10 days.[6] In fact, adequate levels of penicillin in the cerebrospinal fluid can be obtained by giving aqueous procaine penicillin 2·4 mega-units intramuscularly daily together with probenecid 0·5 g by mouth every six hours;[10] however, it is uncertain how long these levels are maintained throughout each 24-hour period.

Patients with advanced neurosyphilis may present various problems in general management.

In cases of *tabes dorsalis* with atonic bladder, if culture of the urine shows the presence of infection, appropriate antibiotics should be given to control it. Sterility of the urine can sometimes be maintained by giving methenamine mandelate (Mandelamine, Warner) by mouth 0·5 g three times daily, and this can be continued for months or years if necessary. If the patient has a distended bladder presenting as an abdominal swelling, urine should be withdrawn slowly through a soft-rubber catheter. Further catheterization may be unnecessary if the patient tries to empty his bladder every four hours, or more frequently, with the aid of manual pressure on the lower abdomen ('bladder drill'). Emptying may sometimes be aided by injecting subcutaneously a parasympathetic stimulator drug, such as carbachol 0·25 mg. But if retention persists, then a self-retaining Foley type of catheter should be inserted, and if necessary it may be left in situ for several weeks. Transurethral resection of the neck of the bladder has proved helpful in some cases.

In cases of *Charcot's arthropathy* a flail joint may have to be supported by a frame or jacket; orthopaedic surgeons do not usually favour operation, but this may occasionally be necessary, for instance, when vertebral collapse occurs with compression of the spinal cord.

In cases of *optic atrophy*, if visual acuity and the extent of the peripheral visual fields diminish rapidly in spite of treatment with penicillin, then some form of fever therapy may be justified although it is unlikely to influence the outcome. The same might be said of corticosteroids.

Less severe *lightning pains* can often be controlled by moderately strong analgesics, but severe intractable pain has led to the giving of narcotics which may cause addiction. It is worth trying the effect of vitamin B_{12}, 1000 μg by injection daily for 10 days, followed by a maintenance dose of the same size given once weekly. Some patients treated in this way have claimed marked improvement in the degree and frequency of the pains. Phenytoin (Epanutin or Dilantin) given by mouth in doses of 100 mg, three times a day, is reported to have diminished or abolished severe attacks of lightning pains in a few cases; corticosteroids are also reported to have given relief as has carbamazepine (Tegretol) in doses of 200 mg by mouth two to four times a day. However, further experience is required before any of these claims can be substantiated. In some severe cases, cordotomy or leucotomy has been considered necessary.

The risk of *perforating ulcers* will be diminished by the patient wearing well-fitting shoes and regular attention by a competent chiropodist. If ulcers develop, bed rest and scrupulous cleansing are usually required for healing to occur.

In cases of *general paralysis*, when there is clinical progression or evidence of continuing activity of infection in tests of the cerebrospinal fluid in spite of repeated treatment with penicillin, malarial therapy may be justified. The aim is to produce 10 to 12 peaks of fever at 41°C (106°F) before termination of the treatment with antimalarial therapy. The fitness of the patient for this treatment should be carefully assessed because it is potentially dangerous.

In cases of *Erb's spastic paraplegia* or of *anterior spinal artery thrombosis*, the general management is that of a paraplegic.

Congenital Syphilis

Congenital syphilis is, of all forms of syphilis, the most preventable. Penicillin administered to a syphilitic pregnant woman is most effective in preventing infection of the fetus, whether it is given early or late in pregnancy. Ten to twelve daily injections of procaine penicillin are almost always adequate, and there are no hazards unless the patient is sensitized to the drug. Provided that adequate treatment is given in the first pregnancy, there seems little risk of transmission of infection if no further treatment is given in later pregnancies. Nevertheless, it is still common practice to give an additional 10-day course of injections of penicillin in the first subsequent pregnancy, as a precaution, unless there is some contraindication.

ESTABLISHED CONGENITAL SYPHILIS. Those who undertake the nursing care of infants suffering from early congenital syphilis must take the necessary precautions to avoid transfer of infection. These infants are often very ill and unable to feed from the breast or bottle, and feeding by tube may be necessary. Special nursing in a separate room or cubicle is essential. For the treatment of established congenital syphilis, penicillin is the effective remedy. Best results are obtained in the early stage of the disease, in the first two years of life. It is good practice to give 500,000 units of penicillin per kg of body weight. Thus, for an infant weighing 4 kg the total dosage would be 2 million units given over a period of 10 days. The patient should be admitted to hospital for treatment. Procaine penicillin, 200,000 units daily for 10 days, is the treatment of choice. It gives good results and saves the extra injections which would be required if crystalline penicillin were used. In the later stages of the disease the scheme of treatment is similar, with the total dosage again based on body weight until dosages the same as those given to adults are reached.

When it is impossible to arrange for admission to hospital or for regular injections to be given, a single dose of benzathine penicillin intramuscularly, 50,000 units per kg of body weight, is likely to be effective. This method should be avoided if possible because of the pain which the injection causes and also because it fails to produce detectable levels of penicillin in the cerebrospinal fluid.[11]

INTERSTITIAL KERATITIS. In cases of interstitial keratitis, suppressive treatment with steroid hormones should be used in addition. A useful routine is to give soluble prednisolone in aqueous suspension (prednisolone disodium phosphate, 0·5 per cent: 'Predsol'), or cortisone ointment (15 mg/g) or both, by local application to the conjunctival sac. The patient is admitted to hospital and the application is made every two hours until the symptoms and signs of the local condition are suppressed; this may take four or five days. The treatment is then continued at intervals of four hours. In severe cases subconjunctival injections of cortisone (10 mg in 0·4 ml) or, preferably, prednisolone (20 mg in 0·4 ml) may be required in addition. The patient stays in hospital for about 10 to 14 days and then continues the local applications at home, every four hours during the day only for four weeks, then eight-hourly and finally twice daily. After another four weeks the treatment can be stopped, although it must be resumed if relapse occurs. This method is likely to give freedom from symptoms, the probability of normal vision and little or no corneal scarring. Local cortisone acetate suspension in normal saline (5 mg/ml), hydrocortisone (5 mg/ml) and prednisone acetate (0·25 per cent) have also been used successfully. In all these cases the pupil must be kept dilated with atropine (atropine drops, 1 per cent, twice daily) throughout the period of treatment because of the associated anterior uveitis.

The value of high doses of penicillin with probenecid (as on p. 155), given in the hope of lessening the risk of recurrence, is uncertain (see p. 170).

SENSORINEURAL DEAFNESS. There is evidence (Hahn, Rodin and Haskins[12]; Morrison[13]) that prednisone, in considerable and prolonged dosage, has produced improvement in some cases of this intractable condition. Commencing dosage was usually 30 mg daily in divided dosage, reduced to 20 mg after one week and thereafter reduced by 2·5 mg each month if progress was satisfactory. The dose was raised again in the event of marked deterioration. Progress was measured by audiometry. Treatment should not be continued for more than one month if there is no clear-cut response.

Alternative Treatment

When a patient is known to be sensitized to penicillin, a different antibiotic should be employed. These drugs and their dosage are described on pages 149 and 151. Most experience has been gained with the tetracyclines, and, except in pregnant women and in children up to eight years of age, these should be the first choice. Erythromycin is also effective. It seems clear that none of these drugs compares with penicillin in effectiveness for the treatment of syphilis and very careful supervision is required of patients for whom it has been necessary to resort to these less effective remedies.

REACTIONS TO TREATMENT

Jarisch–Herxheimer Reaction

This is a focal and systemic reaction which, in some cases, follows the first dose of an antisyphilitic remedy. It was first described following the use of mercury. It occurred commonly after the first injection of an organic arsenical and occurs also with penicillin and other antitreponemal antibiotics. After the first injection of bismuth it is said to be less frequent and less severe. The reaction occurs most frequently and with greatest severity in cases of early syphilis. More than half of these patients experience it. It can be produced by doses as small as 1000 units of penicillin and the reaction is an 'all or none' type of phenomenon,[14] occurring with full force if it occurs at all. Thus, starting treatment with small doses of penicillin would not be expected to prevent it. The systemic reaction occurs from two to twelve hours after the injection, commencing usually with fever, followed by headache, malaise, flushing and sweating. The patient's temperature may be above 38°C (101°F), and occasionally considerably higher. Patients describe the reaction as like an attack of influenza, but it is all over by the next day. In cases of early acquired syphilis the reaction is of no consequence if the patient is warned about it; if not, he may cease to attend for treatment. After therapeutic doses of penicillin the reaction occurs once and is hardly ever repeated. The systemic symptoms are accompanied by local tissue changes. The primary chancre may become more swollen, or a secondary rash may make its first transient appearance. Microscopically, areas of syphilitic inflammation show, as the result of this reaction, temporary cellular infiltration with polymorphonuclear leucocytes.[15] Jarisch–Herxheimer reactions also occur in cases of congenital syphilis and may be a contributory factor in fatalities occurring after commencing treatment of babies.[16]

In the late stages of syphilis the Jarisch–Herxheimer reaction occurs in no more than 25 per cent of the cases except in the presence of general paralysis, when it occurs in over 50 per cent. In the great majority of cases it is very slight, taking the form of a small rise in temperature of which the patient may be unaware. Occasionally, however, serious results have been attributed to this cause such as oedema of the glottis in a patient with gummatous involvement of the larynx, coronary occlusion due to sudden swelling of an infiltration at the opening of a coronary artery, cerebral thrombosis, and rupture of an aneurysmal sac or of a weakened area of the aortic wall. In cases of general paralysis, the Jarisch–Herxheimer reaction most commonly takes the form of a harmless febrile attack. Occasionally there may be an intensification of the psychosis and the patient may injure himself or others. Rarely the reaction has taken the form of one or more epileptiform fits which, on very rare occasions, have terminated fatally. Bismuth does not prevent these reactions. Patients suffering from general paralysis should be admitted to hospital for treatment with penicillin and they may be given appropriate sedation. In cases of tabes dorsalis, severe attacks of lightning pains have been attributed to the Jarisch–Herxheimer reaction.

The possible prevention of this reaction in cases of late syphilis by preliminary treatment with bismuth has been mentioned (p. 148) but it is difficult to explain any effect in this regard if the reaction is of the 'all or none' type. Some physicians[17] have claimed that small doses of steroid hormones, such as prednisone, 5 mg, given before each of the first two injections of penicillin, appear to have been effective in preventing or diminishing the febrile reaction. There is a case for using this method before commencing penicillin in the treatment of general paralysis and the other conditions in which a reaction may be particularly dangerous such as syphilitic aortic disease. It is advisable, however, to use a larger dose, such as 30 to 40 mg of prednisone daily in divided doses. Penicillin may be commenced after two to three days of the treatment and the steroid continued for a further two to three days before tailing it off rapidly.

The mechanism of the Jarisch–Herxheimer reaction is not known. It has been attributed to destruction of treponemes with sudden release of the products of their disintegration producing hypersensitivity effects. The release of leucocyte pyrogens could explain many of the features. These suggestions must be regarded as speculative.

Toxicity of Penicillin

Reactions to penicillin are still few, but its use is so widespread that inevitably more people are becoming sensitized to it. In the United States of America, treatment with penicillin is regarded as one of the commonest causes of fatal anaphylactic shock. In Great Britain reactions due to hyper-sensitivity may be expected in 1 to 5 per cent of patients who receive this treatment. Reactions may be immediate, accelerated or delayed. Immediate reactions take the form of acute anaphylaxis, which has been fatal in some cases. Accelerated reactions occur within 30 minutes to 48 hours and are generally urticarial. Delayed reactions may appear from 48 hours to several weeks after administration of the drug, and they often resemble serum sickness. Common manifestations are pruritus, urticaria and other rashes of the skin including erythema nodosum, arthralgia, effusions into joints, fever and proteinuria. Exfoliative dermatitis and polyarteritis nodosa have been described. An acute psychotic reaction sometimes occurs after aqueous procaine penicillin. This is probably due to the procaine and not a penicillin allergy, and it is likely that the material has entered a blood vessel.

Prevention

The first and essential precaution is to ask the patient whether he has had penicillin before and whether it produced some reaction. Nearly all patients who suffer immediate reactions due to sensitization have received the drug before. If there is a history of sensitivity, penicillin should not be given. The practice of giving antihistamines in the same syringe does not prevent serious reactions. The most that can be hoped for from this is to diminish and shorten the less serious reactions. Patients should also be questioned as to personal or family history of allergic diathesis, such as asthma, hay fever or urticaria, and patients with this history should be given antibiotics with care and restraint and only for the treatment of serious disease. In cases of doubt as to sensitivity, useful information may sometimes be obtained by sensitivity tests. One method[18] which has given useful results is to apply drops of procaine penicillin, 300,000 units per ml, to a skin scratch and to the conjunctival mucous membrane. Itching, redness, oedema and wheal formation of the skin, or itching, watering, redness or oedema of the eye, within 15 minutes, indicate the probability of dangerous sensitization. Unfortunately not all patients who are sensitized give positive tests, but most of those who are subject to anaphylactic reactions do so. Sensitivity tests are not without risk. Even the minute dosage of penicillin used in these tests has caused serious reactions. Two other precautionary methods have been recommended, namely giving the injection low enough in an extremity to permit the application of a tourniquet, and preliminary treatment with corticosteroids. Even with these precautions the risks are probably not justified if sensitization is suspected in cases of syphilis, because other antibiotics can be substituted in treatment. Claims have been made for a preparation called penicilloyl-polylysine, obtained by coupling poly-lysine with penicillinic acid, which when injected intradermally showed some promise as a method of determining the possibility of risk of an immediate reaction to penicillin. The mechanism of its action and its application in 3667 cases has been discussed by Shapiro,[19] who found, however, that over 50 per cent of patients with positive tests but no history suggesting sensitivity had no reaction to penicillin. Lentz and Nicholas,[20] more recently, described experiences with an improved preparation in 5461 cases. The positive tests were more clear-cut than with older preparations and there were few ambiguous results. There were adverse reactions to the test in five cases but none of them serious. By using this test they were able to diminish reactions to treatment with penicillin from 3·5 per cent to 0·1 per cent.

Wide and Juhlin[21] employed a radioimmunological technique to detect antibodies (IgE) to penicilloyl, claiming that this test was a valuable alternative to the more dangerous intracutaneous test with penicilloyl-polylysine for detection of penicillin hypersensitivity of the immediate type.

It is common practice in the United States of America to keep under observation for 30 minutes any patient who has received an intramuscular injection of penicillin.[22]

Treatment of Reactions

ACUTE ANAPHYLAXIS

In cases of acute anaphylaxis, cardiac arrest has occurred occasionally, and this should be treated immediately with external cardiac massage. Those who give injections of penicillin should be instructed in the technique of this procedure and also in methods of artificial respiration. Apart from this, the immediate remedy is adrenaline, 0·6 ml of a 1:1000 solution intramuscularly. The drug acts as a cardiac stimulant and also produces vasoconstriction with rise in blood pressure. If necessary, this may be followed by an intravenous injection of aminophylline, 250 mg in 10 ml of sterile distilled water, which relieves bronchial spasm. The patient's airway should be unobstructed and oxygen should be given if there is respiratory distress. Artificial respiration may be required. Every centre at which numbers of injections of penicillin are given should be equipped with an emergency tray containing the necessary drugs and sterilized syringes and needles together with instructions on the methods of cardiorespiratory resuscitation, ready for immediate use. The immediate treatment may be followed by hydrocortisone solution given by intravenous drip, the initial dose being 100 to 250 mg, followed by 1000 mg during the succeeding 24 hours.

DELAYED REACTIONS

Delayed reactions may be treated with antihistamines such as diphenhydramine hydrochloride, 150 mg daily, or promethazine hydrochloride, 75 mg daily, in divided doses. If necessary, prednisone or prednisolone may be given in dosage of 10 mg four times daily for the first few days; then 7·5 mg four times daily, with gradual reduction of the dose over 10 days. Another measure is to give penicillinase, 800,000 units, by intramuscular injection. This may be repeated after three or four days. However, anaphylactic reactions to penicillinase itself have been reported and it should only be used in selected cases. It has no place in the emergency treatment of acute reactions to penicillin.

FOLLOW-UP AFTER TREATMENT

Early Syphilis

Patients treated for early syphilis should be observed and tested at regular intervals. A good routine is to examine them and perform reagin tests monthly for the first six months after treatment, and then each three months for a further eighteen months. Clinical examination should pay particular attention to moist areas of the skin, especially the perianal region, and to the mouth and throat. Serological tests should include one quantitative estimation which will give a good indication of progress. Reagin tests may become negative within a few weeks, but they can remain positive for four to six months or longer. Provided that the titre is declining this need cause no concern. Two years after treatment, tests should be performed on the cerebrospinal fluid, and if these are negative examination of the cerebrospinal fluid need not be repeated. If at the end of two years the patient is well, serological reagin tests have remained negative and the cerebrospinal fluid is normal, he can be regarded as cured for all practical purposes.

Late Syphilis

In cases of late syphilis, tests of the cerebrospinal fluid should be performed before treatment to determine the presence or absence of asymptomatic neurosyphilis. If they are negative and the patient remains well during the period of observation after treatment, tests of the cerebrospinal fluid need not be repeated. Observation and testing should be carried out as for early syphilis, but the patient should remain under observation indefinitely, attending once a year in cases of latent and gummatous syphilis, and at intervals of three to six months in cases of cardiovascular syphilis, unless the seriousness of the residual condition requires more frequent supervision. Blood tests should be performed, but the fact that they may remain positive at a lower titre, or even at the same titre, is quite to be expected and is not an indication for further treatment. However, a non-reactive FTA-ABS IgM test a year or more after treatment may indicate that inflammatory activity has ceased but the evidence for this is inconclusive (see p. 142).

Assessment of the progress of patients with neurosyphilis after treatment depends upon careful clinical examination and tests of the cerebrospinal fluid. Clinical improvement, if it occurs at all, is likely to be limited to a short period after treatment, and thereafter clinical examination shows irreversible residual changes. Tests of the cerebrospinal fluid should be repeated three and six months after treatment. Assuming that there is no evidence of clinical progression, a decision as to the need for further treatment is usually made according to the principle laid down by Dattner and Thomas, of the Bellevue Hospital, New York,[23,24] and known as the 'Dattner–Thomas concept'. According to this, if the cell count of the cerebrospinal fluid becomes and remains normal, the syphilitic process is no longer active in the central nervous system and no further treatment is required. This is a valuable guide but should not be taken as an absolute rule.

Following successful treatment, the cell count of the cerebrospinal fluid usually returns to normal within three months. If it is still abnormal after six months, further treatment should be given. The amount of protein usually returns to normal within six months, but the fact that it is still above normal at that time is not necessarily an indication for more treatment.[25] Positive Wassermann reaction, or equivalent test, in the cerebrospinal fluid and changes in the colloidal-gold test often persist for years and do not indicate the need for further treatment. In the absence of clinical progression and with tests of the cerebrospinal fluid which become and remain normal, it is nevertheless a wise precaution to perform further tests of the cerebrospinal fluid after a further two years.

The titres of quantitative reagin tests usually fall after treatment, but should they rise further tests of the cerebrospinal fluid should be performed without delay.

REFERENCES

1. PLOTKE, F., EISENBERG, H., BAKER, A. H. and LAUGHLIN, M. E. (1949). *J. vener. Dis. Inf.*, **30**, 252.
2. MOORE, M. B., PRICE, E. V., KNOX, J. M. and ELGIN, L. W. (1963) *Publ. Hlth Rep. (Wash.)*, **78**, 966.
3. MAHONEY, J. F., ARNOLD, R. C. and HARRIS, A. (1943) *J. vener. Dis. Inf.*, **24**, 355.
4. Committee on Medical Research, U.S. Public Health Service and Food and Drug Administration (1946) *J. Am. med. Ass.*, **131**, 271.
5. GUTHE, T., REYNOLDS, F. W., KRAG, P. and WILLCOX, R. R. (1953) *Br. med. J.*, **1**, 594.
6. Morbidity and Mortality Weekly Report (1976) **25**, 101.
7. Committee on Safety of Medicines. Report No. 10. June 1973.
8. FENTON, L. J. and LIGHT, I. J. (1976) *Obstet. Gynec.*, **47**, 492.
9. MOHR, J. A., GRIFFITHS, W., JACKSON, R., SARDAH, H., BIRD, P. and RIDDLE, J. (1976) *J. Am. med. Ass.*, **236**, 2208.
10. DUNLOP, E. M. C., AL-EGAILY, S. S. and HOUANG, E. T. (1979) *J. Am. med. Ass.*, **241**, 2538.
11. KAPLAN, M. J. and McCRACKEN, G. H. (1973) *J. Pediat.*, **82**, 1069.
12. HAHN, R. D., RODÍN, P. and HASKINS, H. L. (1962) *J. chron. Dis.*, **15**, 395.

13. MORRISON, A. W. (1969) *Proc. R. Soc. Med.*, **62**, 959.
14. FARMER, T. W. (1948) *J. Am. med. Ass.*, **138**, 480.
15. SHELDON, W. H. and HEYMAN, A. (1949) *Am. J. Syph.*, **33**, 213.
16. HOLZEL, A. (1956) *Br. J. vener. Dis.*, **32**, 175.
17. DE GRACIANSKY, P. and GRUPPER, C. (1961) *Br. J. vener. Dis.*, **37**, 247.
18. SMITH, V. M. (1957) *New Engl. J. Med.*, **257**, 447.
19. SHAPIRO, J. (1964) *Proceedings of the World Forum on Syphilis and other Treponematoses.* U.S. Public Health Service Publication, No. 997, p. 328.
20. LENTZ, J. W. and NICHOLAS, L. (1970) *Br. J. vener. Dis.*, **46**, 457.
21. WIDE, L. and JUHLIN, L. (1971) *Clin. Allergy*, **1**, 171.
22. SIMPSON, W. G. (1964) *Proceedings of the World Forum on Syphilis and other Treponematoses.* U.S. Public Health Service Publication, No. 997, p. 212.
23. DATTNER, B. and THOMAS, E. W. (1944) *The Management of Neurosyphilis.* London: Heinemann Medical.
24. DATTNER, B., CARMICHAEL, D. M., DE MELLO, L. and THOMAS, E. W. (1952) *Am. J. Syph.*, **36**, 179.
25. HAHN, R. D., CUTTER, J. C., CURTIS, A. C., GAMMON, G., HEYMAN, A., JOHNWICK, E., STOKES, J. H., SOLOMON, H., THOMAS, E., TIMBERLAKE, W., WEBSTER, B. and GLEESON, G. A. (1956) *Archs Derm.*, **74**, 367.

9

Prognosis of Syphilis

In discussing prognosis it is necessary to define what is meant by 'cure' of the disease. It is impossible to determine that the last treponeme has been eliminated from the patient's body, and it is therefore necessary to establish certain arbitrary standards. For patients with *early* syphilis 'cure' means: (*a*) clinical recovery which is maintained to the end of life, (*b*) absence of infectivity to others, and (*c*) persistently negative reagin tests for syphilis of the blood and normal cerebrospinal fluid.

For patients with *late* syphilis, 'cure' means: (*a*) permanent clinical recovery, (*b*) absence of infectivity, and (*c*) normal cerebrospinal fluid.

In the late stages of the disease persistence of positive tests of the blood serum is of no significance in prognosis unless repeated quantitative tests show a rising titre.

PROGNOSIS OF UNTREATED SYPHILIS

The best-known studies of this subject are based on a group of patients who were observed without treatment in Oslo at the turn of the century. Boeck, who was in charge of the Dermatological Clinic at Oslo from 1891 to 1910, believed existing methods of treatment to be ineffective. During these years he observed 2181 patients with primary or secondary syphilis, keeping them in hospital and giving either no treatment or small amounts of mercury and iodides by mouth as placebos. His successor, Bruusgaard,[1] published in 1929 conclusions based on re-examination of a number of these patients and of case reports and post-mortem reports of others. This material was again studied in considerable detail by Gjestland,[2] who reported in 1955. It appeared that the average duration of the manifest course of untreated early syphilis was 4·6 months in women and 3·2 months in men. Nearly a quarter of the patients whose records were studied were known to have experienced infectious relapses, and in some cases there were multiple relapses. Most of the infectious lesions of relapse were in the mouth or in the anorectal region. At a later stage, some form of benign tertiary syphilis developed in about 15 per cent of patients of both sexes and 15 per cent of males and 8 per cent of females had evidence of cardiovascular syphilis. Various types of neurosyphilis occurred in about 9 per cent of males and 5 per cent of females. The final conclusion from this very careful and detailed study was that over 60 per cent of untreated syphilitics went through life with little or no inconvenience as a result of the disease. Contrary to popular belief there was no evidence that benign tertiary syphilis gave any protection against cardiovascular syphilis or neurosyphilis.

PROGNOSIS OF TREATED SYPHILIS

Early Syphilis

The evidence indicates that, with modern methods of treatment, 'cure' of early syphilis by accepted standards is achieved in more than 95 per cent of the cases. *Treponema pallidum* can no longer be found in surface lesions within 24 hours of commencing treatment. The lesions heal promptly, but evidence of their presence, in the way of pigmentation of the skin and enlargement of lymph nodes, may remain for many weeks. In cases of seropositive primary syphilis and of secondary syphilis, the reagin tests may take from 2 to 4 months or even longer to become negative. The specific tests may become negative at the same time or later; more often they remain positive. In cases of early latent syphilis, reagin tests may continue to be positive for considerably longer. Failure of treatment is likely in less than 5 per cent of primary or secondary cases and in many cases it can be difficult to distinguish from reinfection. It may be shown by the appearance of fresh lesions, so-called clinical relapse, which is most likely to occur in the first year after treatment and to take the form of infectious lesions in the mouth and throat or in the perianal region. Relapse may also be indicated by negative reagin tests becoming positive or positive tests becoming progressively more strongly positive, so-called serological relapse. Serological relapse is likely to precede clinical relapse. Clinical relapse may also manifest itself by the birth of a syphilitic infant to a woman who has been treated for early syphilis. The term 'serological relapse' is also used for the case in which a patient who has been treated for early syphilis later shows evidence of active infection in tests of the cerebrospinal fluid.

O'Neill and Nicol[3] have shown that most patients treated for syphilis cease to produce IgM antibody to *Treponema pallidum* in serum quite soon after treatment, usually within months. They suggest that persistent positive results to the IgM FTA-ABS test may indicate inadequate treatment but other workers have described different findings (see p. 142).

Late Latent Syphilis and Gummatous Syphilis

In cases of late latent syphilis the prognosis is excellent and progression or relapse of any kind has been reported only rarely. With gummatous syphilis the prognosis as regards healing and absence of relapse or progression in the future is excellent. Failures have been reported only rarely. As regards the destructive effects of the gumma before treatment is started, this depends, of course, upon the site and duration of the lesion. The disability from neglected lesions may be considerable, especially from widespread destruction of bones of the skull, face or nose and throat, or from portal hypertension which may follow widespread involvement of the liver. In the latter type of case death may follow from haemorrhage due to rupture of an oesophageal varix. Methods by which these conditions can be alleviated have been mentioned (p. 153).

In cases of late syphilis of any kind the results of serological tests during observation after treatment rarely help in indicating the prognosis. Serological tests are likely to remain positive indefinitely after adequate treatment in more than 50 per cent of cases, although in most of them there is some reduction of the quantitative titre. Nevertheless, it is important that these tests should be done during the period of observation because a consistent rise in titre indicates the likelihood of relapse and the need for further treatment. In those cases in which serological tests do become negative, the patients derive considerable comfort from the fact, for it is difficult for them to accept the doctor's assurance that in their particular cases positive tests are of no significance.

Cardiovascular Syphilis

For cardiovascular syphilis the prognosis is hard to assess in individual cases. With *uncomplicated aortitis* the outlook is usually good, and following treatment the patient's life is unlikely to be shortened by syphilis unless a complication supervenes. The prognosis in cases of *aortic regurgitation* depends upon a number of factors. If the condition presents with heart failure, the outlook is poor. Medical care may prolong life considerably, but the patient usually has increasingly frequent episodes of heart failure. If, on the other hand, the condition is diagnosed before symptoms of failure supervene, the outlook may be good, unless the patient's work is heavy and he refuses to change it, or unless some other complication such as aneurysm is present. There is no doubt that to continue a physically strenuous occupation may greatly shorten the duration of life. Age, race, and sex all have a bearing on this prognosis, as already described. *Aneurysmal dilatation* is always a serious complication; and although he may live for years the patient is always in danger of death from rupture of the aneurysm and of serious and possibly fatal complications due to pressure on important structures. Successful surgical treatment may entirely change the prognosis in these cases, but candidates for this treatment must be selected with great care and the risks of operation are always considerable. If possible, some months should elapse after penicillin therapy before surgery is undertaken. The results of erythrocyte sedimentation tests (ESR) may give some indication of the degree of inflammatory reaction still present.

The presence or absence of *coronary ostial involvement* is of great importance in prognosis. Apart from aneurysm the prognosis of cardiovascular syphilitics depends to a great extent upon the state of the myocardium; coronary ostial narrowing is almost certain to damage the myocardium, to an extent which depends upon the degree of narrowing and the rapidity with which it occurs.

At any stage of cardiovascular syphilis a patient may die suddenly. Autopsy examination may reveal coronary ostial occlusion, rupture of an aneurysm, or damage to an aortic valve cusp. A patient may die suddenly in the course of an attack of congestive failure, or even when myocardial damage is well compensated. Sometimes the autopsy findings give no clue to the cause of sudden death.

Neurosyphilis

The prognosis of neurosyphilis clearly depends upon the sites and degree of involvement of the nervous system. Destroyed nerve cells cannot regenerate and residual effects are inevitable. With neurosyphilis resulting from *early syphilis*, the prognosis following adequate treatment and careful follow-up is excellent. The prospects of cure are almost 100 per cent. With *asymptomatic neurosyphilis* in the late stage, prognosis is very good indeed; less than 1 per cent of the cases require further treatment. In many cases of *meningeal syphilis* the outlook is good, with clinical recovery or improvement in more than 50 per cent of cases. The prognosis is least satisfactory in cases of *Erb's spinal spastic paraplegia* and *syphilitic amyotrophy*. In cases of *general paralysis*, at the stage of onset improvement is likely to occur in 80 per cent or more. Of those with simple dementia, over 50 per cent show some improvement; but of those with a paranoid psychosis, only 25 per cent show any improvement. With *tabes dorsalis* the response to treatment is problematical. In cases in which the duration of symptoms has been short and the cell content of the cerebrospinal fluid is high, there may be some improvement in lightning pains, unsteadiness, numbness and tingling, urinary complications and even in impotence in some 50 per cent of cases. The characteristic signs remain unchanged by treatment. The prognosis in cases of *primary optic atrophy* is usually poor. Total blindness is the likely outcome in the course of years, but there is some reason to suppose that adequate treatment may prolong remission and even prevent total blindness.

Congenital Syphilis

In cases of *early* congenital syphilis the prognosis is excellent if the patient survives the early hazards of the illness, the danger of intercurrent infections and the Jarisch–Herxheimer reaction. In *late cases* the prognosis depends upon the existing damage. The stigmata persist for life, and, at this stage, interstitial keratitis, perceptive deafness, and Clutton's joints are probably not prevented by treatment. Reagin tests remain positive in spite of treatment in about 70 per cent of cases, and specific tests behave in general as in late acquired syphilis.

The Cure of Late Syphilis

Cure of syphilis in the sense of elimination of the last *Treponema pallidum* can never be determined with certainty, and the work of Collart, Borel and Durel[4] has raised particular doubts concerning some cases of late syphilis. They were able to demonstrate what appeared to be typical *T. pallidum* of attenuated virulence in the lymph nodes of patients with late syphilis in whose cases the treponemal immobilization test remained positive in spite of adequate or, by usual standards, more than adequate treatment. These findings were confirmed by Yobs, Olansky, Rockwell and Clark.[5] Smith and Israel[6] described four cases with signs suggesting late ocular syphilis or neurosyphilis in which *T. pallidum* were found, although standard serological tests and, in two cases, treponemal immobilization tests were negative. The organisms were found by fluorescent staining in the cerebrospinal fluid in two cases and in the aqueous humour in the other two. In one case of late seronegative syphilis treponemes were demonstrated in liver tissue obtained by biopsy. The same group of workers[7] described two cases of late ocular syphilis from which aqueous humour injected into rabbits produced syphilitic lesions in which the presence of *T. pallidum* was confirmed. Goldman and Girard[8] also found intraocular *T. pallidum* in cases of treated congenital syphilis.

In a study[9] at Moorfields Eye Hospital in London, and at the London Hospital, treponemes were found in cerebrospinal fluid or in aqueous humour from 7 of 21 patients who had had previous antisyphilitic treatment. It seemed likely that the organisms were *T. pallidum*.

Nevertheless, Wilkinson[10] has stated that forms resembling treponemes might be artefacts such as glass spirals or filaments, and Montenegro et al.,[11, 12] reviewing the work of their group, reported that some of the findings previously considered to be treponemes were artefacts, although others were apparently treponemes.

However, it seems probable that these findings are of academic rather than of practical interest. In only a tiny minority of the published cases have the 'treponemes' been proved to be virulent. They may provide an explanation for the continued positivity of the treponemal tests but they do not provide a sufficient reason for altering antisyphilitic treatment except possibly in cases of ocular syphilis, where more prolonged treatment with large doses of penicillin or ampicillin plus probenecid might give better levels in the aqueous humour. However, there is some evidence[13] that the treponemes in these cases are in a quiescent state so that they are, in a sense, indifferent to the effects of penicillin. Certainly there have been recurrences of ocular inflammation after large doses of penicillin plus probenecid. Whether giving large doses for several months would be more effective is not known.

SYPHILIS AND MARRIAGE

In cases of early syphilis patients should be advised to avoid any form of sexual contact until cure can be presumed. Obviously this raises difficulties for the married patient or for one who is due to marry. For the unmarried, marriage should be postponed until satisfactory observation and tests have been completed after two years. For the married patient who has responded well to treatment and whose reagin tests are negative, it is usual to permit married intercourse after six months' observation. If the partner in marriage has also suffered from the infection, response to treatment must be satisfactory in both partners before unprotected sexual intercourse can be resumed. These are counsels of perfection and in practice many patients resume intercourse as soon as they have completed the course of treatment. The risks are small if both partners have been treated, but it is obviously important to prohibit intercourse with a partner who is undergoing observation to ascertain whether infection has occurred.

In cases of late syphilis, marriage can be permitted at any time after successful treatment. If the patient with late syphilis is married and the partner in marriage has not been infected, marital intercourse may safely continue after treatment.

REFERENCES

1. BRUUSGAARD, E. (1929) Archs Derm. Syph. (Berl.), 157, 309.
2. GJESTLAND, T. (1955) Acta derm.-venereol. (Stockh.), 35, Suppl. 34.
3. O'NEILL, P. and NICOL, C. S. (1972) Br. J. vener. Dis., 48, 460.
4. COLLART, P., BOREL, L-J. and DUREL, P. (1962) Annls Inst. Pasteur, 102, 596, 693, 953.
5. YOBS, A. R., OLANSKY, S., ROCKWELL, D. H. and CLARK, J. W. (1965) Archs Derm., 91, 379.
6. SMITH, J. L. and ISRAEL, C. W. (1967) J. Am. med. Ass., 199, 980.
7. SMITH, J. L., ISRAEL, C. W., McCRARY, J. A. and HARNER, R. E. (1968) Am. J. Ophthal., 65, 242.

8. GOLDMAN, J. N. and GIRARD, K. F. (1967) *Archs Ophthal.*, **78**, 47.

9. RICE, N. S. C., DUNLOP, E. M. C., JONES, B. R., HARE, M. J., KING, A. J., RODIN, P., MUSHIN, A. and WILKINSON, A. E. (1970) *Br. J. vener. Dis.*, **46**, 1.

10. WILKINSON, A. E. (1968) *Trans. ophthal. Soc., U.K.*, **88**, 251.

11. MONTENEGRO, E. N. R., ISRAEL, C. W., NICOL, W. G. and SMITH, J. L. (1969) *Am. J. Ophthal.*, **67**, 335.

12. MONTENEGRO, E. N. R., NICOL, W. G. and SMITH, J. L. (1969) *Am. J. Ophthal.*, **68**, 197.

13. COLLART, P., FRANCESCHINI, P., POITEVIN, M., DUNOYER, F. and DUNOYER, M. (1974) *Br. J. vener. Dis.*, **50**, 251.

10

Gonorrhoea

HISTORY

There is some division of opinion as to the antiquity of gonorrhoea, but it is generally believed to have existed from the earliest times. Many believe that the description of 'an issue of seed' in the fifteenth chapter of the Book of Leviticus in the Old Testament, and of the precautions that were to be taken to deal with it, is a reference to this disease.

The causative organism of gonorrhoea, the gonococcus (*Neisseria gonorrhoeae*), was discovered by Neisser in 1879, and the full results of his investigations were published in 1882. Leistikow in 1882 and Bumm in 1885 grew the organism on culture medium and the latter also successfully inoculated the male urethra, producing characteristic symptoms and signs of gonorrhoea. The gonococcal complement-fixation test (GFT) was introduced by Müller and Oppenheim in 1906.

EPIDEMIOLOGY

As with the other venereal diseases, war and its aftermath result in an increase in incidence of this disease to almost epidemic proportions. In 1946 the number of cases of gonorrhoea reported from the clinics in England and Wales was 47,343 (see p. 173). The settled conditions of peace, combined with the effects of new remedies, produced a rapid decline in incidence up to 1954, when the number of cases was 17,536. Since then the trend has been reversed, and the number of cases has risen almost every year. In 1970 the number of reported cases was 54,717 and in 1973, 60,170, but since then the incidence has been fairly static.[1] The rate per 100,000 population in England was 95·6 in 1968, 126·1 in 1973 and for the year ending June 30 1977, 127·1. These figures are taken from the Annual Reports of the Chief Medical Officer of the Department of Health and they do not include cases treated by general practitioners, specialists in private practice or Medical Officers in the Armed Forces.

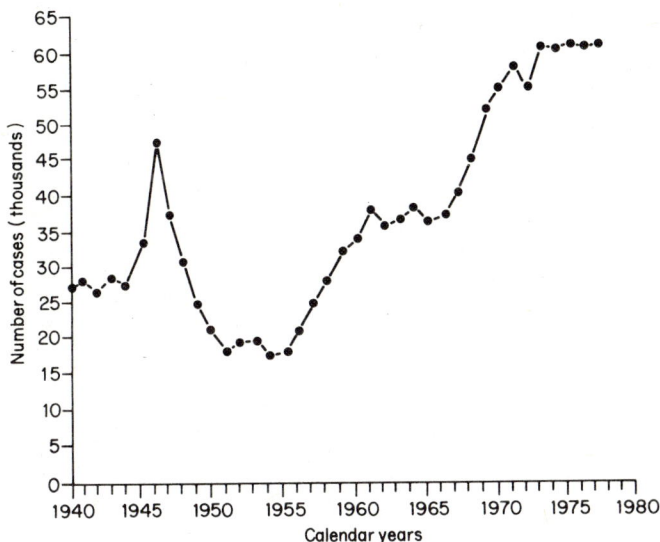

Number of cases of gonorrhoea dealt with for the first time in England and Wales, 1940–1977

Thus, while indicating the trends of rise and fall, they understate the true incidence of the disease but probably by no more than one-fifth. In a study in the United Kingdom in 1971[2] it was shown that 9·8 per cent of infections were acquired by homosexual intercourse. The figure for London was 19·9 per cent. A recent report[3] from the World Health Organization states that there is a large proportion of male homosexuals suffering from gonorrhoea in capital cities or large conurbations in a number of countries. Figures have varied from 10 to 26 per cent.

The numbers of reported cases of gonorrhoea in the United States of America from 1950 to 1977 are shown on p. 174. The rate per 100,000 population was 135·7 in 1956 and 465·9 in 1977, when 1,000,177 cases were reported.[4] However, many cases are not reported and it has been estimated[5] that the true incidence may be over three times that reported, although this may be an overestimate.[6]

An Expert Committee of the World Health Organization reviewed the problem of gonorrhoea and reported in 1963[7]. The Committee recognized that measures to control this disease had failed throughout the world and stated that it had been estimated that the annual number of new cases exceeded 60 to 65 millions. Among the reasons for failure were the increasing resistance of the gonococcus to antibiotics, the short period of incubation which made it difficult to interrupt the chain of transmission, the highly infectious character of the disease combined with lack of immunity and lack of proper education in matters of health and sex of the most vulner-

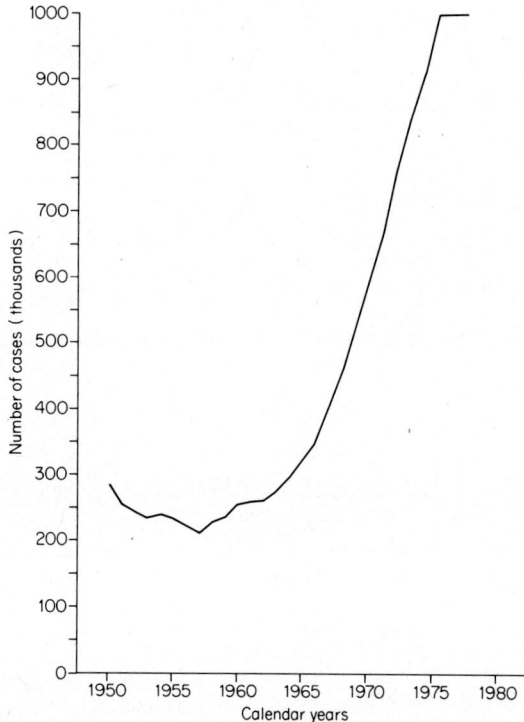

Number of cases of gonorrhoea dealt with in the United States of America, 1950–1977

able members of society—namely young people. For full details of the world-wide problem, reference should be made to that Report (see also Chapter 29) and to the more recent review of the world situation from the same source,[3] based on Technical Discussions held during the Twenty-eighth World Assembly in 1975. The following is a brief review of the factors which seem to have been responsible for the recent increase in most countries.

Causes of Increase in New Cases

INCREASE IN PROMISCUITY. This is the determining factor. In many countries all levels of the population have played their part with considerable contributions from prostitutes, 'good time girls' and practising homosexuals.

INCREASE IN WORLD POPULATION. The rise was said to be 500 millions between 1950 and 1960 and a further increase of 600 millions was expected by 1970. In many countries the numbers of young and sexually active increased disproportionately. A truer picture is obtained by comparing rates per 100,000 population in the various age groups. The World Health Organization[3] has reported a disquieting trend noted in some countries, characterized by steeper rates of increase among young women in the 15 to 19 year old age group.

RAPID INDUSTRIALIZATION. INCREASE IN URBAN POPULATION.
Industrial activity was said to have increased by 50 per cent in some developed countries between 1956 and 1966 and by as much as 200 per cent in some underdeveloped countries during the same years. In Africa and Asia there has been enormous growth of towns and weakening of social control exerted by families and tribal organizations.

MOVEMENTS OF POPULATION. These always result in increase of venereal disease. Migration, expansion in shipping trade, international travel, mobile labour groups and the movement of armed forces have all contributed to the increase.

REJECTION OF TRADITIONAL MORAL PRINCIPLES AND CODES OF BEHAVIOUR, ESPECIALLY BY YOUNG PEOPLE. In some countries reported venereal disease in young people under the age of 20 is as common or more common among females as among males, due in considerable measure, it is supposed, to the increased personal and economic freedom permitted to young women and loosening of family ties at an earlier age.

As might be expected, much venereal disease is found in the slums of large cities among socially disorganized groups with low economic standards. But it is also true that high rates of venereal disease have been reported among university students, notably in Africa and Sweden.

RESISTANCE TO ANTIBIOTICS. The development of resistance to penicillin and some other antibiotics by some strains of gonococci has led to increase in the number of failures of treatment of gonorrhoea, especially in some areas of the Far East.

MODERN CONTRACEPTIVE METHODS. The increase in use of oral gestogen pills and intrauterine contraceptive devices has eliminated fear of pregnancy and has possibly led to increase of sexual activity. Mechanical protectives which give some measure of protection against venereal infection are less used than formerly.

IGNORANCE. Studies in many countries have shown a remarkable lack of knowledge about venereal disease, especially among young people. This deficiency extends to the medical profession. Webster[8,9] studied reports on the teaching of venereal disease throughout the world and found that lack of adequate instruction was widespread, especially concerning epidemiological methods of controlling the disease. It should be noted that there has been at least one report[10] of gonorrhoea transmitted by artificial insemination from a donor.

RESERVOIR OF INFECTION IN WOMEN. Another factor is the 'reservoir' of undiscovered gonococcal infection in the female population. The disparity in numbers of cases in males and females has been accepted by some as a

TABLE I

GONORRHOEA

Sites of Infection and Local and General Complications

Classification	Sites of Direct Infection	Local Complications	General Complications
In Men	Urethra	Anterior Urethra { Tysonitis Paraurethral-duct infection Littritis Periurethral abscess Urethral stricture Cowperitis and abscess of Cowper's gland Posterior Urethra { Prostatitis acute—chronic Prostatic abscess Vesiculitis Epididymitis Trigonitis	Arthritis Dermatitis Anterior uveitis* Myocarditis Endocarditis Pericarditis Meningitis Hepatitis Perihepatitis†
	Anorectum Conjunctivae Oropharynx		
In Women	Urethra	{ Skenitis { Periurethral abscess	Arthritis Dermatitis
	Cervix uteri	{ Salpingo-oöphoritis Parametritis Pelvic abscess Pelvic peritonitis Perihepatitis†	Anterior uveitis* Myocarditis Endocarditis Pericarditis Meningitis Hepatitis
	Bartholin's glands Anorectum Conjunctivae Oropharynx	Bartholin's abscess	
In Children	Vulva and Vagina Anorectum		General complications as in adult
	Conjunctivae	{ Suppurative panophthalmitis and blindness	

* The belief that the gonococcus causes metastatic anterior uveitis is time-honoured. There is, however, good reason to suppose that anterior uveitis occurring in the course of gonorrhoea may be due to associated 'non-specific' infection.

† Perihepatitis arises mainly from local spread from pelvic infection in women, but may occasionally result from bacteraemia in either sex.

true indication of the relative incidence of promiscuity among men and women, but there is evidence that the more intensive the search for contacts, the lower the male : female ratio of cases. According to the World Health Organization Report,[7] in Memphis, Tennessee, the male : female ratio was originally 6 : 1 in certain districts. Intensive contact tracing reversed the ratio to 1 : 1·7. In the United States of America as a whole the ratio dropped from 2·4 : 1 in 1960 to 1·5 : 1 in 1977.[4] In Sweden[11] there has been a continuous decline in the ratio of men to women from 1·7 : 1 in 1961 to 1·1 : 1 in 1976. In England the ratio has fallen from nearly 4 : 1 in 1961 to 1·7 : 1 in 1977. The main reason for the frequency of undiagnosed gonorrhoea in women appears to be that many of them have no symptoms of the disease.

SITES OF INFECTION

The sites of infection and of local and general complications are shown in Table 1.

REFERENCES

1. *A. R. Med. Offr Dept Hlth (Lond.)* (1946–77) London: H.M.S.O. (1947–1978)*.
2. British Cooperative Clinical Group (1973) *Br. J. vener. Dis.*, **49,** 329.
3. *Public Health Papers. No. 65. Social and Health Aspects of Sexually Transmitted Diseases* (1977) pp. 14, 18. Geneva: W.H.O.
4. *S.T.D. Statistical Letter* (1978) United States Department of Health, Education and Welfare, Public Health Service, Center for Disease Control, Atlanta, Georgia.
5. FLEMING, W. L., BROWN, W. J., DONOHUE, J. F. and BRANIGAN, G. W. (1970) *J. Am. med. Ass.*, **211,** 1827.
6. Neisseria Gonorrhoeae and Gonococcal Infections. *Wld. Hlth Org. techn. Rep. Ser.,* Geneva (1978). No. 616, p. 39.
7. WHO Expert Committee on Gonococcal Infections (1963) *Wld Hlth Org. techn. Rep. Ser.,* Geneva, **262,** 4.
8. WEBSTER, B. (1966) *Br. J. vener. Dis.*, **42,** 132.
9. WEBSTER, B. (1972) *Med. Clins N. Am.*, **56,** 1101.
10. FIUMARA, N. J. (1972) *Br. J. vener. Dis.*, **48,** 308.
11. WALLIN, J. (1978) *Br. J. vener. Dis.*, **54,** 24.
* From 1970 the figures in the report are for England only.

11

Anatomy and Histology of the Genital Tract

MALE

(See diagram opposite and Fig. 101, p. 182.)

Urethra

This canal extends from the bladder neck to the external urinary meatus; its length is approximately 20 cm. From the bladder to the symphysis pubis it curves forwards with the concavity upwards; thence to the external meatus the concavity is downwards.

The urethra is divided into three parts: prostatic, membranous, and spongy. The prostatic and membranous parts together form the *posterior* urethra and the spongy portion forms the *anterior* urethra.

PROSTATIC URETHRA

The prostatic urethra lies within the substance of the prostate gland nearer to the anterior than the posterior surface. It is lined with transitional epithelium. It begins at the neck of the bladder and runs downwards and slightly forwards to end at the posterior layer of the triangular ligament (urogenital diaphragm); it is about 3 cm in length. In transverse section the lumen forms an arch; on distension it is wider in its central part. A number of small ducts of the prostatic acini open on to its anterior surface, and on its posterior surface is a longitudinal ridge, the *verumontanum*. On each side of this structure there is a depression, the *prostatic sinus*, into which open the ducts of the middle and lateral lobes of the prostate. In the centre of the verumontanum is a small depression, the *sinus pocularis*, on the lateral edges of which are the two small openings of the *common ejaculatory ducts*.

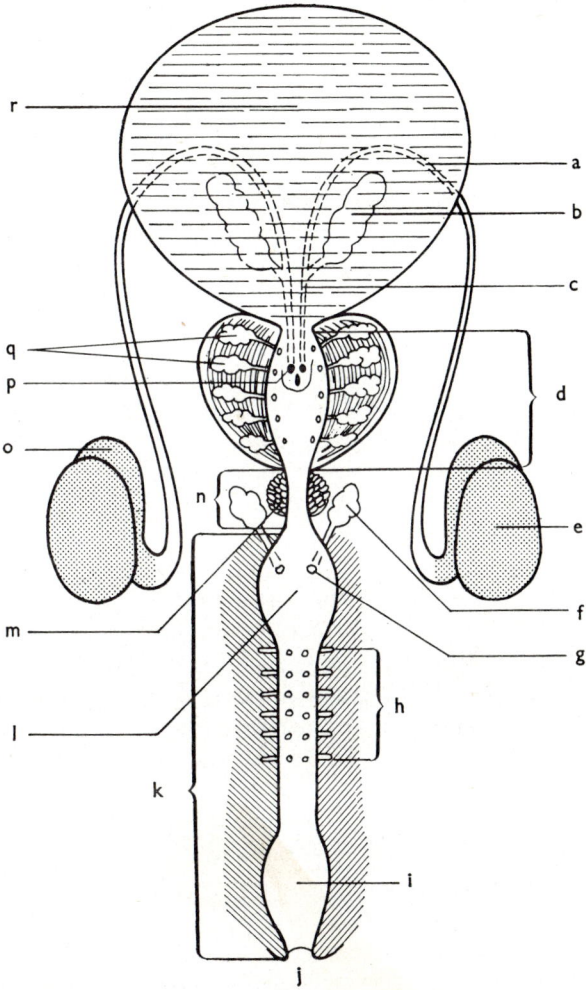

Floor of the Male Urethra

(Redrawn from Burke's adaptation of Pelouze)

a. Vas deferens
b. Vesicula seminalis
c. Ejaculatory duct
d. Prostatic urethra
e. Testis
f. Cowper's gland
g. Orifice of duct of Cowper's gland
h. Littré's glands
i. Fossa navicularis
j. Urinary meatus
k. Anterior urethra
l. Bulb
m. Compressor urethrae muscle
n. Membranous urethra
o. Epididymis
p. Verumontanum
q. Prostatic acini
r. Bladder

MEMBRANOUS URETHRA

The membranous urethra, which is lined with transitional epithelium, lies between the two layers of the triangular ligament, and 2·5 cm below and behind the pubic arch. It extends from the apex of the prostate to the bulb of the spongy urethra. It is only 12 mm in length and is the narrowest part of the urethra, showing in section as a transverse slit. The *glands of Cowper* lie one on either side of its posterior surface. It is surrounded by the compressor urethrae muscle.

SPONGY URETHRA

The spongy urethra is about 15 cm in length and is lined by columnar epithelium, except for the terminal 12 mm, the *fossa navicularis*, which is lined with stratified squamous epithelium. It extends from the anterior layer of the triangular ligament to the external urinary meatus and lies within the *corpus spongiosum*. It is divided into two parts, of which the proximal part is the bulb, which extends from the anterior layer of the triangular ligament to the penile angle. This part of the urethra is dilated and it is fixed by the suspensory ligament of the penis. The ducts of Cowper's glands open on to the floor about 2 cm in front of the anterior layer of the triangular ligament. The distal, or pendulous, part is about 6 mm in diameter. It is free and takes a downward course from the penile angle to the fossa navicularis, where it widens and then narrows again at the external meatus. In section it appears as a transverse slit, except at the meatus, where the slit is vertical. In the roof and sides of the penile urethra are the many ducts of *Littré's glands*, the openings of which are directed forwards. In the roof of the fossa navicularis is a larger opening, the *lacuna magna*. Here and there, several ducts of Littré's glands open together into depressions termed *lacunae of Morgagni*. The ducts are lined by columnar epithelium; the glands normally secrete mucus. The submucosa surrounding the lining of the penile urethra contains longitudinal and circular plain muscle fibres, and the blood vessels and nerves supplying the urethra. Mal-development of the terminal urethra sometimes occurs, with a ventral deficiency termed *hypospadias*.

The Penis

In addition to the structures already described, the penis consists of two masses of erectile tissue, the *corpora cavernosa*, which lie on each side of, and dorsal to, the corpus spongiosum. The terminal part of the latter enlarges to form the glans penis. The glans is covered by the prepuce, the main blood supply of which enters ventrally at the *fraenum preputii*. On either side of the frenum open the ducts of the *glands of Tyson*, which secrete sebaceous material. The *paraurethral ducts* are small blind channels which run parallel to the terminal part of the urethra for varying distances and

open near or within the lips of the external meatus; they are often inconspicuous. The glans penis and under surface of the prepuce are lined with
squamous epithelium.

Prostate Gland

The prostate gland is shaped like an inverted cone, measuring 4 cm by 4 cm
and lying at the base of the bladder. It surrounds the proximal urethra and
rests on the triangular ligament; posteriorly it is in contact with the anterior
rectal wall. It consists of a 'middle' and two lateral lobes and is enclosed by
a fibromuscular capsule. The glandular tissue is of the branched tubular type
and is lined with columnar epithelium. The ducts open into the prostatic
urethra. The common ejaculatory ducts also pass through the prostatic
tissue to open on the floor of the prostatic urethra. The so-called middle
lobe of the prostate is the upper and posterior part of the gland, which is
bounded by the urethra in front and the ejaculatory ducts on either
side.

The *seminal vesicles* are convoluted structures, each approximately 5 cm
in length, and contribute about 60 per cent of the seminal fluid. They lie
between the base of the bladder and the rectum. They are lateral to the
terminal parts of the *vasa deferentia*, which they join at the base of the prostate
to form the common ejaculatory ducts.

The vasa deferentia extend from the lower poles of the epididymes to
the base of the prostate. They are thick-walled tubes, 40 cm in length.
The testicular portion ascends along the back of the epididymis; then it
becomes the main part of the spermatic cord running up to the external
inguinal ring and passing through the inguinal canal. At the internal inguinal
ring it leaves the associated vessels of the spermatic cord and enters the
pelvis. It passes downwards and backwards over the lateral aspect of the
bladder to its posterior surface and anterior to the rectum. It becomes wider
and sacculated and passes inwards to the base of the prostate, where it
dilates to form the ampulla before narrowing to join the duct of the seminal
vesicle and form the common ejaculatory duct.

Testes and Epididymes

The testes and epididymes are contained in the scrotal sac. The testis is an
oval structure and has the epididymis attached to its posterior aspect. The
anterior and lateral surfaces are smooth and covered by the visceral layer
of the *tunica vaginalis*. The body of the testis is enclosed by the fibrous tissue
of the *tunica albuginea*. This covering becomes much thicker beneath the
epididymis, where it forms the *mediastinum testis*. Posterosuperiorly, the
mediastinum testis is pierced by the efferent seminiferous tubules. These
unite to form some 20 larger tubes, the *vasa efferentia*, which in turn form
the upper pole of the epididymis, or *globus major*. Here they unite into a
single canal, the duct of the epididymis, which is a coiled tube some

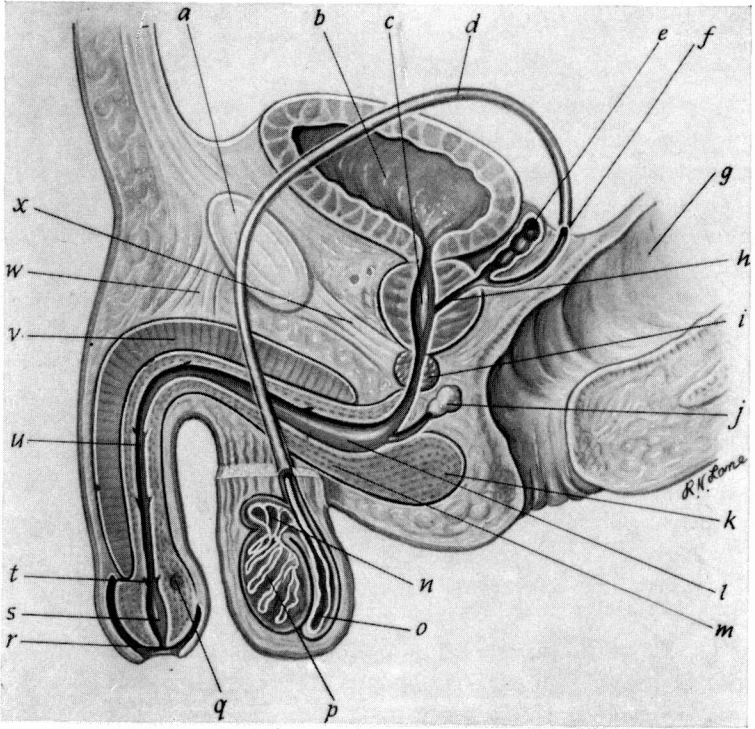

Fig. 101. Sagittal section of male genito-urinary tract.
(*After Burke's adaptation of Pelouze.*)

a. Symphysis pubis
b. Bladder
c. Prostatic urethra
d. Vas deferens
e. Seminal vesicle
f. Ampulla of vas
g. Rectum
h. Ejaculatory duct
i. Compressor urethrae and membranous urethra
j. Cowper's gland
k. Bulb
l. Bulbous urethra

m. Corpus spongiosum
n. Globus major ⎱ of epididymis
o. Globus minor ⎰
p. Testis
q. Tyson's gland
r. Urinary meatus
s. Fossa navicularis
t. Lacuna magna
u. Penile urethra
v. Corpus cavernosum
w. Suspensory ligament
x. Triangular ligament

ii (left) Virtually normal-looking cervix from which the gonococcus was isolated. (right) Proctitis, as seen through a proctoscope.

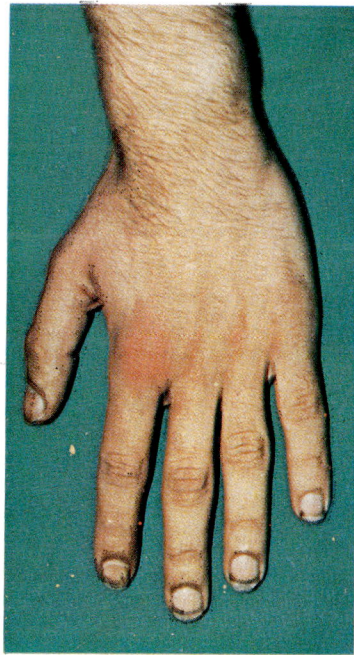

iv Septicaemia—cutaneous lesion.

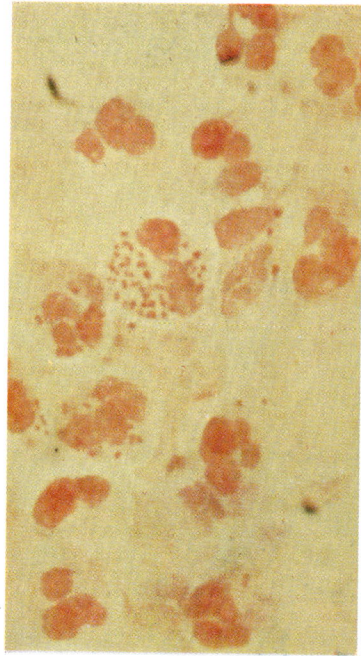

i Gram-stained slide showing gonococci.

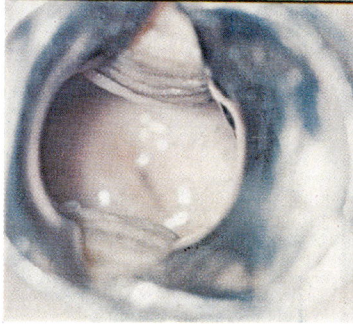

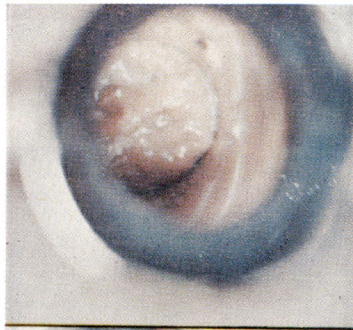

iii Septicaemia—acute arthritis.

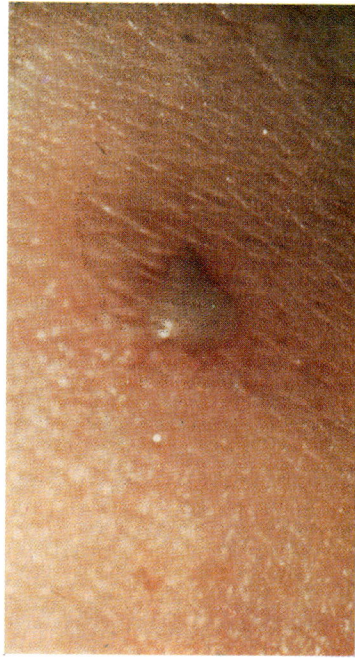

PLATE IV

6 metres in length forming the body and tail of the epididymis; the latter is called the *globus minor*. A groove can be felt between the epididymis and the testis. Occasionally the epididymis is situated anterior to the testis.

Seminal Fluid

The fluid is alkaline and contains numerous fully developed and motile sperms. According to the Farris classification, 185 million or more motile sperms in the complete ejaculum indicates a high degree of fertility; 80–185 million indicates moderate fertility; while fewer than 80 million indicates sub-fertility. However, conception is possible with much lower counts.

Prostatic Fluid

The fresh secretion of the normal prostate is a thin, white, semi-translucent fluid, which is alkaline. Microscopically it is seen to consist of structureless material containing small refractile granules, termed *lecithin bodies*. Laminated bodies, the so-called '*corpora amylacea*', may also be seen. In most normal individuals the secretion contains few polymorphonuclear leucocytes or other white cells.

FEMALE

(Figs. 102, 103 and 104)

Vulva

The vulva or external genital organ of the female consists of the following structures:

(a) The *mons veneris* is a rounded eminence formed by a pad of subcutaneous fatty tissue which lies in front of the pubic symphysis. After puberty it becomes covered with hair.

(b) The *labia majora* are longitudinal folds which extend downwards and backwards from the mons veneris to join posteriorly at the *fourchette* or posterior commissure, which is situated about 2·5 cm in front of the anus. The outer aspects are covered with hair, but the inner aspects are smooth and the skin contains numerous sebaceous glands. The labia majora have a thick layer of subcutaneous fat and they enclose the labia minora. They are the anatomical equivalent of the scrotum in the male.

(c) The *labia minora* are small cutaneous folds which unite above to form the prepuce of the clitoris, and below join at the fourchette.

(d) The *clitoris* lies centrally at the upper junction of the labia minora. It consists of erectile tissue and is the equivalent of the male penis.

(e) The *vestibule* is the space between the labia minora, and into it, from above downwards, open the urinary meatus, the ducts of Bartholin's glands and the vaginal introitus.

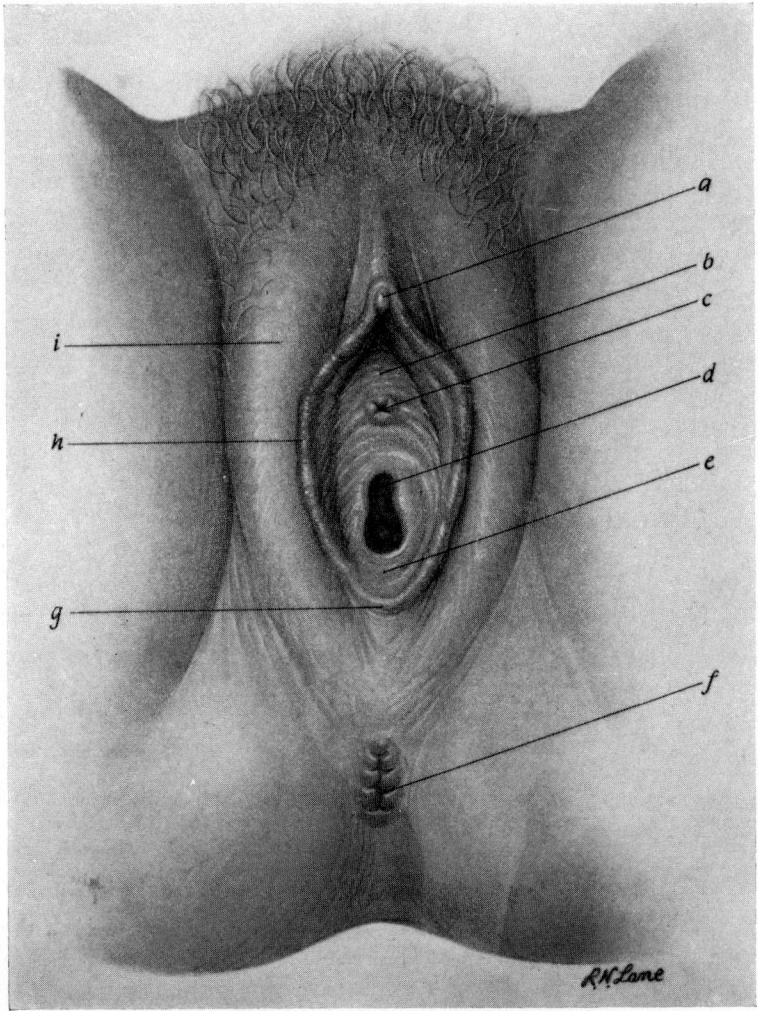

Fig. 102. The vulva. (*After Burke.*)

a. Clitoris	*f.* Anus
b. Vestibule	*g.* Fourchette
c. Urethral opening	*h.* Labium minus
d. Vaginal opening	*i.* Labium majus
e. Hymen	

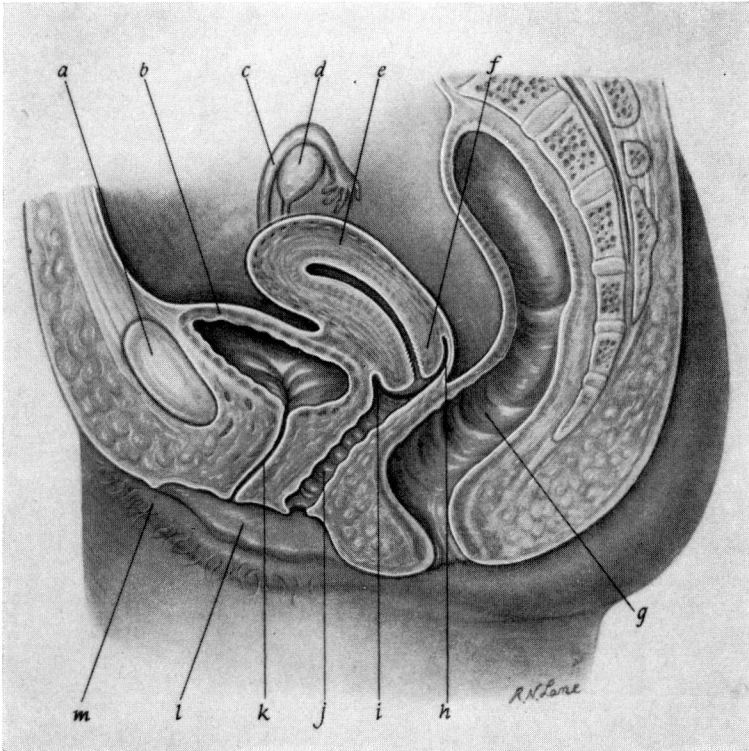

Fig. 103. Sagittal section through female pelvis. (*After Burke.*)

a. Symphysis pubis	*h.* Posterior fornix
b. Bladder	*i.* Anterior fornix
c. Fallopian tube	*j.* Vagina
d. Ovary	*k.* Urethra
e. Uterus	*l.* Labium minus
f. Cervix	*m.* Labium majus
g. Rectum	

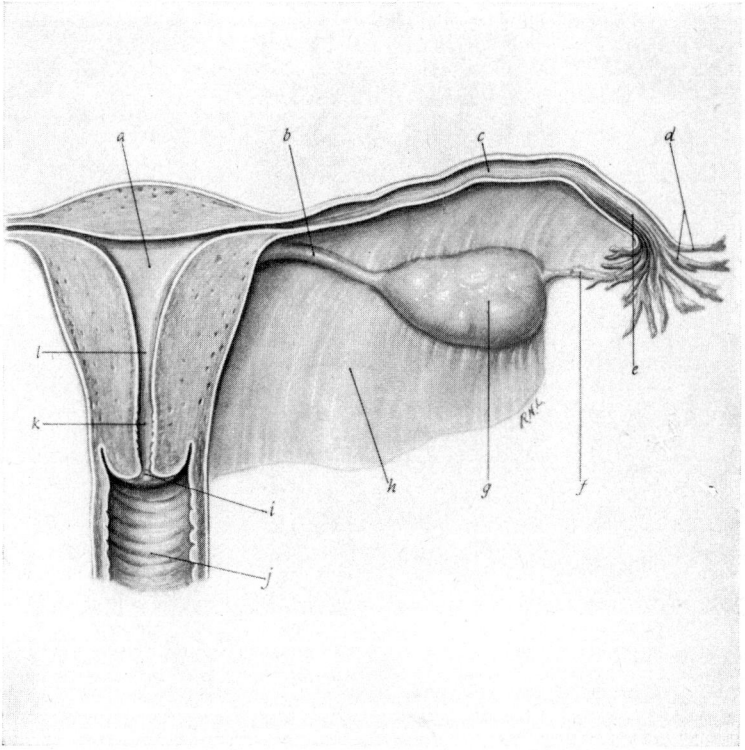

Fig. 104. The uterus and its appendages. (*After Burke.*)

a. Body of uterus	*g.* Ovary
b. Ovarian ligament	*h.* Broad ligament
c. Fallopian tube laid open	*i.* External os cervix
d. Fimbriae	*j.* Vagina
e. Infundibulum	*k.* Cervical canal
f. Ovarian fimbria	*l.* Internal os cervix

(*f*) The *glands of Bartholin* are two in number, and each lies within the lower third of the corresponding labium majus. Each duct opens on the inner surface of the corresponding labium minus at the junction of the upper two-thirds and the lower third. The opening of each duct is covered by a small mucosal fold. The glands are of the tubulo-racemose type and the ducts are lined with columnar epithelium.

(*g*) The *hymen* varies in size and shape; it may be a ring or a fold of mucosa extending up from the fourchette and ending in a concave upper border. It is likely to be ruptured at the first sexual intercourse, but hymenal tags may remain.

Urethra

The female urethra is 4 cm long and extends downwards and forwards from the base of the bladder to the external urinary meatus, at the upper part of the vestibule below the clitoris. It is equivalent to the posterior urethra in the male; it is lined with transitional epithelium in its proximal part and by stratified epithelium distally. It is very distensible. The mucous membrane contains many small glands, resembling the glands of Littré in the male. The ducts are lined by columnar epithelium and open into the urethra.

Skene's glands are situated one on either side of the urinary meatus; the ducts, which are lined with columnar epithelium, open into the vestibule or into the urinary meatus itself, and may be at different levels. The glands are vestigial and serve no useful purpose. They are sometimes involved in genital infection.

Vagina

The vagina is a passage which extends upwards and backwards from the vestibule to end above the terminal part of the cervix uteri, which it surrounds. The anterior wall is 9 cm long but the posterior wall measures 14 cm. The various parts of the cul-de-sac which the vagina forms with the cervix uteri are called the anterior, posterior, and lateral *vaginal fornices*. In cross-section the canal is H-shaped with the walls normally in contact; they are lined by squamous epithelium. The vagina dilates easily, particularly in a posterior direction, where it lies in front of the rectum.

The adult vaginal mucosa is a thick membrane lined by stratified squamous epithelium with a high glycogen content. Normal secretion shows, microscopically, epithelial cells and a large Gram-positive bacillus, the bacillus of Döderlein. The action of this bacillus on the glycogen of the cells produces lactic acid; this is responsible for the acidity of the vaginal secretion (pH 4·5), which is believed to protect against infection. The characteristics of the vaginal mucous membrane are controlled by oestrogenic hormones. Before puberty, the vaginal mucosa is thin, with a low glycogen content; Döderlein's bacilli are absent and the vaginal pH is alkaline. Newborn infants may show the adult type of vaginal mucosa and secretion for a few weeks until their tissues cease to contain oestrogens derived from the mother.

After the menopause the vaginal mucosa gradually becomes thin and atrophic. The glycogen content is less and Döderlein's bacilli are scanty. In consequence the vaginal secretion is less strongly acid, or even alkaline.

Uterus

The uterus consists of two parts, the cervix, or neck, and the body. The *cervix* of the uterus projects into the vagina and, at its terminal point, there is an opening, the *external os uteri*, which appears as a transverse slit enclosed by an anterior and a posterior lip. The opening leads into the *cervical canal*. Part of the cervix lies above the vaginal fornices. The cervical canal is fusiform in shape and at the *internal os uteri* opens into the uterine cavity. The surface of the canal is ridged longitudinally and transversely, like a tree with its branches (*arbor vitae*). Embedded in the tissues of the cervix are many compound racemose glands secreting mucus; they open into the cervical canal. They are lined with columnar epithelium.

The *body* of the uterus is a pear-shaped, muscular structure with a cavity 5 cm wide and 8 cm long. The body of the uterus forms an angle with the cervix, being directed forwards and upwards (anteverted) so that it rests on the bladder. It is suspended from the lateral pelvic walls by two folds of peritoneum, forming the *broad ligaments*; the tissue between the peritoneal folds of these ligaments is termed the *parametrium*. The upper part of the body is termed the *fundus uteri*; at each upper and lateral angle it is joined by a Fallopian tube. The uterine cavity is lined by the thick *endometrium*.

Fallopian Tubes and Ovaries

The *Fallopian tubes* lie in the upper part of the broad ligaments. They open into the upper and lateral angles of the uterine cavity and from these extend laterally for about 12 cm, first through the uterine muscle (*pars uterina*), then forming the narrow *isthmus*, which opens into the broader *ampulla*, and finally into the dilated portion called the *infundibulum*, which terminates in finger-like *fimbriae* opening into the peritoneal cavity in proximity to the ovaries. The tubes are lined by ciliated columnar epithelium which is arranged in longitudinal folds.

The *ovaries* are two oval-shaped organs, each about 5 cm long and attached to the posterior aspect of the broad ligament by a fold (*mesovarium*) and also to the uterus medially by the ovarian ligament. One of the fimbriae of the corresponding Fallopian tube is attached to the lateral pole of each ovary (Fig. 104).

12

Gonorrhoea: Mode of Infection; Diagnostic Methods; Pathology; The Incubation Period

MODE OF INFECTION

Infection nearly always results from sexual intercourse with an infected person. Although the gonococcus can survive in dried exudate on towels, lavatory seats and toilet paper for several hours,[1,2] accidental non-venereal genital infection in adults is extremely rare, if it occurs at all. Infection sometimes occurs in a person who has worn a reliable condom, and is probably the result of genital contact prior to intercourse or of contamination by fingers after intercourse. Infection from anorectal coitus, whether homosexual or heterosexual, is quite common, and it has also been described as resulting from buccal coitus. Accidental infection of female children happens occasionally, although less often than in the past. Epidemics have occurred in children's wards and orphanages, usually through some failure in the nursing care, such as inadequate sterilization of thermometers. Infection also occurs through children sharing beds with or using towels and flannels in common with infected parents. Urethral infection is very occasionally seen in small boys; in the newly born this may conceivably be transmitted from the maternal passages during birth. Infection of older children is presumed to be non-venereal, but it is usually impossible to exclude the possibility that some direct contact with an infectious adult has taken place.

In a prospective study[3] involving United States naval personnel in the Far East the risk of acquiring gonorrhoea per exposure with an infected female was 1 in 5 for whites and 1 in 2 for coloureds. It was uncertain whether this represented a true difference in racial susceptibility because of the many factors involved. The risk of a woman acquiring gonorrhoea from an infected man is probably much greater.

DIAGNOSIS

Gonorrhoea must never be diagnosed without the aid of microscopy and cultural tests. The gonococcal complement-fixation test of blood serum is relatively of very small importance. Of the main members of the Neisserian group, *N. gonorrhoeae* and *N. meningitidis* are pathogenic, but *N. catarrhalis*, *N. pharyngis sicca*, *N. lactamica* and *N. subflava* are usually non-pathogenic. Only *N. gonorrhoeae* is commonly found in the genital tract, but the others occur occasionally. Most members of the group can be differentiated by sugar-fermentation reactions and fluorescent technique (see p. 194), but classification of some species within the genus is difficult and remains incomplete.

Examination by Smear

Material from the site of infection is spread carefully on to a glass slide with a platinum loop; it is fixed by gentle heating, stained with Gram's stain (for details see the Appendix, p. 387) and examined microscopically with a 2 mm oil immersion objective. The diagnosis is made by finding Gram-negative diplococci of typical reniform shape in an intracellular position in polymorphonuclear leucocytes (Plate IV, i). Many other Gram-negative organisms can be found in specimens taken from the female genital tract, and short coliform bacilli, often appearing in pairs and sometimes in an intracellular position, may cause particular difficulty in diagnosis. Organisms of the *Mima* group (now known as *Moraxella* and *Acinitobacter*) may also closely resemble gonococci in Gram-stained smears of secretions. Staphylococci which have been ingested by polymorphonuclear leucocytes and partly digested may lose their Gram-positive reaction and cause confusion, particularly if the slide has been over-decolorized. Smear tests have a high degree of sensitivity in the diagnosis of acute urethral gonorrhoea in men, but in women are likely to be negative in a third or more of cases of cervical infection and in an even higher proportion of urethral and rectal infections.

Examination by Culture

That reliable methods for culturing the gonococcus were superior to microscopical smears in the diagnosis of gonorrhoea in women and of chronic gonococcal infections in men was shown more than 50 years ago in Great Britain by Osmond, Price and others, and has been confirmed in many countries since that time. It is generally accepted that the identity of the organism should be confirmed in culture, not only by the oxidase test but also by sugar-fermentation tests and, in some cases, by serological tests employing fluorescent antibody of proved specificity. Apart from the proved superiority of this method in the female, in both sexes cultural tests constitute the only certain medicolegal proof of gonococcal infection, and will also distinguish cases of acute gonorrhoea from those of primary urethritis due to other Neisserian organisms. They are essential in the diagnosis of pharyngeal gonorrhoea because other *Neisseria* are commonly present.

Techniques of Culture

The difficulties of the technique of culture are reflected in the variety of new media, and modifications of old media, which have been recommended and used from time to time. Some media have given excellent results in the hands of those who have first used them and indifferent or variable results in the hands of others. Batches of the same media have given highly variable results at different times for no obvious reasons. In consequence, there has been constant search for media which could easily be prepared and would give consistent results, in an endeavour to raise the admittedly indifferent standard of cultural work outside certain highly specialized laboratories.

It cannot yet be claimed that such an ideal medium has been discovered, but a good deal of useful information has been acquired.

TRANSPORT MEDIUM—STUART'S MEDIUM

The problem of efficient cultural tests for the gonococcus in clinics and hospitals without the advantage of a first-class bacteriological service on the spot is a perennial one, and has been closely investigated in various countries during the last 35 years. In Great Britain and elsewhere considerable success has been achieved with a simple method described by Stuart[4] in 1946. Stuart believed that the death of the gonococcus by drying was caused by increased speed of oxidation. If the organism could be kept under conditions of reduction, this would not occur. He used small screw-capped bottles filled with 0.3 per cent agar, giving the suitable physical conditions. The agar contained one part in 1000 of thioglycollic acid neutralized with NaOH, and the whole was buffered with 1 per cent glycerophosphate and 1:10,000 calcium chloride. One part per 500,000 methylene blue was added to give evidence of persistence of conditions of reduction, the agar remaining colourless as long as this was satisfactory. The swab containing the specimen for culture was pushed into the bottle, its stem cut off flush with the rim, and the cap screwed down. Stuart's results indicated that by this method the gonococcus remained capable of subculture for up to three or four days, and there was no tendency for excessive growth of contaminants. It was found that the method employing Stuart's medium was also

applicable to the detection of *Trichomonas vaginalis*, which remained alive
and active in the medium. Stuart and his colleagues[5] were able to add an
additional point in technique. It was found that certain batches of agar had
a bactericidal action on *Neisseria*. This action could be neutralized by
charcoal, which, however, could not be incorporated in the medium
without absorbing the methylene-blue indicator. The swabs for taking
specimens were therefore dipped in a 1 per cent watery suspension of
finely ground charcoal before being dried and sterilized. Swabs of secretion
in Stuart's medium should be kept in a refrigerator rather than at room
temperature until they can be taken to the laboratory. Isolation of gonococci
from this transport medium is almost always successful after storage up to
24 hours, but after this time there is a progressive loss.

TRANSGROW MEDIUM

This is a combined medium for the transport and isolation of gonococci.
It is described as a modified Thayer–Martin medium (see below), the principal modification being the addition of trimethoprim lactate to reduce the
growth and swarming of *Proteus* organisms. It is put up as slants of the
medium in screw-capped bottles containing an atmosphere of 10 per cent
CO_2. The surface of the medium is inoculated with a swab, the cap screwed
on tightly and the culture posted to the laboratory, where it is incubated
overnight before examination. This medium has been widely used in the
United States of America but reports as to its efficacy have varied. Various
commercial preparations employing the 'transgrow' principle are now
available.

GROWING MEDIUM

Gonococci are fastidious organisms and usually have to be cultured from
sites with an abundant microbial flora which can easily overgrow gonococci,
especially when these are present in only small numbers. Nevertheless
media such as McLeod's chocolate-agar, serum agar and hydrocele-agar
have stood the test of time and have given useful results. The pH of the
medium must be carefully adjusted to 7·5. Plates or slopes are inoculated
either directly or from the transport medium and are incubated in a moist
atmosphere containing 5 per cent CO_2. Incubation should be at 36°C for
48 hours.

Selective media were introduced by Thayer and Martin,[6,7] who incorporated vancomycin (3 units/ml), sodium colistimethate (7·5 mg/ml) and
nystatin (12·5 mg/ml) into the basal medium used for culture. Vancomycin
inhibits many Gram-positive organisms, sodium colistimethate many Gram-
negative contaminants (but not *Proteus*), and nystatin yeast-like organisms.
The use of this combination of antibiotics greatly facilitates the isolation of
gonococci in primary culture even from such heavily contaminated sites
as the rectum. When examined after 18 hours' incubation gonococcal

colonies tend to be rather small on the selective medium but by 48 hours they usually attain the same size as those grown on plates without added antibiotics. According to Wilkinson[8] it is doubtful whether nystatin serves any really useful purpose in the medium. Most species of *Proteus* can be inhibited by adding trimethoprim to the medium at a concentration of 5 μg/ml. Although selective media have greatly facilitated the isolation of gonococci, there have been reports that a minority of strains, perhaps 3–7 per cent, may fail to grow on selective media. This potential loss is more than counterbalanced by the loss through overgrowth of other organisms on non-selective media.

Four main types of colony have been described, of which only Types 1 and 2 are pathogenic. A fifth type is found occasionally.

OXIDASE TEST

After incubation, plates are removed from the incubator, inspected with a hand lens, and a loopful of freshly prepared oxidase reagent (1·0 per cent aqueous tetramethyl-*p*-phenylene diamine HCl) is added to suspected colonies. Gonococcal colonies turn a pink colour, rapidly deepening to purple, and if picked off quickly can be subcultured. The tetramethyl is preferable to the dimethyl salt as the latter is more toxic. Before a plate is discarded as negative it should be flooded with the reagent to ensure that colonies of gonococci occurring amid those of other organisms are not missed (Fig. 105).

TABLE 2

OXIDASE REACTION OF BACTERIA

Positive	Negative
Neisseria (strong)	Coliform group
Many vibrios (strong)	Salmonellae
Brucellae (moderate)	Corynebacteriae
Haemophilus (weak)	Streptococci
Anthrax and anthracoids (moderate)	Staphylococci
P. mallei (moderate)	Sarcinae
Ps. pyocyanea (moderate)	Anaerobes
Mima polymorpha (some strains)	

The oxidase test has been of great value in the detection of gonococcal colonies in mixed culture; but it must be fully appreciated that it is not a specific test and that positive tests occur with other than gonococcal colonies, including other *Neisseria* (see Table 2).

The great advantage of the reaction is that colonies may show up even though overgrown by other organisms.

FERMENTATION REACTIONS

A pure subculture of the Neisserian organisms must first be prepared. This is inoculated on to four hydrocele-agar slopes containing 1 per cent glucose, maltose, sucrose and lactose respectively. When the slopes are incubated, an indicator (phenol red) contained in the medium demonstrates fermentation (acid formation) by changing from red to yellow.

Table 3 shows the fermentation reactions of the *Neisseria*.

TABLE 3

FERMENTATION REACTIONS OF THE NEISSERIA

	Glucose	Maltose	Sucrose	Lactose
N. gonorrhoeae	+	—	—	—
N. meningitidis	+	+	—	—
N. catarrhalis*	—	—	—	—
N. pharyngis sicca	+	+	+	—
N. lactamica	+	+	—	+

* Now known as *B. catarrhalis* of the genus *Branhamella*.
N. subflava ferments glucose and maltose but fermentation of sucrose is variable.

When examining patients with urogenital infection, only a presumptive diagnosis of gonorrhoea can be made until these fermentation tests have been performed. Some laboratories, however, do not perform fermentation tests and, if they are done, at least three days will elapse before a report is available. Thus in the majority of clinics gonorrhoea is diagnosed and treated on the presumptive findings, with the chance of a 3 per cent error in women and a 1·5 per cent error in men. It is wise to request performance of fermentation reactions in all cases in which legal action for rape, or divorce proceedings, might result.

Fluorescent Antibody Methods[9],[10]

The reagent used for these tests is the globulin fraction of a high titred antiserum against gonococci prepared in rabbits and conjugated with fluorescein isothiocyanate. This unites with gonococci which fluoresce an apple green colour when viewed under ultraviolet light. Two methods are used:

DIRECT FA TEST. The reagent is applied to heat-fixed thin films of secretions. Background fluorescence of leucocytes is usually marked but can be overcome by the use of counterstains such as Rhodamine, Naphthalene Black or Evans Blue.

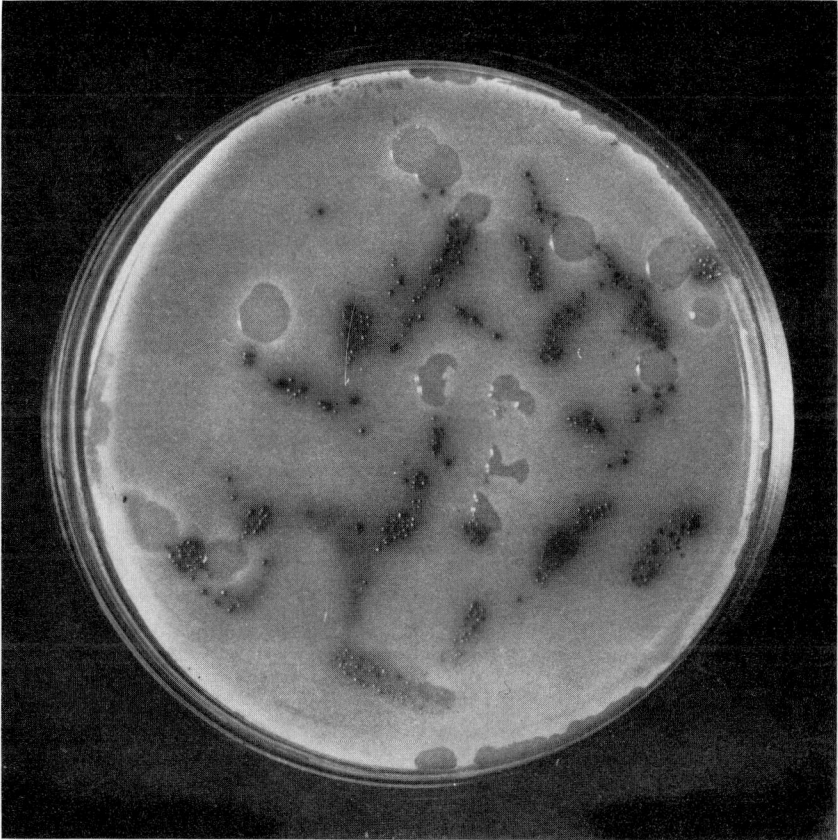

Fig. 105. Gonorrhoea: culture on hydrocele-agar; gonococcal colonies stained with oxidase reagent.

DELAYED FA TEST. Secretions are cultured on slopes of suitable medium overnight and a film of the mixed growth stained with the conjugated antiserum. Most workers have found this the more sensitive technique. The success of these methods depends on the specificity of the antiserum used. Cross-reactions with other *Neisseria* occur, especially with meningococci, and many rabbit sera have antibody to some strains of staphylococci. If these interfering antibodies can be removed, the method appears to be a very useful one.

Tests for Sensitivity of Gonococci to Antibiotics

Most strains of gonococci are still sensitive to penicillin. The proportion of those relatively insensitive varies in different parts of the world and has been particularly high in the Far East. Recently strains have appeared which produce β-lactamase (penicillinase) and are completely resistant to penicillin. Again these strains are particularly prevalent in the Far East (see Chapter 17). Strains relatively insensitive to penicillin usually show diminished sensitivity to streptomycin, tetracycline, spiramycin, erythromycin and cotrimoxazole. Sensitivity determinations should, ideally, be carried out on all strains isolated, but especially on those isolated from apparent treatment failures. Sensitivity to penicillin is best determined by growing gonococci in fluid or solid media into which graded amounts of penicillin have been incorporated and strains requiring 0·125 μg or more for inhibition should be regarded as relatively insensitive. Sensitivity to streptomycin, tetracycline or kanamycin can be determined by the use of disc techniques. Reference strains of known sensitivity should be included in each batch of tests as controls. Advice on obtaining these strains, if not available locally, may be sought from the Director of the WHO Gonococcus Reference Laboratory at the Serum Institute in Copenhagen. It is important to relate local methods of treatment to the changing pattern of sensitivity which strains of gonococci show to antibiotics. It may be accepted as a working rule that more than 5 per cent of failures of treatment is unacceptable and indicates the need for changes in the routine of treatment.

Gonococcal Complement-fixation Test

This procedure employs a standard gonococcal antigen and tests for the presence of circulating antibody. It may be performed as a quantitative test. In its original form, suspensions of gonococci or crude extracts were used

Fig. 106. Gonorrhoea. 1A and 1B. Negatively stained preparations of piliated (1A, p) and non-piliated (1B) gonococci (× 40,000). 2. Freeze-fracture freeze-etch preparation of gonococci showing adherent pili (p) on the organism's surface, which appears to be composed of subunits giving a pebbled texture. The arrows point to pits or holes in the outer membrane of the cell wall (× 140,000). (*Illustrations kindly provided by Dr John Swanson, from The Gonococcus, edited by R. B. Roberts (1977). Reprinted by permission of John Wiley & Sons, Inc., New York.*)

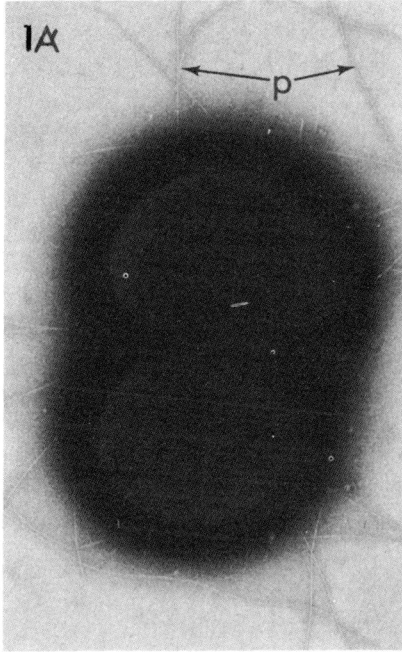

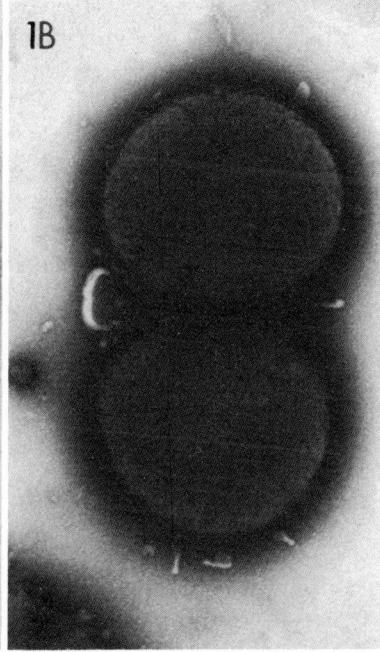

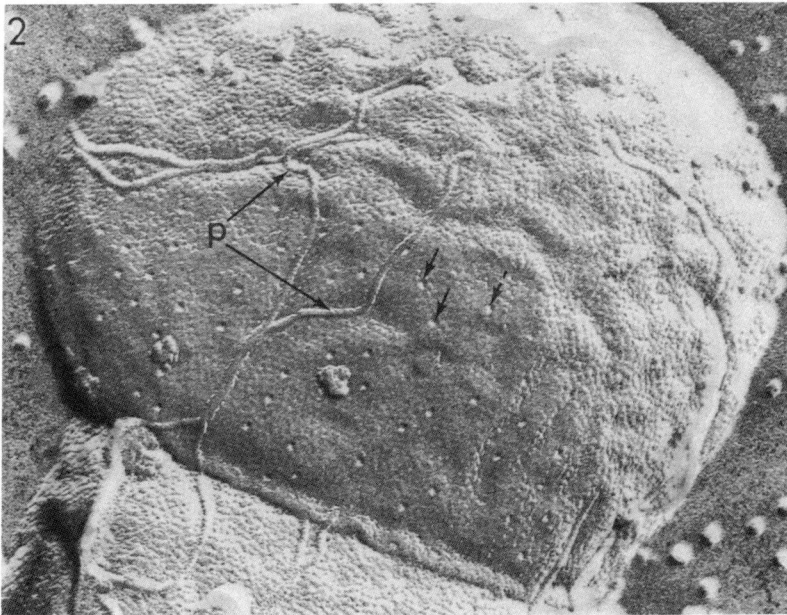

as antigens, but the specificity of the test was open to suspicion because of the occurrence of cross reactions with antibodies to other organisms of the *Neisseria* group. The test only became positive after the infection had lasted for some time or if complications were present. It also often remained positive, sometimes for very long periods, after apparently effective treatment. A positive fixation test alone is not sufficient to warrant a diagnosis of gonorrhoea, but in the absence of a past history of gonococcal infection, especially when a contact is known to have gonorrhoea, a positive fixation test suggests the possibility of such infection, and further efforts should be made to isolate the gonococcus. It is clear, therefore, that the test has only limited value and is not suitable for application to low-risk groups, in which the proportion of false-positive results will be higher.

More recently, attempts have been made to develop tests using more chemically defined fractions of gonococci by methods other than complement-fixation, as, for instance, antigens adsorbed to inert particles such as bentonite or to red cells. Fluorescent antibody techniques have also been employed and tests using gonococcal pili as antigen. Although sensitivity has been increased by these procedures, in most instances an appreciable incidence of unexplained positive results has been found in sera from apparently healthy individuals. At present there is no sensitive and specific serological test of practical use for gonorrhoea although such a test is urgently needed.

Serum Immunoglobulins in Cases of Gonorrhoea

Scott and Rasbridge[11] estimated immunoglobulin level in 39 cases of uncomplicated gonorrhoea in men. Although most of the results fell within the normal range, mean levels for IgG, IgA and IgM were significantly higher than in a normal control group. It was not possible to relate the change to any characteristic feature of the disease. McMillan et al.,[12] using an immunofluorescent technique, found that IgG antibodies to gonococcal antigen predominate, but IgM and IgA antibodies may also be present early in the course of the infection.

PATHOLOGY

In the urogenital tract, infection tends to spread along mucosal surfaces. The gonococcus has a predilection for columnar epithelium, which it attacks and penetrates, producing a marked polymorphonuclear response in the submucosa. Both transitional and stratified squamous epithelium are more resistant to the organism. Thus in the male the urethra, Littré's and Cowper's glands, the prostate, seminal vesicles and epididymes are the common sites of involvement; and in the female the glands of Skene and Bartholin, part of the urethra and the urethral glands, the cervix and

Fallopian tubes are prone to infection. The rectum is susceptible in both sexes, but the bladder, the upper urinary tract, the preputial sac, the vulva, the vagina and the uterus are less often involved. In untreated cases resolution of the infection depends on two factors, the building up of local-tissue immunity and adequate drainage. In glandular tissue, drainage may be impaired by inflammatory oedema of the gland ducts.

Recent studies by electron microscopy[13, 14] have shown that virulent gonococci possess hair-like structures on their surfaces known as 'pili' or 'fimbriae' (Fig. 106). It has been suggested that these pili are required for successful attachment of the organism to the host cells. However, piliated gonococci are seen much less frequently in pus than in cultures.[15]

INCUBATION PERIOD

This may vary from one to ten days, although in most cases it is five days or less. Occasionally, incubation periods of a month or more have been described, but the likely explanation is that, in the early stages, the symptoms have been so slight that they have failed to attract the patient's attention. Because of the absence or paucity of symptoms in many females and passive homosexuals there is often no ascertainable incubation period in such cases.

REFERENCES

1. ELMROS, T. and LARSSON, P-Å. (1972) Br. med. J., 2, 403.
2. GILBAUGH, J. H. and FUCHS, P. C. (1979) New Engl. J. Med., 301, 91.
3. HOOPER, R. R., REYNOLDS, G. H., JONES, O. G., ZAIDI, A., WIESNER, P. J., LATIMER, K. P., LESTER, A., CAMPBELL, A. F., HARRISON, W. O., KARNEY, W. W. and HOLMES, K. K. (1978) Am. J. epidem., 108, 136.
4. STUART, R. D. (1946) Glasg. med. J., 27, 131. See also WHO Expert Committee on Gonococcal Infections (1963) Wld Hlth Org. tech. Rep. Ser., Geneva, 262, 22.
5. MOFFETT, M., YOUNG, J. L. and STUART, R. D. (1948) Br. med. J., 2, 421.
6. THAYER, J. D. and MARTIN, J. E. (Jr.) (1964) Publ. Hlth Rep. (Wash.), 79, 49.
7. THAYER, J. D. and MARTIN, J. E. (Jr.) (1966) Publ. Hlth Rep. (Wash.), 81, 559.
8. WILKINSON, A. E. (1973) Personal communication.
9. DEACON, W. E., PEACOCK, W. L. (Jr.), FREEMAN, E. M. and HARRIS, A. (1959) Proc. Soc. exp. Biol. Med., 101, 322.
10. DEACON, W. E., PEACOCK, W. L. (Jr.), FREEMAN, E. M., HARRIS, A. and BUNCH, W. L. (1960) Pub. Hlth Rep. (Wash.), 75, 125.
11. SCOTT, A. J. and RASBRIDGE, M. R. (1972) Br. J. vener. Dis., 48, 133.
12. McMILLAN, A., McNEILLAGE, G., YOUNG, H. and BAIN, S. R. (1979) Br. J. vener. Dis., 55, 5.
13. JEPHCOTT, A. E., REYN, A. and BIRCH-ANDERSON, A. (1971) Acta path. microbiol. scand., Section B., 79, 437.
14. SWANSON, J., KRAUS, S. J. and GOTSCHLICH, E. C. (1971) J. exp. Med., 134, 886.
15. NOVOTNY, P., SHORT, J. A. and WALKER, P. D. (1975) J. med. Microbiol., 8, 413.

13

Gonorrhoea in the Male

ACUTE GONORRHOEA : ACUTE URETHRITIS

(Fig. 107)

The patient complains of a burning sensation in the urethra with discomfort on passing urine. The degree of discomfort and dysuria varies but the symptoms are seldom severe. Within 24 hours the patient becomes aware of a purulent urethral discharge at the external urinary meatus, or he may notice stains on his underclothes. He usually feels quite well but there may be slight constitutional disturbance. If the infection has reached the posterior urethra, which it is likely to do within 10 to 14 days if no treatment is given, the patient may complain of increasing dysuria, of some frequency of micturition and perhaps of strangury. In a severe attack there may be a few drops of blood at the end of micturition, but considerable haematuria is rare. There may also be general symptoms such as headache, malaise, increased pulse rate, and pyrexia (which is usually slight but may reach 40°C). Occasionally involvement of the posterior urethra occurs earlier and may appear to be present from the onset of the disease. On examination, the urethral discharge is likely to be profuse, yellow or yellowish-green and purulent. It is important to be sure that it comes from the urethra and not from under the prepuce. The lips of the external urinary meatus are swollen and oedematous and the mucous membrane surrounding the meatus is reddened. There may be slight tender enlargement of inguinal lymphatic nodes. The urine examined by the two-glass test gives a rough index of the extent of spread of infection. The patient passes separate specimens of urine into two glasses. In cases of anterior urethritis the first specimen is cloudy or hazy with pus and, provided that it has been adequate to wash pus from the anterior urethra, the specimen in the second glass is clear. The presence of haziness due to pus in the second specimen suggests involvement of the posterior urethra. Useful information from this test is limited to cases in which the posterior urethra is heavily infected. For greater accuracy it is necessary to apply the three-glass test, in which the anterior urethra

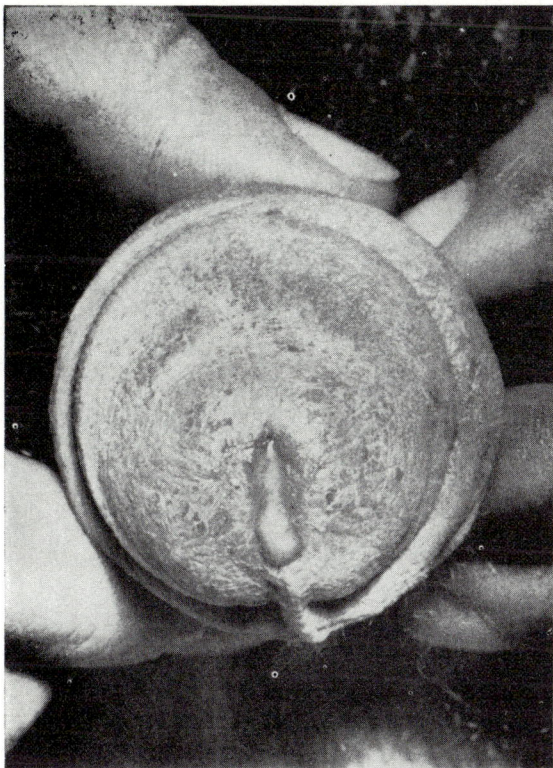

Fig. 107. Gonorrhoea
(male): urethritis.

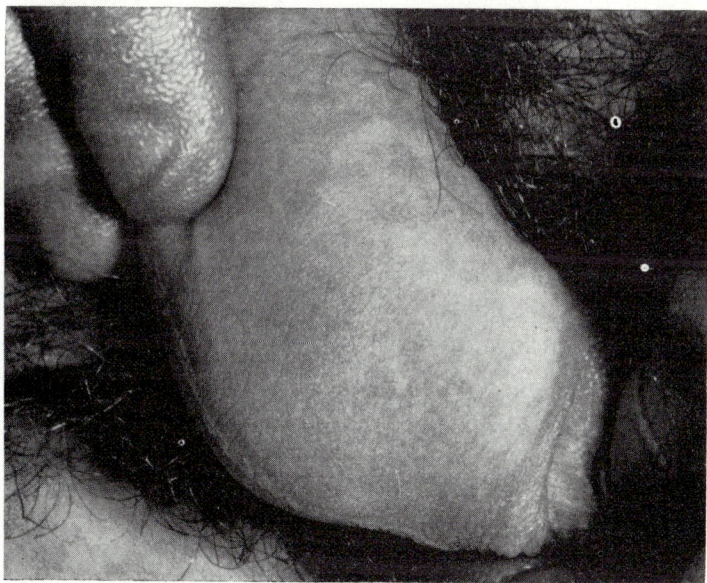

Fig. 108. Gonorrhoea (male): periurethral abscess.

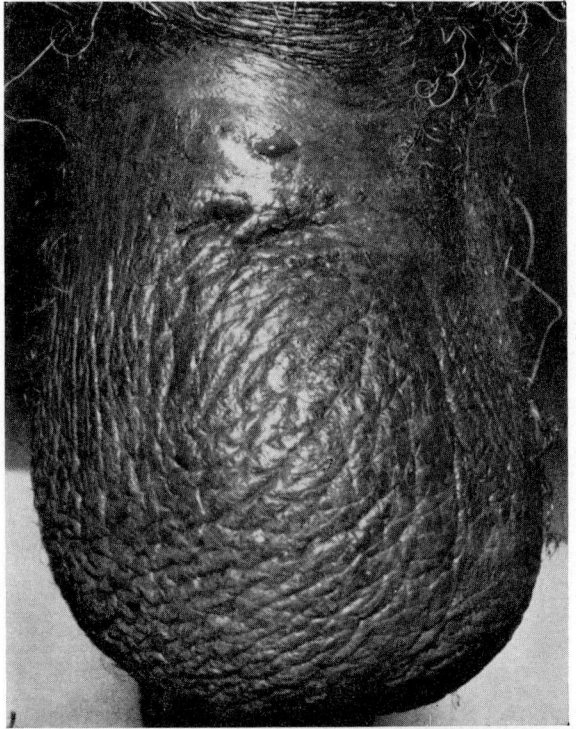

Fig. 109. Gonorrhoea
(male): perineal fistula.

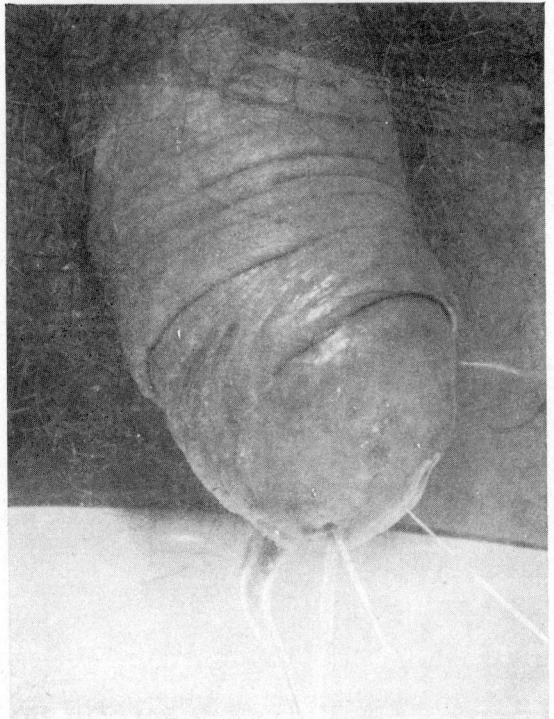

Fig. 110. Gonorrhoea
(male): 'watering-can'
fistulae seen during
micturition.

is irrigated with colourless antiseptic solution, such as 1:8000 oxycyanide of mercury, until the washings contained in the first glass are seen to be clear. The patient then passes urine into two separate glasses. If the first of these contains pus, the posterior urethra is infected. If there is pus in the other glass, the infection has extended to the bladder and purulent material has become mixed with urine contained in the bladder.

In some cases the condition is mild, with only slight or moderate amounts of mucopurulent discharge.

ASYMPTOMATIC INFECTION. This is common in females (see p. 215) but the fact that it occurs in males is less fully appreciated. Pariser, Farmer and Marino[1] drew particular attention to this possibility in a study of 115 male contacts of females with gonorrhoea: 98 had no symptoms, but the gonococcus was demonstrated in 26 of them by delayed fluorescent antibody tests of urethral secretion or urine. Handsfield et al.[2] isolated the gonococcus in culture from the urethrae of 59 out of 2628 enlisted men of the United States Army, who admitted to having had intercourse. About two-thirds of these men had just returned from Vietnam. There were 40 (1·5 per cent) who had asymptomatic infection. The most recent intercourse had been two weeks ago or more in 26 of the cases. The authors suggested that the high proportion of relatively resistant strains of gonococci first seen on the West Coast of the United States may have been due to the importation of these strains by asymptomatic military personnel from Vietnam and sensitivity studies on the organisms supported this view. However, recent work[3] has shown an association between asymptomatic urethral infection and infection by strains of gonococci that require arginine, hypoxanthine and uracil for growth and this particular AHU 'auxotype' is generally sensitive to penicillin. In the United States this auxotype is also found appreciably more often in white than in coloured patients.[4] In another survey[5] in the United States 1·9 per cent of 2064 boys aged 12 to 16 years entering a youth detention centre in New York were found to be harbouring gonococci although asymptomatic.

Local Complications of Acute Urethritis

The following are the possible sites of local complications in the male (Figs. 108 and 109): (*a*) the parafrenal glands of Tyson; (*b*) preputial sac; (*c*) paraurethral ducts; (*d*) median raphe; (*e*) ducts and glands of Littré and lacunae of Morgagni; (*f*) subepithelial tissue of the urethra; (*g*) periurethral tissues; (*h*) Cowper's ducts and glands; (*i*) prostatic ducts and the prostate gland; (*j*) common ejaculatory ducts and seminal vesicles; (*k*) vasa deferentia and the epididymes.

TYSON'S GLANDS

Infection of these glands is not a common complication. It may occur when the prepuce is long and hygiene is faulty. There are no symptoms and the signs are inconspicuous unless the duct becomes obstructed and an abscess forms. An abscess of Tyson's gland appears as a red, moderately tender swelling on one side of the frenum. It may open on the surface and discharge pus containing gonococci. It is not easily mistaken for a periurethral abscess, which is deeply situated and is more likely to present in the midline.

PREPUTIAL SAC AND PENILE SKIN

Gonococcal balanitis is uncommon. It may occur in uncircumcised patients with profuse gonorrhoeal urethral discharge and occasionally it is associated with shallow ulceration, usually in the region of the frenum. The occurrence of a pustular lesion on the penile skin due to direct implantation of gonococci is rare; in most case reports of this condition urethral discharge has been absent.

PARA-URETHRAL DUCTS

Infection of these ducts can only be diagnosed by close and careful inspection of the glans penis and external urinary meatus. On pressure, a small bead of pus may be seen at the opening of the duct, the margins of which may be reddened and slightly swollen. Sometimes the openings are within the lips of the meatus.

MEDIAN RAPHE

Infection of defects in the median raphe on the ventral surface of the penis is occasionally seen. Pus can be expressed from one or more openings leading to sinus tracts which may be swollen. There may or may not be associated urethral infection.

DUCTS AND GLANDS OF LITTRÉ AND THE LACUNAE OF MORGAGNI

Gonococcal infection of the urethra inevitably involves the ducts of the urethral glands of Littré and the lacunae of Morgagni. Involvement of the former is shown by the presence of 'threads' in the first glass of urine in the two-glass test. The threads are casts of the ducts, and if examined under the microscope they are seen to consist of epithelial cells and numerous pus cells. Littritis of itself gives rise to no symptoms, but if ducts of the glands become blocked small follicular abscesses may form in the wall of the urethra.

SUBEPITHELIAL TISSUES OF THE URETHRA

In all cases of acute gonococcal urethritis the organisms penetrate into the submucous tissue of the urethra and give rise to an inflammatory response. When the infection is severe the inflammatory reaction may be very considerable, particularly in the neighbourhood of infected Littré's glands and of the lacunae of Morgagni. This may lead to inflammatory hyperplasia in the submucous tissue, with the formation of so-called soft infiltration. This is not usually diagnosed during the stage of acute urethritis but may be discovered by urethroscopy either during tests for cure or when seeking a cause for a persisting residual non-gonococcal discharge. In such a case fibrous stricture may develop irrespective of treatment with antibiotics.

PERIURETHRAL ABSCESS (see Fig. 108, p. 201)

A more severe form of invasion of subepithelial tissue may result from fusion of a number of follicular abscesses, with the formation of a large peri-urethral abscess extending into the subepithelial tissues and beyond. Such an abscess usually opens into the urethra but sometimes it points on the surface. Occasionally an abscess tracks for some distance in the corpus spongiosum. The patient complains of pain and swelling at the site of the abscess, and, if the swelling is submucosal, there may be some disturbance of micturition. Infiltration of the corpus spongiosum may lead to painful erections with ventral angulation of the penis (chordee). On examination there is a tender swelling, at first firm but later fluctuant. The most likely sites are the fossa navicularis and the bulb. From the fossa navicularis the abscess may point in the region of the frenum, giving rise to a deep-seated, tender nodule with much oedematous swelling of the surrounding tissue. When in the bulb, the abscess may point on the skin surface at the root of the penis, or at the upper part of the scrotum. The overlying skin may be involved and become adherent and reddened. The abscess breaks down to form a sinus discharging pus, in which it may, or may not, be possible to find the gonococcus. Urinary fistula has resulted occasionally and this is more likely if the condition is treated by free incision and drainage rather than by aspiration. Like most other acute complications this manifestation has practically disappeared as the result of modern methods of treatment (see Fig. 109, p. 202).

COWPER'S DUCTS AND GLANDS (see Fig. 114, p. 211)

If gonococcal infection involves the ducts of Cowper's glands without spreading to the glands, there are no additional symptoms to attract the patient's attention, but if infection reaches the glands there is likely to be abscess formation. The patient complains of aching or throbbing pain in the perineum with a sense of fullness and heat; and there may also be pain on defaecation and added frequency of micturition. His temperature may be 37·5° or 38·5°C. Acute retention of urine due to irritative spasm of the compressor urethrae muscle is not uncommon. Cowperitis may also be associated with a pre-existing stricture distal to the openings of the ducts. The abscess usually points in the perineum, but may track for some distance before reaching the surface. The condition is almost always unilateral and is detected by rectal examination with the forefinger in the rectum and the thumb on the perineum, a procedure which must be performed with the greatest gentleness. By this means, the triangular ligament, between the layers of which the gland lies, is compressed between finger and thumb. Palpation on either side of the median raphe enables finger and thumb to be closely approximated on the non-infected side, but on the side of the abscess there is wide separation and acute tenderness on attempted pressure. Such an abscess is apt to be mistaken for a perianal or ischiorectal abscess due to unrelated causes, especially if the patient conceals the fact of his recent gonococcal infection.

THE PROSTATIC DUCTS AND THE PROSTATE GLAND

Infection of the ducts of the prostate gland is likely to occur in the course of gonococcal infection of the posterior urethra, but gives rise to no characteristic symptoms. If the infection spreads to the glandular acini the condition may remain symptomless, or it may give rise to symptoms and signs suggesting acute prostatitis. In less severe cases, the parenchyma of the prostate only is involved; but if the infection is more severe the process may extend to the interstitial tissues. If one or more ducts become blocked, the patient is likely to develop a prostatic abscess.

Acute prostatitis due to this infection is now very rare. Following the evidence of spread of infection to the posterior urethra the patient begins to complain of general malaise, perineal aching and, perhaps, suprapubic discomfort. On examination he may have a temperature of 38° or 39°C. On rectal examination the prostate is tender, swollen and indurated. Involvement may be limited to one lateral lobe or both may be affected. The condition may subside under treatment, in which case residual chronic prostatitis may remain, or it may progress to form a prostatic abscess.

Prostatic abscess. With abscess-formation, the symptoms of acute prostatitis become more severe, with increased frequency, terminal dysuria, pain in the perineum, suprapubic pain and rectal discomfort. The patient may complain of pain on defaecation and perhaps of rectal tenesmus. Acute retention of urine may ensue, due to spasm of the compressor urethrae muscle. The urethral discharge may lessen in amount or may temporarily cease. The patient is ill, with headache, malaise, and fever which may reach 40°C. Rectal examination reveals a large, tense and very tender swelling which bulges into the rectum and rises into the pelvis. In some cases it may seem to fill the whole pelvis. With or without treatment, such an abscess is likely to open into the posterior urethra with profuse discharge of pus per urethram and prompt relief of symptoms. Occasionally it opens into the rectum with resulting gonococcal proctitis (Plate IV, ii, right). In other cases the pus may track in various directions and then usually forms an abscess which opens on the skin surface, in the perineum or elsewhere.

COMMON EJACULATORY DUCTS AND SEMINAL VESICLES

Acute infection of the common ejaculatory ducts extending to the seminal vesicles may occur in acute posterior urethritis, and is then almost always associated with acute prostatitis. Acute infection of the seminal vesicles is likely to invade the whole thickness of the wall and extend to the perivesicular tissue, causing the vesicle to become adherent to the upper surface of the prostate. Rarely the common ejaculatory duct or the seminal duct has been known to become blocked, and to give rise to abscess formation in the seminal vesicle. The symptoms and signs of acute infection of the seminal vesicles are those of the associated acute posterior urethritis and prostatitis. High fever and urgency of micturition are common. The association of acute vesiculitis and terminal haematuria used to be common, and it was even suggested that such haematuria in the course of gonococcal infection was pathognomonic of acute infection of the seminal vesicles. The probable truth is that the passing of blood is an indication of severe infection in which, in the absence of prompt and effective treatment, involvement of all the structures communicating with the posterior urethra is almost certain. Occasionally, in such cases, the semen is bloodstained, and there may be frequent erections and ejaculations. If rectal examination is done—a procedure which requires the utmost care and gentleness in the acute stage—one or both seminal vesicles may be felt as elongated, swollen, sausage-shaped masses extending upwards and outwards from the centre of the upper border of the prostate. They may be extremely tender and, exceptionally, it may be possible to palpate the distended ampullae of the vasa deferentia medial to them. More commonly the borders of the vesicular swellings are ill-defined and indistinguishable from the enlarged and indurated prostate to which they are firmly adherent. It used to be thought that acute infection of the seminal vesicles was particularly likely to be followed by acute metastatic complications of gonorrhoea, such as arthritis, tenosynovitis, 'rheumatism' and anterior uveitis. It is impossible to give a judgment on this point now because acute vesiculitis is, for practical purposes, no longer seen and because, in the past, there was no clear distinction between the metastatic complications of gonorrhoea and those due to associated Reiter's disease.

VASA DEFERENTIA AND THE EPIDIDYMES (see Fig. 113, p. 211)

Once a common complication of gonorrhoea, epididymitis is now seen less often occurring in about 1 per cent of cases. How infection reaches the epididymis from the urethra is an open question. There is not much to suggest infection by the blood stream, but some have thought that infection occurs by lymphatic spread or by surface continuity along the mucous membrane of the vas deferens. The most generally accepted view is that of Pelouze, who believed that infection occurred as the result of the retro-grade passage of infected urine from the urethra along the lumen of the vas deferens to the epididymis. The onset of the condition used, commonly, to be determined by trauma or increase in pressure in the posterior urethra resulting from mismanagement of treatment or from the patient's indiscretions. Thus, excessive pressure in urethrovesical irrigations, too frequent irrigations, or the use of irrigating fluid which was too hot or too strong sometimes resulted in epididymitis. Similarly, prostatic massage or urethral instrumentation applied too vigorously or too early might produce the same effect. Sexual or alcoholic indulgence or vigorous exercise with the bladder full were also determining causes. The condition is usually unilateral, but if both sides are involved affection of one side precedes that of the other. Usually the first complaint is of pain and tenderness at the lower pole of the epididymis on the affected side. Occasionally the initial pain is felt along the course of the vas deferens, which may give rise to abdominal symptoms. If the pain is right-sided it may simulate appendicitis. In other cases the pain and tenderness affect the vas deferens in the spermatic cord above the epididymis. As the condition progresses, the pain becomes more intense and may be agonizing. It may involve the whole epididymis and spread up into the spermatic cord, the whole area being acutely tender. The patient's temperature is raised to 38 to 40°C. Headache and malaise are associated. If the patient has symptoms of acute urethritis they may be relieved at the onset of epididymitis and the urethral discharge may diminish in amount and even cease temporarily. On examination the corresponding side of the scrotum is swollen and reddened. There may be oedema of the overlying skin. On palpation, the globus minor and perhaps the whole epididymis is swollen, infiltrated and exquisitely tender. There is likely to be an associated hydrocele of the tunica vaginalis; this obscures the body of the testis and because of its tenseness may be mistaken for enlargement of the testis. Abscess formation with discharge of pus on the surface is rare. On recovery there is usually residual fibrous thickening of the globus minor. Blockage of the lumen of the epididymis is almost certain, and if the condition is bilateral the patient will almost certainly be sterile.

CHRONIC GONORRHOEA

It is open to question whether chronic gonorrhoea in males now truly exists in the respect that there are chronic inflammatory processes due to the activity of the gonococcus. There are sequelae which may follow acute gonorrhoea if treatment is neglected in the early stages, or if the case is one which proves refractory to treatment. In these cases it is rare to find the gonococcus and the sequelae cannot be differentiated from those which frequently follow non-gonococcal urethritis. There is reason to suppose that an appreciable number of patients who contract gonorrhoea contract at the same time 'non-specific urethritis'. The modern tendency is to attribute most of the sequelae of treated gonorrhoea to associated infection of this kind. Nevertheless, even now there is evidence that gonorrhoea may persist in asymptomatic form, as shown by the fact that some patients who have apparently responded well to treatment of acute gonorrhoea with antibiotics relapse within a few days or a few weeks. Of course, many of these patients will have been reinfected, but in some cases reinfection seems unlikely.

Sequelae

The sequelae may take various forms.

CHRONIC LITTRITIS may remain after the subsidence of follicular abscesses in the urethral wall. On palpation of the urethral wall over a straight sound, these areas may be palpated as small, firm nodules. In such cases the first glass of urine in the two-glass test is likely to contain some pus threads. On urethroscopy, the openings of the ducts may be seen to pout and to show reddening.

SOFT INFILTRATION OF URETHRAL WALL. If the subepithelial tissues of the urethra have been severely involved there may be soft infiltration of the urethral wall. On urethroscopy, such an area may be detected by the pale, smooth appearance of the overlying mucous membrane with surrounding hyperaemia. The affected tissues show faulty dilatation with gentle air insufflation.

FIBROUS STRICTURE. At a later stage fibrous stricture may be present (Figs. 111 and 112), and in such a case the mucous membrane of the affected area is white and bloodless and shows irregularity of the surface on air distension, varying in degree according to the extent of the lesion. In severe cases of long standing there may be gross narrowing of the canal. Leucoplakia of the mucous membrane is seen occasionally, usually in association with long-standing stricture. The normal urethra frequently shows a number of semilunar folds; these are distinguishable from strictures by the normal pink colour and softness of the mucosa and the fact that they offer no resistance to the passage of an instrument. Sometimes there is obvious cystic dilatation of a common opening of Cowper's ducts on the floor of the urethra, the orifice revealing a large cavity or being seen as a pouch with a narrow, bloodless margin, which may resemble a fibrous stricture. Such a condition is sometimes thought to be due to inflammatory changes but is almost always the result of congenital abnormality. Infection may, of course, be superimposed. Stricture formation may involve only part of the urethral circumference at any point, or it may be annular. If the annular type of stricture is strictly localized it forms a 'diaphragmatic stricture', but if it affects a segment of the urethral wall it forms a 'tubular stricture'. Stricture is most commonly found in the bulb, but it may be near the meatus or in other parts of the penile urethra. In the presence of a narrow tubular stricture or multiple strictures the urethroscope tube is unlikely to pass beyond the distal extremity of stricture formation. If more detailed information is thought to be expedient it may be obtained by a urethrogram. If the patient has suffered from a periurethral abscess which has opened on the surface, there will be localized thickening and scarring at the site of the abscess and, if there is a urethral stricture distal to the area of abscess

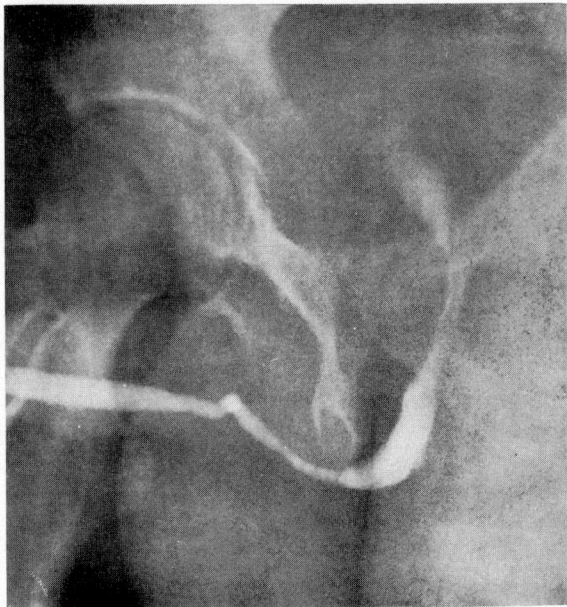
Fig. 111. Gonorrhoea (male): urethral stricture (urethrogram).

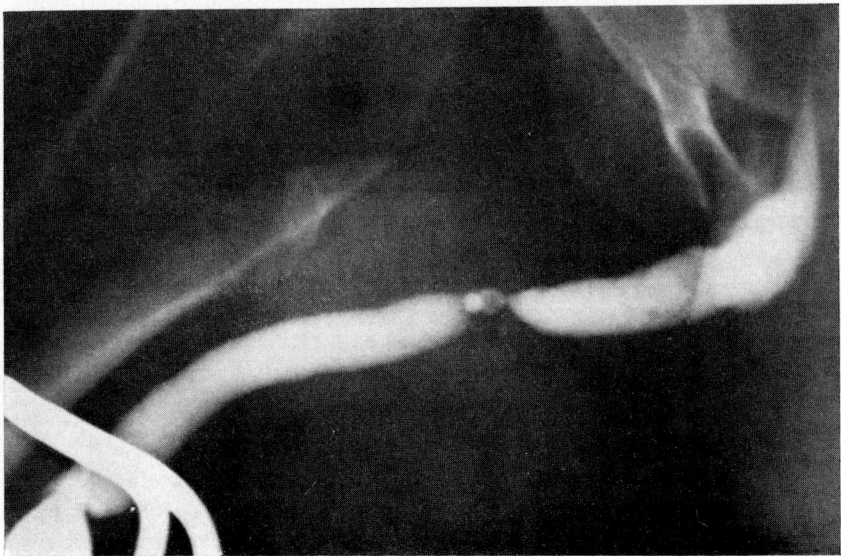
Fig. 112. Gonorrhoea (male): urethral stricture (urethrogram).

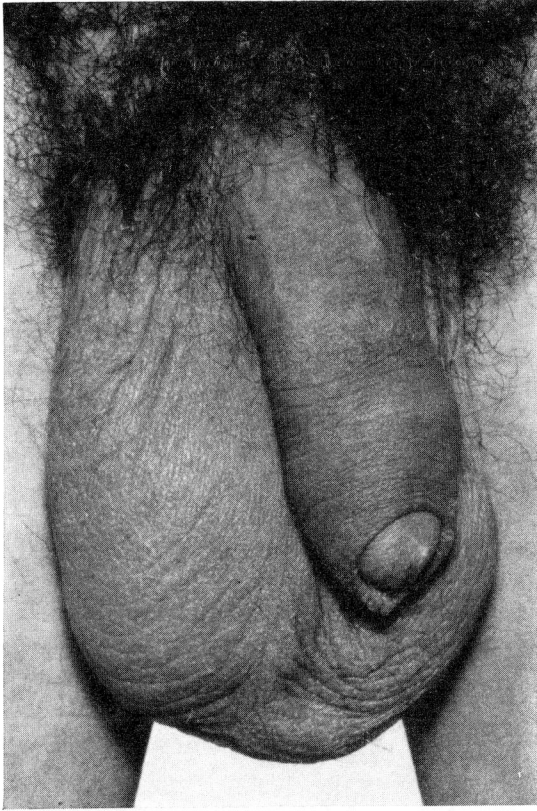

Fig. 113. Gonorrhoea
(male): right
epididymitis.

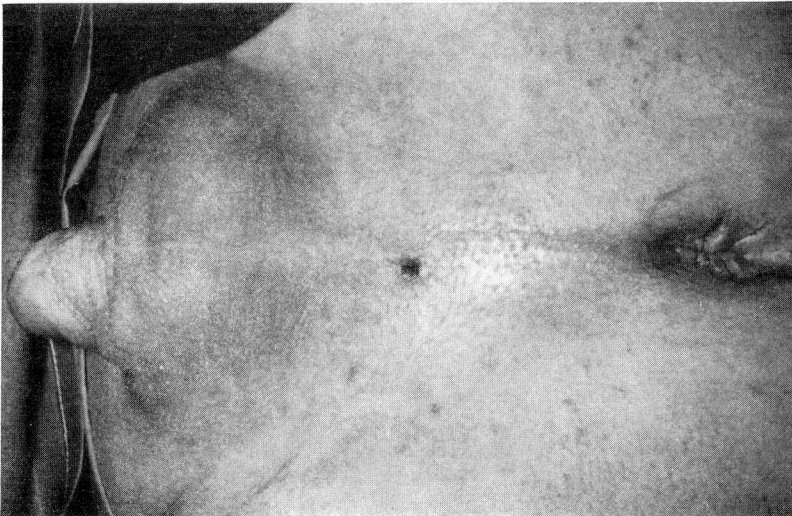

Fig. 114. Gonorrhoea (male): abscess of right Cowper's gland
discharging through sinus in perineum.

formation, there may be a persistent urinary fistula or multiple fistulae (see Fig. 110, p. 202).

CHRONIC COWPERITIS. Chronic inflammation of Cowper's gland is found occasionally. The patient may complain of morning discharge and aching pain or feeling of weight in the perineum. On microscopical examination the discharge is found to consist of mucus with polymorphonuclear leucocytes, secondary organisms and epithelial cells. The morning urine contains mucus and purulent threads. On rectal examination with the forefinger below the prostate and the corresponding thumb on the perineum, it may be possible to feel one or both glands at the side of the median raphe. In size the infected gland varies from that of a small pea to that of a chestnut, and on pressure there may be considerable tenderness. It is not always possible to distinguish the outline of the gland, but the fact that it is infected may be deduced from the abnormally wide separation of thumb and forefinger and from the tenderness on pressure. Persistent symptoms due to this cause may be wrongly attributed to chronic prostatitis.

CHRONIC PROSTATITIS is the commonest sequela of urethral infection of any kind. Owing to modern methods of treatment it is considerably less common after acute gonorrhoea than it used to be. It will be considered in detail as a complication of non-gonococcal urethritis (see pp. 280 and 284).

CHRONIC SEMINAL VESICULITIS is fairly commonly associated with chronic prostatitis. Symptoms may be absent or may be identical with those of chronic prostatitis. Morning 'gleet' may be present, and there may be frequent seminal emissions. The patient may also complain of painful erections. On palpation, the walls of one or both vesicles may be slightly thickened, but the outlines of the organs are easily distinguishable. In other cases there may be marked induration at the sites of the vesicles, but the outlines are not detectable owing to chronic perivesicular inflammation. Microscopical examination of the contents of the vesicles expressed by digital massage in cases in which the ducts are not blocked shows numbers of polymorphonuclear leucocytes and granular debris, with spermatozoa, surrounded by structureless mucinous material. The spermatozoa are sometimes absent, or relatively few in number, and frequently show degenerative changes.

CHRONIC EPIDIDYMITIS may persist after an acute attack. There is palpable nodular thickening of variable extent affecting, in most cases, the globus minor. This may be a purely fibrous nodule, the end result of an inflammatory process which has terminated; or it may indicate the persistence of a chronic inflammatory condition. Such a nodule may be symptomless, although the patient is usually aware of its presence. Sometimes it gives rise to continuous or intermittent pain of an aching character. Occasionally there may be subacute exacerbations of epididymitis, giving rise to local pain, swelling and tenderness. Other symptoms are those of associated chronic prostatitis and vesiculitis, and signs of these conditions are usually to be found.

REFERENCES

1. PARISER, H., FARMER, A. D. and MARINO, A. F. (1964) Sth. med. J. (Bgham, Ala.), **57**, 688.
2. HANDSFIELD, H. H., LIPMAN, T. O., HARNISCH, J. P., TRONCA, E. and HOLMES, K. K. (1974) New Engl. J. Med., **290**, 117.
3. CRAWFORD, G., KNAPP, J. S., HALE, J. and HOLMES, K. K. (1977) Science, **196**, 1352.
4. KNAPP, J. S., THORNSBERRY, C., SCHOOLNIK, G. A., WIESNER, P. J., HOLMES, K. K. and THE COOPERATIVE STUDY GROUP (1978) J. infect. Dis., **138**, 160.
5. HEIN, K., MARKS, A. and COHEN, M. I. (1977) J. Pediat., **90**, 634.

14

Gonorrhoea in the Female

ACUTE GONORRHOEA

Sites of Infection

The common sites of gonococcal infection of the female genital tract are the urethra and the cervix uteri. The anorectum is also involved in about half the cases and occasionally is the only site where infection is found (vide Chapter 15). Urethral infection invariably spreads to the small urethral glands, but the bladder is affected much less often. Periurethral infection is rare, but occasionally a large periurethral abscess may bulge through the anterior vaginal wall. After puberty the vaginal mucous membrane seems resistant to this infection but it is an open question whether gonococcal vaginitis occurs in the vaginal fornices. Sometimes the mucous membrane in this area is reddened and bathed in pus from which the gonococcus can be grown. Whether this indicates local gonococcal infection or the presence of infectious secretion from the cervix is uncertain; but it is also true that the gonococcus can be found in secretion from the vaginal vault of a pre-menopausal patient who has undergone hysterectomy.[1] In from a third to one-half of cases there is associated trichomonal vaginitis, which is responsible for the redness of the vaginal wall and purulent secretion and may sometimes render the accurate diagnosis of gonorrhoea more difficult.

The cervix shows endocervicitis which results in infection of the cervical glands. As a sequela of this infection blocking of the gland ducts may result in the formation of chronically infected retention cysts, the so-called follicles of Naboth, which may be seen on the vaginal portion of the cervix. Spread of infection from the cervix to the Fallopian tubes probably occurs by extension over the surface of the endometrium, although lymphatic spread is possible. In the puerperium the gonococcus may spread directly through the uterine wall at the site of the placental attachment, to cause parametritis. Once infection has reached the Fallopian tubes, both of which may be involved, the organism invades the lining epithelium and spreads to the submucosa. The cavity of the tube is filled with pus, and pus oozes from the fimbriated extremity. The serous surface of the tube is covered with exudate. Gonococcal salpingitis may lead to various other pelvic complications. The fimbriated end of the tube may become blocked and the tube becomes distended with pus, the condition known as pyosalpinx. The pus which has exuded from the tubes produces pelvic peritonitis; this occasionally spreads to cause general peritonitis, or a pelvic abscess may form in the pouch of Douglas. Occasionally pus from the fimbriated end of the tube infects a ruptured ovarian follicle. The tube becomes adherent to the ovary, the central area of which quickly breaks down to produce a tubo-ovarian abscess. The exudate covering the serous surfaces soon organizes and there may be fibrous adhesions between pelvic organs and intestines. In the absence of treatment, and sometimes in spite of treatment, pelvic infection is likely to have permanent residual effects. The gonococcus soon disappears from the secretions and pus is replaced by clear fluid of low protein content, producing either a hydrosalpinx or a tubo-ovarian cyst; the adhesions contract further and rarely fibrous bands may constrict the small intestine, leading to intestinal obstruction. If both tubes are blocked the patient will be sterile. Damage to the lining membrane of patent tubes increases the risk of ectopic pregnancy.

Clinical Characteristics of the Uncomplicated Infection

Symptoms are absent or insufficient to attract the patient's attention in about 50 per cent of cases of uncomplicated gonorrhoea in the female.[2] The majority of infected women attending for diagnosis and treatment do so because their male contacts have developed gonorrhoea;[3] others may attend because of symptoms due to associated infestation with *Trichomonas vaginalis*.

URETHRITIS

The main symptom is dysuria, described by the patient as a scalding or burning pain when passing water. Women, unlike men, do not usually notice urethral discharge. Appreciable vaginal discharge is unlikely unless the cervicitis is very severe or there is associated trichomonal infestation. On examination, after cleansing the vulva, it may be possible to massage a yellow purulent discharge from the urethral orifice by pressing the gloved finger from above downwards on to the urethra through the anterior vaginal wall. For this part of the examination it is important that urine should not have been passed for two to three hours; even so, urethritis may not be obvious. The external urinary meatus may be reddened with oedematous lips, but this is the exception rather than the rule.

CERVICITIS

Cervicitis is often symptomless, but patients may complain of low backache or of a vague feeling of lower abdominal discomfort. In severe cases, profuse, purulent cervical secretion may cause the patient to complain of vaginal discharge. On examination, using a Cusco bi-valve speculum, cloudy mucoid, mucopurulent or purulent cervical secretion is seen flowing from the external os. The infected cervical secretion varies in appearance and may sometimes look like normal clear mucus (see Plate IV, ii). There may be reddening around the external os and the area of mucous membrane may sometimes show 'acute erosion' with bright red erythema and oedema. Such appearances are not, of course, distinctive of gonococcal infection and in many cases the appearances are normal or show only a simple non-inflammatory erosion.

PROCTITIS
This is described on p. 226.

Local Complications
The following are possible sites of local complications in females: (a) Skene's glands, (b) Bartholin's glands, (c) vulva, (d) bladder, and (e) pelvic organs.

SKENITIS
The two small paraurethral glands of Skene lie one on each side of the terminal 2 cm of the urethra, and the ducts open beside or just inside the urinary meatus. When the glands are infected a small bead of pus may be expressed from the duct by massage, as described in examination for urethritis. Sometimes a small abscess forms in one of these glands and it may be felt through the anterior vaginal wall as a small indurated mass to one or other side of the terminal urethra. Other forms of periurethral abscess are rare (Fig. 115).

BARTHOLINITIS
The glands of Bartholin lie in the lower third of each labium majus and the ducts open on the inner surface of each labium minus at the junction of the lower and middle third. The duct becomes infected and from it infection may extend to the gland. The patient complains of pain accompanied by tenderness and swelling, or of an 'abscess down below', causing difficulty in walking (Fig. 116). On inspection there is marked swelling and forward projection of the vulva on the affected side, and an inflammatory mass with reddening of the overlying skin is found in the lower part of the labium majus. On gentle palpation, with the thumb on the outer surface of the labium majus and the index finger in the vaginal introitus, the extent of the swelling and tenderness is evident, and gentle pressure may express a small bead of pus from the duct opening. This may not be possible, if, as often happens, the duct is blocked by the inflammation. If the condition

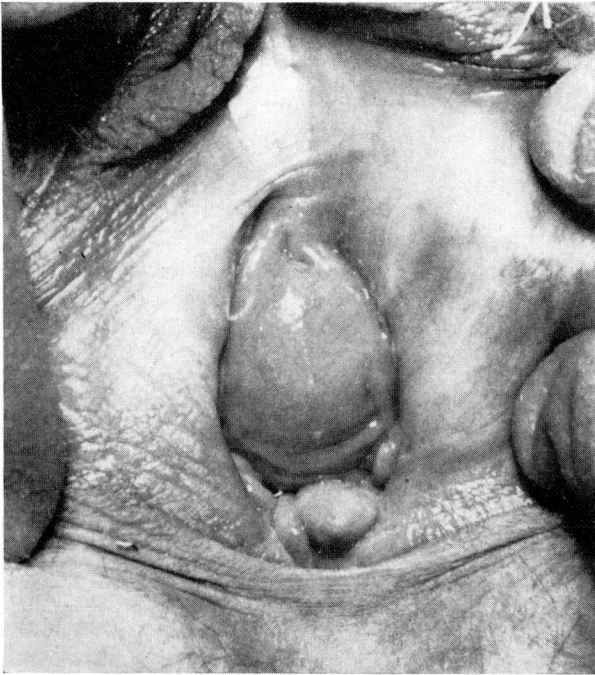

Fig. 115. Gonorrhoea (female): urethritis with periurethral abscess.

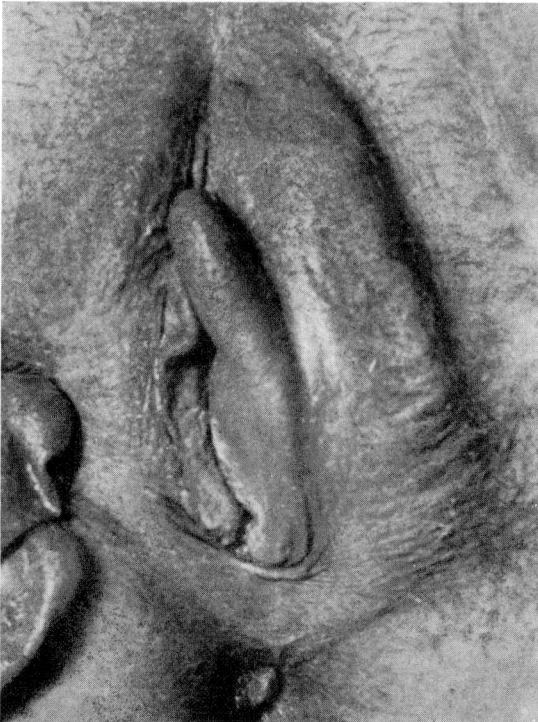

Fig. 116. Gonorrhoea (female): Bartholin's abscess with vulval oedema.

has progressed to abscess formation, fluctuation of the mass will be felt. The abscess may have opened through the mucous membrane of the inner surface of the labium minus or, occasionally, on the outer surface of the labium majus.

VULVITIS

Acute vulvitis due to gonorrhoea is rare in adults. On inspection the labia may be grossly oedematous with pus oozing from between the labia minora. There may be intertrigo and excoriation of thighs and groins. Its presence is more likely to suggest associated trichomonal infestation or infection with *Candida albicans*. The patient complains of marked discomfort and swelling of the vulva which is worse on movement. If *Candida albicans* is present there may be vulval irritation which is sometimes intense.

CYSTITIS

Mild trigonitis is not uncommon, in which case the patient will complain of some urinary frequency. On the other hand severe cystitis with marked frequency, strangury and terminal haematuria is rare. Infection of the upper urinary tract is very rare.

PELVIC INFECTION

When a patient is found to be suffering from symptoms and signs suggesting pelvic infection, the first step in diagnosis is to examine likely sites of gonococcal infection and to establish or exclude the presence of such infection by appropriate laboratory tests.

A patient with gonococcal infection of pelvic organs is likely to present with acute lower abdominal pain of a spasmodic type, which may have begun a day or two after her last menstrual period. She complains of nausea and may have vomited; she may complain of anorexia and headache. If there have been attacks of similar pain over a period of weeks or months, the patient may complain of menorrhagia and dysmenorrhoea of the congestive type; she may also complain of dyspareunia. On examination there may be localized tenderness in either or both iliac fossae on deep palpation; if the tenderness is marked there may also be some lower abdominal guarding and rigidity. Signs of generalized peritonitis are rare. On bimanual pelvic examination there is pain on moving the cervix and marked tenderness in either or both lateral fornices. Sometimes the symptoms and signs are minimal.[4]

The patient usually has fever but the temperature is rarely above 39°C; the pulse rate may be increased. Blood examination may show a polymorphonuclear leucocytosis of varying degree. The erythrocyte sedimentation rate is often raised. There may be a microcytic type of anaemia if there has been menorrhagia. The complement-fixation test for gonorrhoea is often, but not invariably, positive.

When the patient has salpingitis it may not be possible to feel a definite mass in the lateral vaginal fornix of the affected side, but if a pyosalpinx has developed, a tender fluctuant mass is palpable. Infection of the parametrium should be suspected when gonorrhoea is diagnosed in the puerperium; then a wedge-shaped, tender mass may be felt to extend outwards from the side of the uterus to the pelvic wall. When the ovary is involved a large, tender and fluctuant tubo-ovarian abscess may be felt in the lateral fornix. The presence of a tender, boggy mass in the pouch of Douglas suggests a pelvic abscess. The presence of pelvic peritonitis is judged from the degree of systemic reaction and from the presence of lower abdominal rigidity and the sign of 'rebound tenderness'. Perihepatitis may be associated (see p. 223) and may be more frequent than has been supposed.[5]

It is often very difficult to differentiate between the various types of gonococcal pelvic inflammation, and bimanual examination under general anaesthesia may sometimes be necessary. When material is obtained from the pelvic organs at operation or laparoscopy or by culdocentesis, the gonococcus may be isolated in less than half the cases with proven cervical infection.[6,7] Associated chlamydial infection or secondary infection by aerobic and anaerobic organisms of the normal vaginal flora[7,8] may play a part in the patient's condition.

CHRONIC GONORRHOEA

This condition is always difficult to diagnose because in the course of time, in untreated cases, the gonococcus tends to disappear from the secretions; if the organism cannot be isolated in smear or culture, the signs and symptoms cannot be distinguished from those of non-gonococcal infection of the genital tract. Some presumptive evidence may be obtained either from a definite past history of gonorrhoea in the patient or her male consort, or from a positive complement-fixation test for gonorrhoea. It should be emphasized that such a positive test is not alone sufficient to warrant a diagnosis of gonorrhoea. Strong support for the diagnosis may occasionally be obtained by evidence that she has recently infected a male partner, but too much reliance should not be placed upon histories with problems of this kind in which both partners may be seeking to apportion blame. As with male patients, diagnosis in the chronic stage is complicated by the fact that the patient may have contracted non-gonococcal infection at the same time as gonorrhoea.

Patients complain of few symptoms, although they may have chronic backache. The most likely residual signs are those of chronic cervicitis with granular erosion, mucopurulent secretion and perhaps retention cysts of the cervix (Nabothian follicles). Erosion, however, is a common finding in otherwise healthy women, particularly those taking oral contraceptives.

Mild chronic urethritis, skenitis or proctitis may also be present. There may be cystic swelling of a Bartholin's gland. Some of these patients have recurrent acute or subacute attacks of bartholinitis or Bartholin's abscess, a condition which is very likely to recur unless the gland is excised or 'marsupialized' (see p. 246) as soon as the acute attack is subsiding. Removal between attacks is usually not feasible because the gland is no more than a fibrotic remnant which cannot easily be identified. Fluid obtained from the gland during a recurring attack does not contain the gonococcus and it is likely that the recurring condition is really due to non-gonococcal infection. Chronic trichomonal vaginitis is sometimes associated with these various manifestations. Urethral stricture formation in the female is very rare.

The after-effects of untreated gonococcal pelvic infection cause much chronic invalidism in women, who tend to get recurrent attacks of salpingitis with lower abdominal pain and low-grade pyrexia. Dyspareunia, dysmenorrhoea, irregularities of the menstrual cycle and menorrhagia are common. The latter may lead to chronic microcytic hypochromic anaemia. These women suffer from chronic ill-health and may become depressed and embittered with life. Patients who have had bilateral salpingitis may be sterile as a result of loss of tubal patency; this is particularly likely after multiple attacks.[9] For those in whom the tube remains patent there is an increased risk of ectopic pregnancy. On examination there may be lower abdominal tenderness; bimanual examination often reveals that the cervix is pulled to one side by fibrous adhesions and the uterus may be bound down in a retroverted position. The cystic masses of chronic hydrosalpinx or of chronic tubo-ovarian cyst may be felt in one or both lateral fornices. Laparoscopy may aid in accurate diagnosis.

REFERENCES

1. JUDSON, F. N. and RUDER, M. A. (1979) Br. J. vener. Dis., 55, 434.
2. NICOL, C. S. (1948) Br. J. vener. Dis., 24, 26.
3. DUNLOP, E. M. C. (1963) Br. J. vener. Dis., 39, 109.
4. SPARKS, R. A. and DAVIES, A. J. (1976) Br. J. vener. Dis., 52, 178.
5. LITT, I. F. and COHEN, M. I. (1978) J. Am. med. Ass., 240, 1253.
6. THOMPSON, S. E. and HAGER, D. (1977) Sex. transm. Dis., 4, 105.
7. ESCHENBACH, D. A., BUCHANAN, T. M., POLLOCK, H. M., FORSYTH, P. S., ALEXANDER, E. R., LIN, J-S., WANG, S-P., WENTWORTH, B. B., McCORMACK, W. M. and HOLMES, K. K. (1975) New Engl. J. Med., 293, 166.
8. CHOW, A. W., PATTEN, V. and MARSHALL, J. R. (1979) Am. J. Obstet. Gynec., 133, 362.
9. WESTRÖM, L. (1975) Am. J. Obstet. Gynec., 121, 707.

15

Metastatic Gonorrhoea; Oropharyngeal Gonorrhoea; Proctitis; Conjunctivitis

METASTATIC GONORRHOEA

The literature of the past contains many reports of haematogenous spread of gonorrhoea to sites remote from the focus of infection. The metastatic complications described include arthritis, anterior uveitis, meningitis, endocarditis, myocarditis, pericarditis, hepatitis and perihepatitis.

Gonococcal Arthritis

True gonococcal arthritis is a purulent arthritis leading to destruction of the articular surfaces of the joint and resulting in ankylosis. This is now uncommon to the point of rarity, but it was probably more common in the past when methods of treatment were less satisfactory and more traumatic. The past incidence is uncertain as it is now believed that arthritis in the male occurring in association with gonococcal urethritis is most often due to associated Reiter's disease, and not to the gonococcus.[1] The diagnosis of gonococcal arthritis is now unlikely to be acceptable unless the gonococcus can be isolated from the joint fluid, but in times past arthritis occurring in a patient with gonorrhoea was generally assumed to be gonococcal. The clinical picture of true gonococcal arthritis is usually that of involvement of a large joint, often of an upper limb and now more commonly in a female, with onset in the third or fourth week of the infection. The condition presents acutely, with high fever, and severe pain in the affected joint, much increased by attempted movement. The skin overlying the joint is hot and red and there is swelling which outlines the synovial cavity. Aspiration produces thick, purulent material in which the gonococcus can be seen by smear and culture is positive. The joint surfaces are destroyed, and narrowing of the joint space, due to destruction of the cartilage, can be seen in X-rays taken at an early stage.

Gonococcal Septicaemia

There is, however, a form of gonococcal septicaemia which has been described on a number of occasions in recent years, but seldom by venere-ologists. It has been suggested[2,3] that there are two distinct syndromes resulting from the entry of the gonococcus into the blood stream. The first is a serious illness in which endocarditis is present and from which myo-carditis, pericarditis and meningitis[4] may follow; the second and more common presentation is a relatively benign condition in which bacteraemia is generally transient. It is more common in women than in men and characterized by intermittent fever, pain in joints and rashes. Pregnancy, particularly the second half, is a well-known precipitating factor; in the non-pregnant woman it is more likely to begin during or just after men-struation.[5] The rash usually appears at the onset of the condition; it may occur in crops and recur with each bout of fever. The lesions in the skin (Plate IV, iv) usually number between 5 and 20 and are widely distributed, tending to affect the distal parts of the limbs, particularly near joints. The lesions are discrete, from 1 mm to 2 cm in diameter, and begin as pinpoint erythematous macules, passing rapidly through papular, vesiculopustular and haemorrhagic stages. They can be seen in various stages of development and in some cases bullae can be found. The fully developed lesion is raised, slightly umbilicated, and its centre consists of dirty grey necrotic tissue with an irregular haemorrhagic border surrounded by erythema. In the early stages the lesions are tender but usually not painful. Healing occurs in three to four days, sometimes with residual brownish discoloration, but significant scarring is rare. Fever tends to be intermittent and to vary from 37·8° to 39·4°C. Sometimes it is absent. After an initial asymmetrical polyarthralgia most patients have objective evidence of periarticular or articular involve-ment, most often affecting two or three joints. The joints likely to be affected are the wrists, knees, ankles, elbows and small joints of the hands (Plate IV, iii). Tenosynovitis may be associated. There may be overt or laboratory evidence of involvement of the liver. The gonococcus is usually found in the genital tract, much less often in cultures of blood and of joint fluid and only very occasionally in cultures from skin lesions. However, using immunofluorescent staining methods gonococci can be demonstrated in material from skin lesions in the majority of cases.[6,7] Thus, in a number of reported cases the diagnosis has not been proved beyond question, but the clinical picture seems to be characteristic and conforms closely with that found in proven cases. The rash has to be distinguished from that of meningo-coccal septicaemia, *Moraxella* septicaemia and low-grade staphylococcal septicaemia, in which identical lesions may be found. Similar rashes have been described in association with gonococcal endocarditis and it is important to remember that any patient with gonococcal septicaemia is at risk from this complication.

The syndrome is rarely seen initially by venereologists,[8] perhaps because the genital infection is so often asymptomatic and the patient therefore presents in departments of rheumatology, dermatology, general medicine or units for infectious disease. In Seattle, U.S.A.,[9] disseminated gonococcal infection is the leading cause of acute arthritis in those aged 15 to 35 years.

There is evidence[10] that the organisms concerned have particular nutritional requirements for growth in culture and it has been suggested that the varying incidence of gonococcal septicaemia may be determined by the relative frequency of the 'AHU auxotype' in different areas. However, in some areas different auxotypes predominate in gonococcal septicaemia. The organisms are also resistant to the complement-dependent bactericidal action of normal human serum.[11] In addition to bacterial dissemination immune complexes have been found and may play a part in the pathogenesis of the disease.[12]

Patients with gonococcal septicaemia should be admitted to hospital. The condition is described as responding well to penicillin, which is usually given in large doses, and to other antibiotics effective against the gonococcus. Wolff et al.[13] gave 1 mega unit of benzyl penicillin intramuscularly every six hours for seven days, followed by phenoxymethylpenicillin by mouth, 500,000 units six-hourly for nine days. Oral penicillin cannot be relied upon. Good results have been obtained with ampicillin by mouth.[8] A suitable regimen would be an initial dose of 2 g together with 1 g of probenecid followed by 0·5 g of each every 6 hours for 10 days. Fortunately the strains of gonococci isolated from patients with gonococcal septicaemia are nearly always highly sensitive to penicillin.[14] In pregnancy the choice of drugs is limited; pregnant women who give a history of severe allergy to penicillin, so that cephalosporins are contra-indicated, may be given erythromycin for 10 days, preferably intravenously for the first three days (see p. 238).

Meningitis and endocarditis require high dose intravenous penicillin for up to four weeks. Chloramphenicol may be justified in the case of a patient with meningitis who has a history of serious allergic reaction to penicillin (see p. 237).

Gonococcal Perihepatitis

This condition, sometimes called the 'Fitz-Hugh–Curtis[15,16] syndrome', has been regarded as limited to females but a similar case was described in a man by Kimball and Knee.[17] Most cases in females are probably the result of direct extension from the pelvis to the perihepatic area, but some may arise from bacteraemia. Spread by way of retroperitoneal lymphatics has also been suggested.[17] Usually the patients give a history of pelvic inflammatory disease which may be recent or of some standing, but in some cases the pelvic infection has been asymptomatic. The onset may be sudden with pain in the right upper abdomen and sometimes in the right shoulder, increased by deep breathing, coughing or bending of the trunk. The patient has fever, nausea and sometimes vomiting. The area of abdominal pain is acutely tender and, if the presence of genital infection is not suspected, the findings may suggest acute cholecystitis or, perhaps, acute pyelonephritis, pleurisy, subphrenic abscess, renal calculus or even perforated peptic ulcer. Laboratory findings are not especially helpful. The erythrocyte sedimentation rate is likely to be raised. The gonococcal complement-fixation test may become positive. X-ray of the chest may show a small pleural effusion on the right. Genital examination is likely to show evidence of cervicitis and salpingitis with, perhaps, urethritis, and the gonococcus is likely to be found if antibiotics have not yet been given. As a residual effect so-called violin-string adhesions may occur between the surface of the liver and the anterior abdominal wall and the diaphragm. Lassus and Kousa[18] have described a case with an associated eruption characteristic of 'gonococcaemia' in which the gonococcus was cultured from urethra and cervix and from the blood. The condition responds well to penicillin. Lassus and Kousa gave 12 million units of benzyl penicillin intramuscularly daily for three days, followed by 2·4 million units of procaine penicillin daily for six days.

Anterior Uveitis and Iridocyclitis

Occurring in the course of gonococcal infection, or following in later years as a recurrent condition, anterior uveitis and iridocyclitis are now considered to be due to associated Reiter's disease, and it is open to question whether true metastatic gonococcal iritis ever occurs. If the complement-fixation test for gonorrhoea is positive in the blood serum in such a case, it indicates no more than the likelihood that the patient has suffered from gonorrhoea at some time or other in the past.

OROPHARYNGEAL GONORRHOEA

In the past gonococcal infection of the mouth and throat has been regarded as rare. There is good reason to believe that it is becoming more common.

Large series of cases have been reported from Denmark,[19] Norway,[20] Sweden[21] and the United States of America.[22] Among patients suffering from gonorrhoea the frequency of pharyngeal gonorrhoea was about 5 per cent in heterosexual males, 10 per cent in females and 20 per cent in homosexual males. Infections of the pharynx alone were found in all these series and cases of dissemination from this site have been noted.[19, 22] Pharyngeal infection has been reported from several other countries, including Holland,[23] Australia,[24] and the United Kingdom.[25, 26] A particularly high frequency of isolated pharyngeal infections has been found in pregnant women.[27, 28] Although acute pharyngitis or tonsillitis may occur symptoms have usually been slight or absent and there seem to be no characteristic features of the clinical condition. In fact, in many cases the mouth and throat appear normal. The organism has to be differentiated from the meningococcus and other members of the Neisserian group. Often response to standard treatment has been inadequate.[19-21, 23] The most suitable treatment for these cases has yet to be determined but single-dose regimens cannot be relied on, except perhaps 4·8 mega units of procaine penicillin intramuscularly with 1 g of probenecid by mouth.[22] A single injection of 4 g of spectinomycin gave poor results.[22] Bro-Jørgensen and Jensen[19] obtained good results with co-trimoxazole, 2 tablets three times daily for one week, Wiesner et al.[22] with tetracycline hydrochloride, 2 g daily for five days, and Hallqvist and Lindgren[21] with ampicillin, 1 g four times daily for three days, or cephalexin, 0·5 g four times daily for five days. Combining either of these last two regimens with probenecid, 0·5 g four times daily, should make them even more effective. In the United States of America, good results have been obtained by giving an initial dose of 3·5 g ampicillin and 1 g probenecid on the first day followed by 500 mg ampicillin four times a day on each of the succeeding two days.[29]

ANORECTAL GONORRHOEA

MALES

Gonococcal proctitis in males nearly always results from anal coitus in passive homosexuals. It has also occurred through the opening of a prostatic abscess or abscess of Cowper's gland into the anorectal lumen, and has been described as the result of accidental transference of infection on thermometers, enema nozzles and rubber gloves or finger stalls. In many cases the infection gives rise to no symptoms and the evidence of it is found on routine examination. Advice may be sought because of anal warts (see p. 362) or because a sexual partner has been infected with gonorrhoea. In a few cases the onset may be acute with the complaint of burning pain in the anorectum, tenesmus and pain on defaecation. There may be blood and mucopus in the stool. In other cases the onset is less acute, with the complaint of moisture or irritation round the anus. Perianal abscess, ischiorectal abscess or anal fissure are rarely found in association with this condition. On proctoscopy, the rectal wall may be red and oedematous and bleed easily. Pus, or mucopus, is usually evident on the surface of the rectum. There may be infiltration and rarely erosion of the mucous membrane. If ulceration is present concomitant herpes simplex infection or syphilis should be considered. In the less acute cases the signs of inflammation are fewer, but there are streaks of mucopus on the rectal wall and in the columns of Morgagni. In some cases, however, the naked-eye appearances are virtually normal, with minimal exudate. Diagnosis depends on identification of the gonococcus in smears from the secretion, and on isolation of the organism by culture. Cultures are fairly successful, but over-growth with organisms of the colon group is quite common. This can, however, be diminished by the use of Thayer–Martin selective medium (see p. 192). The gonococcal complement-fixation test is of little or no help in the diagnosis of this condition.

FEMALES

Involvement of the anorectal region is found in 30 to 60 per cent of females with gonorrhoea but usually it gives rise to no symptoms. In about 5 per cent it is the only site from which the organism is isolated. Patients sometimes complain of rectal discharge with discomfort on defaecation or of rectal bleeding. Proctitis is usually caused by a spread of infection from the genital tract. It is often due to flow of vaginal discharge or menstrual blood over the everted anal mucosa during defaecation, and infection of this area is, therefore, more likely in the presence of profuse discharge due to associated trichomonal vaginitis. Sometimes infection occurs as the result of anal coitus, and the patient should be asked a direct question to exclude this possibility when gonococcal proctitis has been diagnosed. On proctoscopy, frank pus or mucopus may be seen on the rectal wall (see Plate IV, ii, right) or on the surface of faecal masses. There may be oedema and reddening of the rectal mucosa, but ulceration is rare. As with males, if ulceration is present the possibility of concomitant herpes simplex infection, syphilis or lymphogranuloma venereum should be considered (see p. 260). In many cases the signs are minimal, the infection being diagnosed by routine culture.

GONOCOCCAL CONJUNCTIVITIS

This is rare in adults. It results from direct contamination of the eye with gonococcal pus by fingers or towels, and is therefore likely to be due to gross carelessness or lack of hygiene. The source of infection may be the patient's own genital tract or it may be transferred from a sexual partner. If the infection is recognized and treated promptly, full recovery is the rule, but in neglected cases corneal ulceration and panophthalmitis may result in blindness.

REFERENCES

1. HARKNESS, A. H. (1949) *Br. J. vener. Dis.*, **25**, 185.
2. ABU-NASSAR, H., HILL, N., FRED, H. L. and YOW, E. (1963) *Archs intern. Med.*, **112**, 731.
3. O'SULLIVAN, E. P. (1964) *Br. med. J.*, **1**, 1508.

4. SAYEED, Z. A., BHADURI, U., HOWELL, E. and MEYERS, H. L. (1972) *J. Am. med. Ass.*, **219**, 1730.

5. HOLMES, K. K., COUNTS, G. W. and BEATY, H. N. (1971) *Ann. intern. Med.*, **74**, 979.

6. BARR, J. and DANIELSSON, D. (1971) *Br. med. J.*, **1**, 482.

7. TRONCA, E., HANDSFIELD, H. H., WIESNER, P. J. and HOLMES, K. K. (1974) *J. infect. Dis.*, **129**, 583.

8. SEIFERT, M. H., WARIN, A. P. and MILLER, A. (1974) *Ann. rheum. Dis.*, **33**, 140.

9. HOLMES, K. K. (1977) *Asian. J. infect. Dis.*, **1**, 63.

10. KNAPP, J. S. and HOLMES, K. K. (1975) *J. infect. Dis.*, **132**, 204.

11. SCHOOLNIK, G. K., BUCHANAN, T. M. and HOLMES, K. K. (1976) *J. clin. Invest.*, **58**, 1163.

12. WALKER, F. C., AHLIN, T. D., TUNG, K. S. K. and WILLIAMS, R. C. (1978) *Ann. intern. Med.*, **89**, 28.

13. WOLFF, C. B., GOODMAN, H. V. and VAHRMAN, J. (1970) *Br. med. J.*, **2**, 271.

14. WIESNER, P. J., HANDSFIELD, H. H. and HOLMES, K. K. (1973) *New Engl. J. Med.*, **288**, 1221.

15. FITZ-HUGH, T. (1934) *J. Am. med. Ass.*, **102**, 2094.

16. CURTIS, A. H. (1930) *J. Am. med. Ass.*, **94**, 1221.

17. KIMBALL, M. W. and KNEE, S. (1970) *New Engl. J. Med.*, **282**, 1082.

18. LASSUS, A. and KOUSA, M. (1973) *Br. J. vener. Dis.*, **49**, 48.

19. BRO-JØRGENSEN, A. and JENSEN, T. (1973) *Br. J. vener. Dis.*, **49**, 491.

20. ÖDEGAARD, K. and GUNDERSEN, T. (1973) *Br. J. vener. Dis.*, **49**, 350.

21. HALLQVIST, L. and LINDGREN, S. (1975) *Br. J. vener. Dis.*, **51**, 395.

22. WIESNER, P. J., TRONCA, E., BONIN, P., PEDERSEN, A. H. B. and HOLMES, K. K. (1973) *New Engl. J. Med.*, **288**, 181.

23. STOLZ, E. and SCHULLER, J. L. (1974) *Br. J. vener. Dis.*, **50**, 104.

24. NEWNHAM, W. A., WALKER, W. R. and FOGARTY, P. (1975) *Med. J. Aust.*, **2**, 470.

25. McMILLAN, A. and YOUNG, H. (1978) *Sex. transm. Dis.*, **5**, 146.

26. SHAHIDULLAH, M. (1976) *Br. J. vener. Dis.*, **52**, 168.

27. CORMAN, L. C., LEVISON, M. E., KNIGHT, R., CARRINGTON, E. R. and KAYE, D. (1974) *J. Am. med. Ass.*, **230**, 568.

28. STUTZ, D. R., SPENCE, M. R. and DUANGMANI, C. (1976) *J. Am. vener. Dis. Ass.*, **3**, 65.

29. DICAPRIO, J. M., REYNOLDS, J., FRANK, G., CARBONE, J. and NISHIMURA, R. (1978) *J. Am. med. Ass.*, **239**, 1631.

16

Gonorrhoea in Children

GENITAL INFECTION

Genital gonorrhoea is relatively rare in children; it is much more often found in girls than in boys.

An infected boy may be brought by the parents because he has complained of dysuria, or because they have noticed signs of discharge on his under-clothes. Infection is usually accidental in families with poor standards of hygiene. It may have occurred at school, and the possibility of some kind of sexual contact must be considered. Complications of the urethritis are exceptional. Sexual assault may result in gonococcal proctitis.

In girls before the age of puberty the vaginal mucosa is more susceptible to gonococcal infection than that of the adult (see p. 187). Thus gonococcal infection usually presents as an acute vulvovaginitis.[1] The child may complain of soreness or of dysuria, but often advice is sought because the mother has noticed discharge on the child's underclothes. Rarely the condition is so mild that it goes unnoticed by both mother and child. The usual cause of infection is sharing a bed or bath towel or flannel with infected parents, but sometimes there is a history of sexual assault. Occasionally in the past there have been outbreaks of infection transmitted from one child to another by inadequate sterilization of thermometers, by toilet articles used in common or possibly even by freshly contaminated fingers, in hospital wards or children's homes.

On examination, the child is generally found to have an acute purulent vaginitis with some inflammation of the vulva, but sometimes the signs are minimal. It is usually very difficult to assess whether urethritis is also present; proctitis is not uncommon. Tests should be taken with a platinum loop or swab without the use of speculum or proctoscope. Complications of any kind are very unlikely, but response to treatment is not always as prompt and satisfactory as in the adult.

TREATMENT

Female children who are suffering from genital gonorrhoea may require to be admitted to hospital and isolated from other children. Nursing precautions must be taken against transference of infection. Immediate response to penicillin and other appropriate antibiotics is good. Treatment is that described for adults (see Chapter 17), with lesser dosage according to age and body weight. In some of these cases there is a tendency to relapse, and it is therefore advisable to continue with penicillin or ampicillin by mouth after the initial injection has been given.

OPHTHALMIA NEONATORUM

This was formerly the commonest cause of blindness in children. Now it is a relatively uncommon condition and, if promptly recognized and treated, causes no damage to sight. In 1914 it was made a notifiable disease in England and Wales under the Public Health (Ophthalmia Neonatorum) Regulation of that year. The law defines it as: 'A purulent discharge from the eyes of an infant starting within 21 days of birth.' Probably no more than 5 to 15 per cent of cases of ophthalmia neonatorum are now due to the gonococcus,[2] but this is the most dangerous cause as regards potential damage to the eye. In London chlamydial ophthalmia neonatorum may be over five times more common;[3] in Atlanta, Georgia, U.S.A.,[2] chlamydial infection was found to be twice as common, accounting for 28·5 per cent of cases, and there was reason to believe that the true frequency was appreciably greater.

PROPHYLAXIS

The principles of preventive treatment are: to cure the disease in the mother during pregnancy, or failing this to treat the mother in the early stages of labour, and to treat the child's eyes after delivery.

There is no doubt that the most effective method of prevention is to diagnose and treat the disease in the mother during pregnancy. Unfortunately the precaution of examining and testing for gonococcal infection is not generally observed in antenatal clinics. The need for this in areas where the prevalence of gonorrhoea is high has been shown by several workers. For example, in two studies in the United States of America[4,5] the infection was found in 5·7 per cent and 5·5 per cent of antenatal patients respectively. However, routine screening of antenatal patients in the United Kingdom has produced far fewer cases.[6,7]

The time-honoured procedure for prevention is Credé's method, which has two stages. The first is to wipe the eyelids and eyelashes of the infant free from pus or any organic matter with a swab, as soon as the head is born and before the eyes are opened. The second stage, which is carried out as soon as practicable after the child is born, consists in instilling one or two drops of antiseptic into each conjunctival sac. For many years the antiseptic of choice was 1 per cent silver nitrate, but certain organic silver preparations, namely Protargol 5 per cent and Argyrol 20 per cent, seem to have been less irritating and just as effective. In recent years the view has gained ground that conjunctival antiseptics are ineffective and potentially irritating, and that the second stage of Credé's method should not be employed for prophylaxis. Nevertheless silver nitrate is still used in some parts of the world with apparent success[2] and elsewhere antibiotics have been substituted. The recommended preparations include crystalline penicillin in concentration of 10,000 units to the millilitre, chlortetracycline solution 0·5 per cent, and erythromycin ointment 5 mg/g. Quaternary ammonium compounds (e.g. Desogen-Geigy, 0·5 per cent) have also been recommended and so have intramuscular injections of penicillin. The value of any of these procedures in prophylaxis is hard to assess.

It should be remembered that the gonococcus may be present in other sites. Gonococci have been isolated from material obtained by orogastric aspiration in newborn babies,[8] particularly where there has been early rupture of the membranes. All of the babies had had prophylaxis against ophthalmia neonatorum; none developed conjunctivitis, but many of them had evidence of sepsis, including pneumonia, although this was not proved to be gonococcal. The organism has also been recovered from the rectum and the external ear canal.

CLINICAL MANIFESTATIONS (Figs. 117 and 118)

The incubation period of gonococcal ophthalmia neonatorum is usually one to four days but can be as long as 13 days.[9] The affected eye becomes red and inflamed. The lids are swollen, and pus is seen oozing from between the lids. If the lids are parted, pus under pressure may spurt out; the inner surfaces of the lids are red and oedematous and there is considerable injection of the scleral conjunctiva. The eye is painful and there is marked photophobia. There may be enlargement of the pre-auricular nodes. If no treatment is given, the cornea becomes involved with cellular infiltration, oedema and ulceration. In severe cases the eye may be destroyed. If corneal ulceration occurs, some residual damage to sight is inevitable.

TREATMENT

Infants with gonococcal ophthalmia neonatorum should be admitted to hospital and treated without delay. They require isolation and special precautions to prevent transference of infection. If only one eye is affected, the other should be protected with a Buller's shield or pad and bandage. The conjunctivitis responds well to local instillations of crystalline penicillin in watery solution, in concentration of 10,000 units to the millilitre. Treatment should be immediate and intensive. Pus is swabbed away with moist pieces of cotton wool, and one or two drops of penicillin solution are instilled into the conjunctival sac every minute until the discharge has ceased, which may take anything from half an hour to three hours. An accepted routine is then to repeat the treatment every five minutes for half an hour, every half-hour for three hours, hourly for six hours and then every two hours for 24 to 48 hours. A much simpler method is to use drops

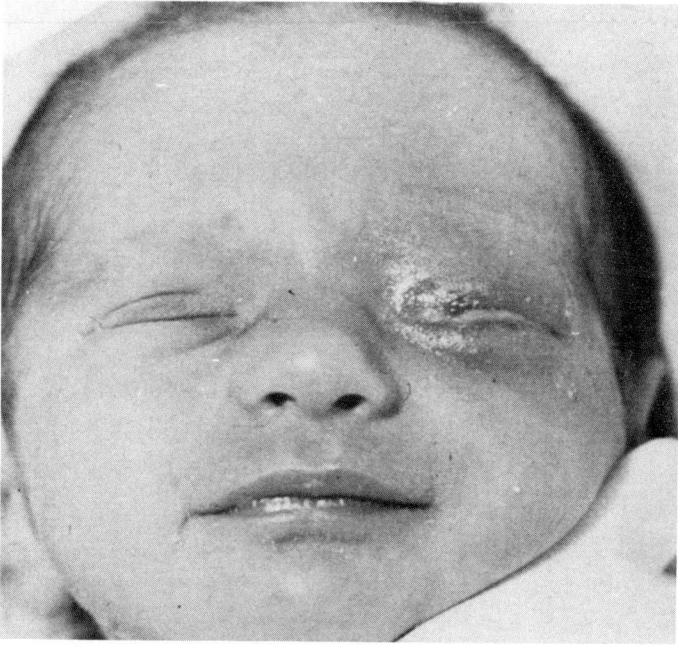

Fig. 117. Gonorrhoea: ophthalmia neonatorum.

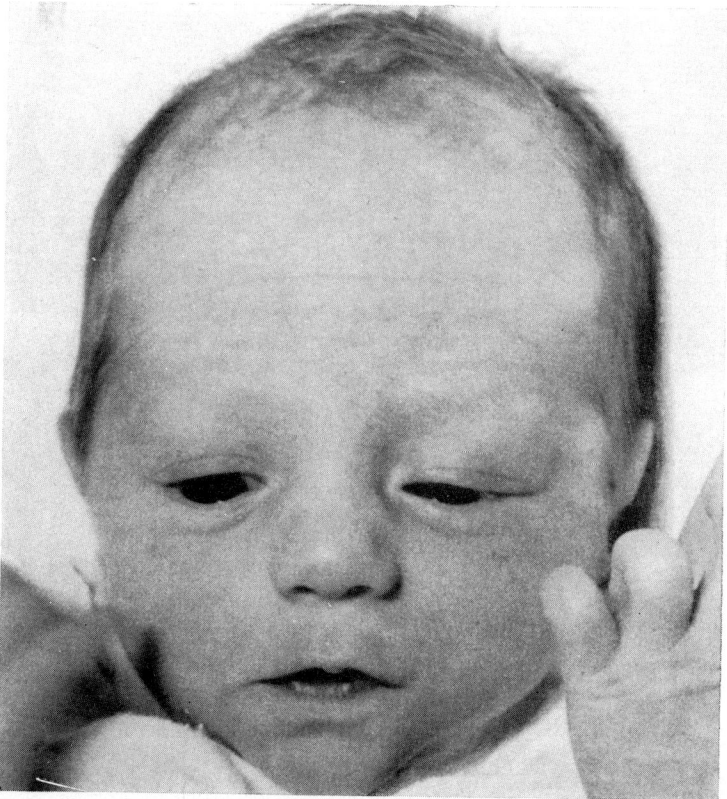

Fig. 118. Gonorrhoea: ophthalmia neonatorum—after treatment.

of crystalline penicillin in much stronger concentration, namely 1 million units per millilitre.[10] The conjunctiva is flooded with the drops again after 15 minutes and then after each feed for 3 days. If there is any evidence of damage to the cornea the pupil should be kept dilated with eye drops containing 1 per cent of atropine. Because of the risk that the organisms may be present in other sites[8] or that dissemination may have occurred, penicillin should also be given by injection. One method is to give 200,000 units of crystalline penicillin intramuscularly, every six hours for three days. As an alternative Dunlop[10] has recommended procaine penicillin 300,000 units intramuscularly daily for three days. The United States Public Health Service recommends systemic treatment for seven days.[11]

Meningitis and Arthritis

These complications may occur in children as in adults. Meningitis complicating ophthalmia neonatorum has been described[12] and also a case of fatal fulminating meningitis with the Waterhouse–Friderichsen syndrome (adrenal haemorrhage) in a three-month-old baby.[13]

REFERENCES

1. SERSIRON, D. and ROIRON, V. (1967) Br. J. vener. Dis., **43**, 33.
2. ARMSTRONG, J. H., ZACARIAS, F. and REIN, M. F. (1976) Pediatrics, Springfield, **57**, 884.
3. DUNLOP, E. M. C. (1975) In: Recent Advances in Sexually Transmitted Diseases, ed. R. S. Morton & J. R. W. Harris. p. 290. London: Churchill Livingstone.
4. KRAUS, G. W. and YEN, S. S. C. (1968) Obstet. Gynec., **31**, 258.
5. CAVE, V. G., BLOOMFIELD, R. D., HURDLE, E. S., GORDON, E. W. and HAMMOCK, D. (Jr.) (1969) J. Am. med. Ass., **210**, 309.
6. CASSIE, R. and STEVENSON, A. (1973) J. Obstet. Gynaec. Br. Commonw., **80**, 48.
7. SPARKS, R. A., WILLIAMS, G. L., BOYCE, J. M. H., FITZGERALD, T. C. and SHELLEY, G. (1975) Br. J. vener. Dis., **51**, 110.
8. HUNTER, H. H., HODSON, W. A. and HOLMES, K. K. (1973) J. Am. med. Ass., **225**, 697.
9. SCHOFIELD, C. B. S. and SHANKS, R. A. (1971) Br. med. J., **1**, 257.
10. DUNLOP, E. M. C. (1977) Clin. Obstet. Gynec., **4**, 451.
11. Gonorrhea: CDC Recommended Treatment Schedules (1979) Sex. transm. Dis., **6**, 38.
12. BRADFORD, W. L. and KELLEY, H. W. (1933) Am. J. Dis. Child., **46**, 543.
13. SWIERCZEWSKI, J. A., MASON, E. J., CABRERA, P. B. and LIBER, M. (1970) Am. J. clin. Path., **54**, 202.

17

Treatment and Prognosis of Gonorrhoea

TREATMENT

General Measures

The efficacy of modern remedies has diminished the need for the strict regulation of diet and activity which was once considered essential. Nevertheless, patients should be strongly advised to assist prompt and satisfactory recovery by refraining from alcohol and vigorous physical exercise. In most cases these restrictions are only necessary for the first 10 to 14 days after treatment is started. All patients infected with gonorrhoea should refrain from sexual intercourse until they have completed a satisfactory period of observation and tests (see pp. 246–8).

Sulphonamides

The introduction of sulphonamides resulted in a notable advance in methods of treatment of gonorrhoea, after they had been shown to be effective by Dees and Colston in 1937.[1] Nevertheless, in the course of years it became clear that, although more effective and less toxic derivatives became available, the proportion of failures of this treatment was increasing. The most striking evidence on this point came from troops fighting in the Italian campaign in 1944, when Campbell[2] noted a sudden and disquieting change in the results obtained with sulphonamides. Less than 25 per cent of the patients responded satisfactorily to the standard courses of chemotherapy, and a good many of them relapsed. The introduction of penicillin for the treatment of gonorrhoea caused a virtual abandonment of sulphonamides for the treatment of this disease and, in consequence, there is little evidence on the incidence of 'sulphonamide resistance' in later years. However, an investigation in London in the period 1946 to 1947,[3] in which patients were given 25 to 28 g of sulphathiazole over periods of five to seven days, showed a recovery rate of only 14 per cent. There is now some evidence that many strains of gonococci are sensitive to sulphonamides in vitro, but in view of past experience and the availability of better and less toxic remedies, this form of treatment is not to be recommended.

Co-trimoxazole (Sulphamethoxazole-Trimethoprim)

Csonka and Knight[4] found that the action of sulphonamides against the gonococcus was apparently potentiated by the concurrent administration of trimethoprim, an antifolic acid agent. The combination gave success in 93 per cent of cases whereas sulphonamide alone gave only 31 to 33 per cent of successes. The combination is available in single tablets (Septrin, Bactrim) each containing 400 mg of sulphamethoxazole and 80 mg of trimethoprim. There have been some variations in the dosage employed and some variations in the reported results, but the general experience has been that this is an effective remedy for gonorrhoea. Good results have been obtained by giving four tablets daily in a single dose for five days,[5,6] four tablets twice daily for two days,[7,8] and five tablets twice on the first day and once on the second.[8] Excellent results were obtained in Denmark with two doses of five tablets with an interval of eight hours,[9] but a more recent report from the same country[10] described results which were not quite so good. In Thailand[11] even three doses each of five tablets at 12-hour intervals have recently given poor results.

Single doses have been employed by Rahim[12] in England, who treated 1223 patients each with a single dose of eight tablets, with a success rate of 96 per cent. In a more recent trial[13] in the United States of America, however, a single dose of nine tablets gave a cure rate of only 77 per cent. In another trial[14] two doses of eight tablets with an interval of 24 hours gave better results than a single dose of eight tablets.

Rodin and Seth[6] found evidence of cross-resistance between penicillin and co-trimoxazole as early as 1972 and this was noted again[15] in the same laboratory in 1974. This has also been observed in the United States of America.[13] Thus it might be predicted that in areas with a high prevalence of strains with reduced sensitivity to penicillin, results of treatment with co-trimoxazole will be less satisfactory. Patients who have already failed to respond to penicillin would be particularly likely to do the same with co-trimoxazole and it is probably best avoided in such cases.

This remedy seldom causes toxic effects and can be very useful in the cases of patients known or believed to be sensitive to penicillin. It has no effect on *Treponema pallidum* and therefore will not mask incubating syphilis.

Penicillin

The treatment of gonorrhoea with penicillin has slowly evolved in the past 30 years. There has been a gradual reduction of sensitivity of the gonococcus to the remedy so that the dose of penicillin has had to be increased. Strains of gonococci with MICs of 0·125 μg per ml or more of penicillin are generally considered to be of reduced sensitivity and most patients whose infections do not respond to penicillin harbour strains requiring significantly higher MICs than those found in patients who are cured. The change in sensitivity of the organism has progressed at different rates in different parts of the world so that treatment effective in Europe would be much less so in the Far East. In that area antibiotics can often be bought without prescription and their indiscriminate use has probably been a major factor in producing increased resistance. There is evidence from some countries, for example England[16] and the United States,[17] that since 1970 the trend towards increasing resistance has stopped or even been reversed. Treatment trials reported from one area are relevant to another only if it is known that the patterns of sensitivity are similar. A recent and very important development has been the occurrence of strains of gonococci which produce β-lactamase (penicillinase) and these again occur with greatest frequency in the Far East. Penicillin and ampicillin will be of no value in the treatment of infection due to these strains.

There has been extensive experience of the treatment of gonorrhoea with penicillin and ampicillin. The addition of probenecid is widely used to achieve higher and more prolonged blood levels. For strains which do not produce β-lactamase the following schedules have produced satisfactory rates of cure in various parts of the world:

1. Aqueous procaine penicillin 2·4 mega units intramuscularly in a single injection with 1 or 2 g of probenecid by mouth just before the injection.[15]

2. Aqueous procaine penicillin 4·8 mega units intramuscularly, divided into two doses and injected into each buttock at the same visit, with 1 or 2 g of probenecid by mouth just before the injection. This dose of penicillin is that recommended by the United States Public Health Service.[18] Appreciably better results were obtained with 2 g of probenecid than with 1 g in the treatment of American servicemen in Thailand.[19]

3. One or 2 g of probenecid by mouth followed after 15 to 60 minutes by a single injection of 5 mega units of benzyl penicillin made up with 8 ml of 0·5 per cent lignocaine solution to prevent local pain.[19, 20]

4. Four mega units of fortified procaine penicillin (3 mega units of aqueous procaine penicillin and 1 mega unit of benzyl penicillin) with 1 or 2 g of probenecid 30 minutes before the injection.[21]

Schedules 2, 3 and 4 are particularly suitable in countries where the majority of strains show reduced sensitivity to penicillin. Schedule 4 has given good results in Thailand, where there is a high proportion of such strains, but very recent results are less good because of the advent of β-lactamase-producing strains.[11]

Penicillin by mouth cannot be relied on and oral therapy with ampicillin has superseded this.

Ampicillin

Ampicillin by mouth has been widely used for the treatment of gonorrhoea in the past decade, especially in Scandinavia. It has usually been combined with probenecid and the results have been comparable with those obtained with intramuscular procaine penicillin and probenecid. The following schedules employing single doses have given good results.

1. Ampicillin 2 g by mouth together with 1 or 2 g of probenecid.[15,22-24]
2. Ampicillin 3·5 g by mouth together with 1 g of probenecid. This is the regimen recommended by the United States Public Health Service,[18] but in the United States it has been slightly less effective than 4·8 mega units of procaine penicillin intramuscularly with 1 g of probenecid.[25] It is likely that 2 g instead of 1 g of probenecid would improve the results.[19]

The first schedule gave good results in Thailand until the recent advent of β-lactamase-producing strains.[11,21] This is perhaps surprising in view of the predominance of relatively resistant strains there and the experience in the United States of America with larger doses of ampicillin. Possibly the smaller size of Thai individuals could explain this. Another method which has found favour in Scandinavia is to give 1 g of ampicillin and a further 1 g five hours later. This has given results comparable to those obtained with a single dose of 2 g of ampicillin and 1 g of probenecid.[22,23]

Pivampicillin Hydrochloride

This is an ester of ampicillin which is said to be better absorbed than ampicillin, into which it is rapidly hydrolysed in the body. It has given serum concentrations considerably higher than those obtained with corresponding doses of ampicillin. Excellent results have been obtained in Scandinavia with single doses by mouth of four capsules each of 350 mg together with 1 g of probenecid.[26-28] Two doses, each of three 350 mg capsules, given with an interval of five to six hours have also given good results.[29]

Talampicillin Hydrochloride

This is another ester of ampicillin which also produces higher serum concentrations than ampicillin. Single doses by mouth of 1·5 g combined with 1 or 2 g of probenecid have given excellent results in England.[16,30]

Amoxycillin

This is a comparatively new semi-synthetic penicillin with a spectrum of activity similar to that of ampicillin. So far there have been relatively few trials of this drug. In London, Willcox[31] found the optimum schedule to be an initial dose of 2 g followed by a second dose of 1 g five hours later, which gave a 98 per cent cure rate. Price and Fluker[32] obtained excellent results with single doses of 3 g. In a more recent trial in London[33] 1 g of amoxycillin with 1 g of probenecid gave a cure rate of 86 per cent, compared with 94 per cent with 3 g of amoxycillin with 1 g of probenecid. However, the two groups were rather small in numbers and the difference in the results was not statistically significant. In Seattle, U.S.A.,[34] a single dose of 3 g of amoxycillin alone was effective in 95 per cent of cases and in Winnipeg, Canada,[35] 3 g of amoxycillin with 0·5 g of probenecid gave a cure rate of 95 per cent. The dosage recommended by the United States Public Health Service[18] is 3 g amoxycillin with 1 g probenecid.

Streptomycin

At first, streptomycin gave good results in the treatment of gonorrhoea when given intramuscularly in single doses of 1 or 2 g. Unfortunately strains of gonococci resistant to streptomycin appeared, and they have increased in number. Resistance to streptomycin is usually complete, that is to say the organism resists any concentration of streptomycin that it is possible to produce in the patient's body. There is evidence, also, that strains of gonococci which are partially resistant to penicillin are often completely resistant to streptomycin. Streptomycin is now so uncertain in its effect that it is no longer recommended as a remedy for gonorrhoea.

Chloramphenicol

Good results have been claimed from the administration of this drug by mouth in single doses of 1 to 3 g. However, it is a potentially dangerous drug because of its toxic effects upon the bone marrow and, because other and safer remedies are available, it should not be used for the treatment of gonorrhoea. The one exception might be a patient with meningitis who is allergic to penicillin.[18]

The Tetracyclines

There seems little to choose in effectiveness between the members of this group of drugs. Tetracycline and oxytetracycline are probably a little more effective than chlortetracycline and the minor toxic effects are less. Treatment failures correlate with resistance to the drug. It should be noted that strains of gonococci which show reduced sensitivity to penicillin are also more likely to be less sensitive to tetracycline. Good success rates have been obtained in the United States of America[25, 36] with tetracycline by mouth, 1·5 g initially, followed by 0·5 g four times daily for four days, totalling 9·5 g. Judson and Rothenburg,[37] however, found that the initial loading dose is unnecessary, equally good results having been obtained with the same total dosage given over four and a half days without the loading dose. At present the United States Public Health Service[18] recommends 0·5 g tetracycline hydrochloride four times daily for five days. Tetracycline is best taken an hour before or two hours after meals and should not be taken with milk or milk products, which could affect absorption. Toxic effects of the tetracyclines are few and seldom severe. Some patients suffer from mild gastrointestinal disturbances. Occasionally severe and even fatal cases of staphylococcal enteritis have been described. Exposure to bright sunlight may cause a rash in a patient taking tetracycline and should be avoided.

Tetracycline in single doses is unlikely to be effective. However, some of the newer derivatives of tetracycline, notably doxycycline and minocycline, have been more successful in this regard in the United Kingdom and Europe, where single oral doses of 300 mg of either drug have generally produced cure rates of over 90 per cent. In the United States, on the other hand, where strains of gonococci are likely to be less sensitive to tetracycline than in Europe, unsatisfactory results have been obtained with this treatment and treatment with single doses is not recommended by the United States Public Health Service.[18] Poor results have also been reported from Australia.[38] Söltz-Szöts and Kokoscha,[39] in Austria, gave 2 doses of doxycycline by mouth, each of 300 mg with an interval between doses of eight hours, to each of 100 women, with no failures. Two doses each of 300 mg of doxycycline with an interval of one hour between doses have given good results in the United States of America.[40, 41] The results with two doses seem to warrant further study. The only side effect of these large doses appears to be nausea and vomiting. According to Masterton and Schofield[42] these can easily be prevented by the concurrent administration of 50 ml of milk or by using the syrup instead of capsules.[43]

Some claims have been made for another member of the tetracycline group, methacycline, in the treatment of gonorrhoea. However, Wiesner et al.[40] obtained poor results with single doses of 1200 mg of this drug. They point out that many patients with gonococcal infection which does not respond to tetracycline become asymptomatic whilst still harbouring the organism, and they suggest that sub-curative doses of tetracycline may be an important factor in the development of resistance in the United States of America.

Erythromycin

Early reports on the use of this remedy were favourable but there have been few recent trials. Brown et al.,[44] in the United States of America, treated 152 men suffering from urethral gonorrhoea with either erythromycin base or the estolate, giving 1·5 g initially by mouth and then 0·5 g four times daily for four days. The failure rate with the base was 23 per cent and with the estolate 24 per cent, despite the fact that the latter proved to have an average activity in the serum which was nearly twice as high as that with the base. If these findings are confirmed this drug would seem to have little place in the treatment of gonorrhoea. However, it might have to be used for pregnant women with a history of severe allergy to penicillin, so that cephalosporins are contra-indicated, but the estolate should not be given. In such cases it might be preferable to give 750 mg four times daily for seven days after the initial dose of 1·5 g; intravenous erythromycin, 0·5 g every six hours, could be given if there is gonococcal septicaemia. Cross-resistance with penicillin has been reported.[45]

Spiramycin (Rovamycin)

There have been few reports on the use of this drug, also. Like erythromycin it belongs to the macrolide group of antibiotics. Heinke et al.,[46] in Germany, obtained a success rate of 83·7 per cent with single doses of 2·5 g. With two doses each of 2·5 g with an interval of three hours the success rate was 94·8 per cent. Toxic effects are uncommon.

Kanamycin

This aminoglycoside antibiotic has been shown to be highly effective and has the advantage that it seems to have no effect on syphilis. Wilkinson et al.[47] treated 341 men suffering from gonorrhoea, giving single intramuscular injections of 2 g, two injections each of 1 g in one day or the same on successive days. The failure rate was only 2 to 3 per cent. Hooton and Nicol[48] gave single injections of 2 g of the drug to 138 women suffering from gonorrhoea with success in 96·4 per cent of cases. Keys et al.[49], working in United States Navy bases in the Far East, gave single injections, each of 2 g, to 105 men suffering from urethral gonorrhoea with success in 92 per cent of cases. Fluker and Hewitt[50] used the same dose in the treatment of 100 homosexual men with rectal gonorrhoea. The failure rate was 15·5 per cent, but this compared favourably with the results with 100 similar cases treated with single injections of 1·8 mega-units of procaine penicillin, in which the failure rate was 27·1 per cent. However, the assessment was made purely on the basis of Gram-stained smears.

Kanamycin must be used with care because of the occasional toxic effects upon the 8th nerve and on the kidneys. It should not be used for patients with impaired hearing or with evidence of dysfunction of the kidneys. It is also expensive and therefore unsuitable for routine use. It has a place as a substitute for penicillin if the patient is sensitized to the latter or if the organism is relatively resistant, or if the patient may be suffering from syphilis of which the diagnosis has not been confirmed.

Spectinomycin Hydrochloride

This aminocyclitol antibiotic has been extensively tested in the past decade with uniformly good results reported from various parts of the world. It is well tolerated in single doses of 2 or 4 g, the latter given as 2 g in each buttock. A large-scale cooperative trial in the United States of America,[25] using 2 g for males and 4 g for females, gave a failure rate of approximately 5 per cent in each series. Although the manufacturers recommend giving 2 g to males and 4 g to females, equally good results have been obtained by giving 2 g to females;[51, 52] the United States Public Health Service,[18] in fact, recommends giving 2 g to both sexes. Very occasionally highly resistant strains have been recovered from patients[53, 54] but in general treatment failure does not correlate with sensitivity to the drug in vitro. At present spectinomycin should be reserved for the treatment of patients allergic to penicillin and those who have failed to respond to other drugs, so that it may be hoped that the development of resistant strains will be delayed. However, it may be necessary in the future to use it as a routine in areas where β-lactamase-producing gonococci become prevalent. The U.S. Public Health Service[18] recommends its use for pregnant women who are allergic to penicillin, but its safety for the fetus has not been established. Spectinomycin has some treponemicidal activity and could possibly mask syphilis. Apart from slight local discomfort in some cases, toxic effects have been negligible.

Cephalosporins

Cephaloridine. Single doses of 2 g intramuscularly have given good results in Europe.[39, 55, 56] However, the same dose used in the United States Navy in the Far East[49] gave a cure rate of only 84 per cent. Blood levels of cephaloridine are not enhanced by probenecid.

Cephazolin. Single doses of 2 g intramuscularly have given variable results in the United States of America, success rates varying between 75 per cent[57] and 90 per cent.[58] Blood levels of cephazolin are enhanced by probenecid but Duncan[59] had 6 failures in the cases of 25 men treated with 2 g of cephazolin and 1 g of probenecid.

Cephradine given in two intramuscular injections of 2 g with an interval of 8 hours gave excellent results in Athens.[60]

Cefuroxime is a new semi-synthetic cephalosporin derivative. It is of particular interest because unlike most other cephalosporins it is unaffected by β-lactamase. Price and Fluker[61] obtained excellent results using either 1 g or 1·5 g intramuscularly combined with 1 g of probenecid by mouth in the treatment of 110 men suffering from urethral gonorrhoea. There was only one failure among the 85 patients seen at least once after treatment. At the present time it seems best to hold this drug in reserve for the treatment of patients known or believed to be harbouring β-lactamase-producing strains of gonococci. So far few patients with such strains have been treated with cefuroxime but Arya et al.[62] found that all eight of their cases given 1 g intramuscularly without probenecid were cured. Other cephalosporin derivatives resistant to β-lactamase have been developed and are likely to prove useful. These include *cefoxitin* and *cefotaxime*.

Cephalexin is a semi-synthetic cephalosporin derivative which is given by mouth. Willcox and Woodcock[63] treated 102 men suffering from gonorrhoea, giving two doses each of 2 g with an interval of five hours; 82 remained under observation and there were 12 failures (14·6 per cent). Single doses of 3 g with 1 g of probenecid gave a failure rate of 13 per cent. In the Far East, Brownlow et al.[64] had a failure rate of 50 per cent after single doses of 5 g but Landes et al.,[65] in the United States of America, obtained a cure rate of 96 per cent with single doses of 5 g plus 2 g of probenecid. On the whole the results with one or two doses of this drug have been indifferent, but if it is used it is probably best in combination with probenecid.

Rifampicin

Single doses of 900 mg of this antibiotic given by mouth for the treatment of gonorrhoea have generally produced cure rates of 85 to 90 per cent. Because of the comparatively low cure rate and evidence of rapid development of resistance of the gonococcus to the remedy,[66] it is not recommended for the treatment of gonorrhoea. It is, of course, a valuable anti-tuberculous drug and is best reserved for use with that condition. It has no action on *T. pallidum*.

Gentamicin

Felarca et al.,[67] in the Philippines, treated men suffering from gonorrhoea with intramuscular injections of varying dosage of this relatively new antibiotic. They noted a direct relationship between the size of the dose and the proportion of cures. Of those who received the larger dose, namely 280 mg, 34 out of 37 remained under observation and all were said to be cured. Of 180 patients treated, two developed a slight rash and two complained of severe local pain. Hantschke et al.,[68] in Germany, treated 62 patients, of whom 48 were women and 14 men, giving single intramuscular injections amounting to 5 mg per kg of body weight. Treatment was successful in 58 cases, giving a cure rate of 94 per cent. There were no side effects. This antibiotic, like kanamycin, belongs to the aminoglycoside group, which is known to cause vestibular and auditory damage, especially when given to patients with impaired renal function. The drug was given only to patients with satisfactory audiometric and caloric tests and with normal levels of blood urea nitrogen and serum creatinine. There was no evidence of ototoxicity in the patients treated. Single injections of 240 mg have given cure rates of 85 per cent[69] to 92 per cent.[70] Gentamicin has no effect on *T. pallidum*. The indications for its use are similar to those for kanamycin but it seems to be not quite so effective.

Recommendations

It will be seen that the treatment of gonorrhoea, which until recently many regarded as a simple matter, has become complicated by some deterioration in the effectiveness of the main remedies, by a rise in the number of patients who are sensitized to them, by a multiplicity of new remedies and by variations of experience, not only in different areas of the world but also of different observers working in the same area. It is a disease which lends itself to a good routine of treatment but the fact remains that no treatment is effective in all the cases and that some give an appreciable proportion of failures. From the epidemiological standpoint any method of treatment which gives more than 5 per cent of failures must be regarded as ineffective. Proper management of these cases requires stringent observation and tests for cure and continuous assessment to ensure that methods which have proved effective remain so.

The following recommendations are believed to be valid for routine use in the circumstances existing at the present time. Cases in which treatment fails require special study and individual management.

1. Penicillin by injection combined with probenecid by mouth in the dosages given on p. 235.

2. Ampicillin and probenecid by mouth in the dosages given on p. 236. The larger doses should be used in areas with a high proportion of relatively resistant strains. As 2 g of probenecid seems to be well tolerated this is preferable to 1 g for routine use.

For patients allergic to penicillin one of the following is likely to be effective:

a. Kanamycin 2 g intramuscularly.

b. Spectinomycin 2 g intramuscularly.

c. Co-trimoxazole 8 tablets by mouth initially with another 8 after 24 hours, or 4 tablets twice daily for 2 days or once daily for 5 days (these schedules are likely to give better results in Europe than in the United States of America or the Far East).

d. Tetracycline 500 mg by mouth four times daily for 5 days or doxy-cycline 300 mg initially, preferably with milk, and a further 300 mg two to four hours later after food. Tetracycline itself should not be taken with dairy products.

Cephaloridine 2 g intramuscularly may be used justifiably if the patient has suffered only a mild delayed reaction to penicillin but, because of the risk of cross-allergy, it should be given only if other alternatives are unsuitable.

For patients who have failed to respond to one of the standard doses of penicillin or ampicillin it is probably preferable to use spectinomycin or kanamycin because of the evidence of cross-resistance with tetracycline and co-trimoxazole.

If treatment failure is associated with a β-lactamase-producing strain of gonococci then spectinomycin 2 g intramuscularly or cefuroxime, 1 g intramuscularly plus probenecid 2 g by mouth, should be used. Kanamycin 2 g or cefoxitin 2 g intramuscularly plus probenecid 2 g by mouth is also likely to be effective. In Europe a combination of spectinomycin, 2 g intramuscularly, and co-trimoxazole, 8 tablets by mouth with another 8 after 24 hours, may be expected to give a cure rate of virtually 100 per cent with these strains at the present time and would be justifiable treatment in these cases.

Pharyngeal gonorrhoea does not respond as well as anogenital gonorrhoea to the standard methods of treatment. Its treatment is discussed on p. 225.

β-lactamase (Penicillinase)-producing Strains of Gonococci

Late in 1975, strains of gonococci began to appear which were completely resistant to penicillin. This resistance was due to the possession of a plasmid containing a gene responsible for β-lactamase production, possibly acquired from ampicillin-resistant *H. influenzae* or *Enterobacteriaceae*. Most of the strains seemed to have originated in the Far East and West Africa, but they have now been reported from many parts of the world. In Liverpool, some strains appeared in February 1976 and soon accounted for 9 per cent of isolates.[71] However, very few of these strains were found after November 1976.[62] In certain cities in the Philippines 30 to 40 per cent of gonococcal infections are due to β-lactamase-producing strains and up to 50 per cent of gonococcal infections of United States military personnel in the Philippines are due to the strains.[72] Forty-three per cent of the Far Eastern strains but none of those from West Africa have an additional conjugative plasmid which transfers the β-lactamase R factor to other gonococci and this may explain the relatively high prevalence of penicillinase-producing gonococci in the Far East.[73] The Far Eastern strains are also more likely to be relatively resistant to tetracycline.[73] Isolates have been obtained from patients with salpingitis, bartholinitis, epididymitis and disseminated gonorrhoea.[71, 72]

Ideally all gonococcal isolates should be tested for β-lactamase production and this is essential for those obtained from patients who have failed to respond to treatment. As already mentioned, the best treatment for infections due to β-lactamase-producing gonococci is either spectinomycin or cefuroxime. Several hundred cases have been treated with 2 g of spectinomycin with a failure rate of less than 4 per cent.[74] None of the treatment failures failed to respond to a second injection of 4 g of spectinomycin. So far very few cases have been treated with cefuroxime but it seems likely to be very effective.[62]

Patients with complicated infections will require multiple daily doses, such as 1 g cefuroxime intramuscularly or intravenously plus 0·5 g probenecid by mouth, each given four times daily, or spectinomycin two to four times daily.

Unfortunately those penicillins which are unaffected by β-lactamase are not very active against the gonococcus. It is obvious that intensive contact tracing should be undertaken in these cases if the spread of β-lactamase-producing strains is to be controlled.

Treatment Without Diagnosis

The diagnosis of gonorrhoea in the female can present difficulties, especially when the disease is of some standing. In consequence, there are some venereologists who advocate the use of treatment without accurate diagnosis in some circumstances. They would give treatment to female consorts of men known to have gonorrhoea, even though evidence of gonococcal infection cannot be found. Similarly they are disposed to treat women with clinical signs of disease which may be gonorrhoeal but in whose secretions no gonococci are found. The objections to this kind of procedure are less than in cases of suspected syphilis but, again, the procedure is a violation of a fundamental principle, 'diagnosis before treatment', and the indications should be carefully considered. Any departure from the rule should be regarded as an undesirable expedient, and this kind of action should never be undertaken as a substitute for detailed and careful investigation of the patient's condition. It is bad for the patient, because it leads to anxiety and uncertainty; it is bad for the clinician because, if practised extensively, it leads to careless work and deterioration of standards. It may give rise to medicolegal difficulties. In spite of these objections, routine treatment of contacts is recommended by the United States Public Health Service.[18]

Treatment of Complications in the Male

Acute Complications

Acute complications are now quite uncommon and most of them respond well to antibiotics, although these may need to be given in larger dosage and for longer periods than for uncomplicated disease. These cases require individual management and it is not practicable to advocate a settled routine. Occasionally the following additional measures may be required.

Periurethral abscess may need to be aspirated until antibiotic therapy has produced its full effect. Surgical incision and drainage should be avoided if possible because of the danger of urinary fistula.

If infection of *Tyson's glands* or *paraurethral ducts* proves resistant to systemic remedies, destruction of the gland or duct with the electro-cautery may be necessary. This, or sometimes excision, may also be required for a *median raphe* infection.

If an abscess of *Cowper's gland* has opened on the surface leaving a dis-charging sinus in the perineum, the fistulous tract and the gland may need to be excised (see Fig. 114, p. 211).

In cases of spasmodic retention of urine in association with *prostatic abscess* or infection of Cowper's glands, relief may be achieved with an injection of morphine 15 mg followed by a hot bath. Catheterization should be avoided if possible, but if it becomes necessary a Jacques rubber catheter (18 F) should be passed. Hot rectal douching with water at 43°C may sometimes help to relieve pain and congestion and may be given two or three times daily. Alternatively, and more conveniently, hot sitz baths can be taken by the patient four or five times a day. Antibiotics should be given in high dosage for seven days or more.

In cases of *acute epididymitis*, as well as giving an appropriate antibiotic, support for the scrotum should be given with a 'jockstrap' or a well-fitting suspensory bandage. Prompt relief of pain is likely to follow the administra-tion of phenylbutazone, 200 mg three times daily by mouth, but this drug can occasionally give rise to serious side effects and indomethacin, 50 mg three times daily, would be a safer alternative.

True *gonococcal arthritis* requires admission to hospital and prompt antibiotic therapy in high dosage, such as 1 mega-unit of benzylpenicillin every six hours for at least seven days together with probenecid 0·5 g six-hourly, to which it responds well. Delay may lead to destruction of the joint surfaces. The treatment of gonococcal septicaemia is described on p. 223.

Anterior uveitis occurring in association with gonorrhoea is well controlled by topical treatment with steroid hormones (see p. 306). The pupil should be dilated with atropine. Systemic treatment with antibiotics should be given for the gonococcal infection of the urethra, but it has no demonstrable effect on the uveitis. Associated non-gonococcal infection is the likely cause.

Patients with acute complications should be admitted to hospital and be kept completely at rest in bed until the pain is relieved and the temperature is normal. The affected areas should be palpated and manipulated as little as possible. Prostatic massage should *never* be performed in the presence of an acute complication. No additional local treatment is required for gonococcal proctitis, in most cases.

Chronic Complications

Chronic complications are usually residual from gonococcal infection and probably related to associated non-gonococcal infection. They are considered in detail in Chapters 21 and 22.

Patients with *urethral strictures* require dilatation with bougies followed by curved metal sounds in most cases. Meatotomy, meatoplasty, internal urethrotomy or urethroplasty may be required in cases of difficulty. The latter procedures and subsequent management should be left to the genito-urinary surgeon.

Treatment of Complications in the Female

Acute Complications

As in the male most acute complications respond well to antibiotics. No special treatment is required for acute *skenitis* but an abscess of *Bartholin's gland* may be treated by repeated aspiration through a wide-bore needle, to relieve pain. It is best to insert the needle through normal skin lateral to the abscess after infiltration with a small amount of lignocaine. It may be necessary to incise and drain the abscess, but this should be avoided if possible because it increases the difficulty of finding and excising the gland in the chronic stage.

If the patient has *pelvic infection* due to gonorrhoea she should be confined to bed, preferably in hospital. She should have a light diet with plenty of fluids, and analgesics should be given for the relief of pain. Constipation can be relieved with contact laxatives and, if necessary, with enemata. Penicillin should be given intramuscularly, starting with benzylpenicillin 1·0 mega-unit plus 0·5 g of probenecid by mouth, both given six-hourly until there has been clear-cut improvement. This is followed by procaine penicillin 2·4 mega-units plus probenecid 2 g daily for a total of 10 days. As an alternative to procaine penicillin, ampicillin 0·5 g with probenecid

0·5 g may be given by mouth four times daily. If the clinical response is incomplete the patient may also have associated non-gonococcal salpingitis and should then be given tetracycline 0·5 g four times daily or doxy-cycline 200 mg daily for 14 to 21 days. Sometimes, metronidazole is added to deal with anaerobic organisms. Effective dosage is likely to be 400 mg three times a day. Surgical intervention is hardly ever necessary, but it is sometimes undertaken through mistakes in diagnosis, which are probably avoidable by proper examination of, and tests from, the genital organs. In recent years laparoscopy has been helpful in difficult cases. Occasionally it may be necessary to drain a pelvic abscess through the pouch of Douglas or abdominally.

The treatment of gonococcal septicaemia is considered on p. 223.

Chronic Complications

These are likely to be due to non-gonococcal genital infection and they are considered under that heading. A Bartholin's cyst or recurrent Bartholin's abscess should be treated surgically by excision or 'marsupialization'. The literature and technique of the latter procedure has been reviewed by Hutfield.[75] If Skene's ducts are the sites of chronic infection they may need to be destroyed with the electrocautery. Chronic cervicitis persisting after the treatment of gonorrhoea is almost always due to non-gonococcal infection. Patients who suffer from recurrent or chronic pelvic inflam-mation are usually relieved by rest, tetracyclines, metronidazole for anaerobic organisms and pelvic short-wave diathermy. Unfortunately the condition is prone to recurrence and surgical removal of inflamed pelvic organs may ultimately be required.

Treatment of Children

This is discussed in Chapter 16.

PROGNOSIS OF GONORRHOEA

Cases of uncomplicated infection treated early have an excellent prognosis for prompt and complete recovery. Difficulties and dangers arise from neglect to seek advice and from associated non-gonococcal genital infection. Severe complications, especially pelvic infection in women, may lead to recurrent illness and chronic ill-health if diagnosis and treatment are delayed. Meningitis and endocarditis can endanger life.

Tests for Cure

In order to determine the cure of gonorrhoea and the absence of associated non-gonococcal infection, it is essential to observe patients closely and to perform various tests for latent infection over a period of time.

CHANCROID   GRANULOMA INGUINALE

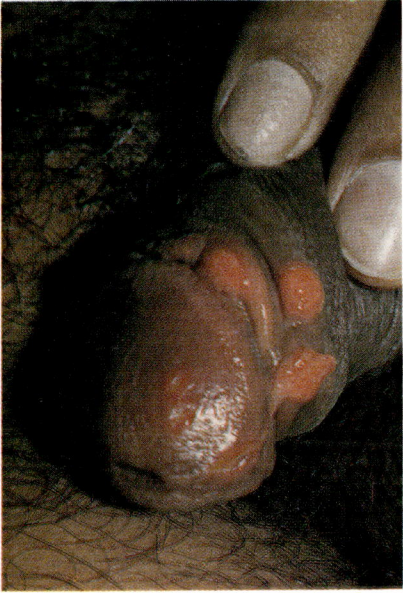

i Multiple chancroidal ulcers on the penis.

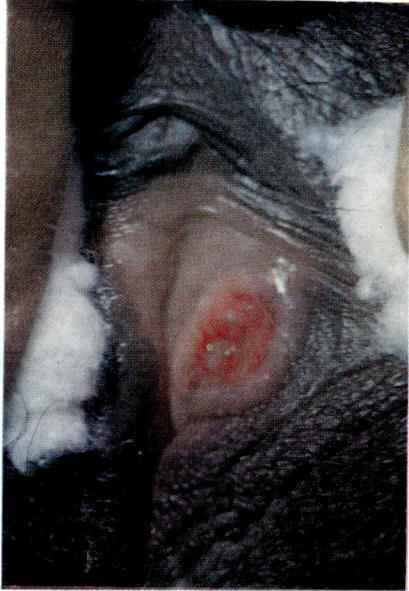

ii Early lesion of granuloma inguinale on vulva.

REITER'S DISEASE

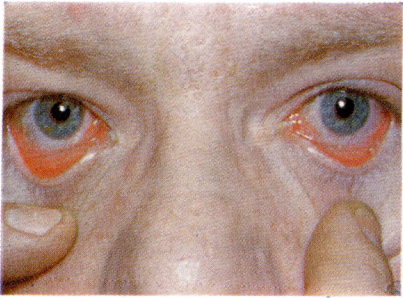

iii Bilateral conjunctivitis.

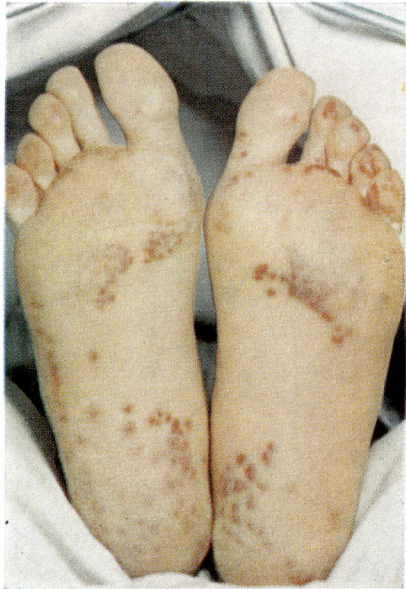

v Keratoderma blennorrhagica of soles of feet.

PLATE V

Male Patients

A man who has been treated for acute gonorrhoea should be seen on or before the third day after treatment, if possible in the early morning before the first urine is passed. If this is not possible he should hold urine for at least three hours before he is seen. Urethral secretion is examined microscopically for presence of gonococci and sent for culture, and the urine is examined by the two-glass test. The third or fourth day after treatment is the optimum time for an examination for signs of persisting infection due to strains of gonococci which are partially resistant to penicillin; the patient harbouring such organisms may or may not have symptoms or signs of urethritis, depending, to a certain extent, on the degree of antibiotic resistance. Smear and culture should be repeated after another seven days. In most cases treatment will have been successful, but even so there is likely to be some mucoid or mucopurulent urethral secretion which, microscopically, shows leucocytes, epithelial cells and few or no secondary organisms. The urine may be slightly hazy with pus, or may show threads. If cure is complete these signs should disappear in the course of ten days or so. If they persist the possibility of associated non-gonococcal infection has to be considered. This is a common occurrence and must be treated (see p. 281). The patient is seen once more after another two weeks and tests of urethral secretion and urine are repeated. If treatment has been delayed, or response to treatment slow, the condition of the prostate, seminal vesicles and Cowper's glands should be investigated in due course by palpation per rectum and prostatic fluid expressed by digital massage and examined microscopically. If it contains an excess of polymorphonuclear leucocytes the patient may have chronic prostatitis. The anterior urethra should also be inspected by urethroscopy in these cases, especially for evidence of stricture. There is a modern tendency to omit investigation of the prostate and seminal vesicles even when the indications mentioned are present. This, perhaps, reflects the fact that prostatitis is less common than it used to be and that the treatment of chronic prostatitis is unsatisfactory (see p. 284). Nevertheless it is important to know that the patient has chronic prostatitis, whether treatment is undertaken for it or not. The condition can have an important bearing on his future health. Finally, after three months blood is taken for serological tests for syphilis. If all these tests are satisfactory the patient may be discharged as cured.

If the patient was treated with penicillin or some other drug which has antitreponemal activity, some venereologists like to repeat the blood tests at the end of a further three months in case the antibiotic has delayed the appearance of evidence of syphilitic infection. Others, as the result of experience, have thought this to be an unnecessary precaution.

Not all patients are willing to submit themselves to this routine; in fact, more than half the patients treated at clinics absent themselves soon after their symptoms are relieved. Every effort should be made to impress upon these patients the importance of complete observation and tests.

Female Patients

A woman who has been treated for gonorrhoea should be examined and tested on the third day and then twice more at weekly intervals with the last test preferably after a menstrual period. Tests include smears and cultures from urethra·and cervix. A fresh preparation of the vaginal fluid is examined for *Trichomonas vaginalis* and a stained smear for *Candida albicans*. Rectal smears and cultures should be taken after treatment if the patient originally had evidence of anorectal infection for sometimes this is the only site at which failure of treatment is evident. Serological tests for syphilis are performed as for men. A careful bimanual examination of the pelvic organs should be made once or twice during the period of observation. If all tests are negative after three months, the patient can be discharged as cured.

REFERENCES

1. DEES, J. E. and COLSTON, J. A. C. (1937) *J. Am. med. Ass.*, **108**, 1855.
2. CAMPBELL, D. J. (1944) *Br. med. J.*, **2**, 44.
3. DUNLOP, E. M. C. (1949) *Br. J. vener. Dis.*, **25**, 81.
4. CSONKA, G. W. and KNIGHT, G. J. (1967) *Br. J. vener. Dis.*, **43**, 161.
5. CARROLL, B. R. T. and NICOL, C. S. (1970) *Br. J. vener. Dis.*, **46**, 31.
6. RODIN, P. and SETH, A. D. (1972) *Br. J. vener. Dis.*, **48**, 517.
7. SVINDLAND, H. B. (1973) *Br. J. vener. Dis.*, **49**, 50.
8. LAWRENCE, A., PHILLIPS, I. and NICOL, C. S. (1973) *J. infect. Dis.*, **128**, suppl. 673.
9. ULLMANN, S., NIORDSON, A. M. and ZACHARIAE, H. (1971) *Acta derm.-vener. (Stockh.)*, **51**, 394.
10. NIELSEN, A. O. and NISSEN, E. K. (1977) *Ugeskr. Laeg.*, **139**, 393.
11. PANIKABUTRA, K., (1978) Personal communication.
12. RAHIM, G. (1975) *Br. J. vener. Dis.*, **51**, 179.
13. ELLIOTT, W. C., REYNOLDS, G., THORNSBERRY, C., KELLOGG, D. S., JAFFE, H. W., BROWN, S. T., ARMSTRONG, J. and REIN, M. F. (1977) *J. infect. Dis.*, **135**, 939.
14. BRATHWAITE, A. R. (1975) *Can. med. Ass. J.*, **112**, 405.
15. TAYLOR, P. K. and SETH, A. D. (1975) *Br. J. vener. Dis.*, **51**, 183.
16. AL-EGAILY, S., DUNLOP, E. M. C., RODIN, P. and SETH, A. D. (1978) *Br. J. vener. Dis.*, **54**, 243.
17. JAFFE, H. W., ZAIDI, A. A., THORNSBERRY, C., REYNOLDS, G. H. and WIESNER, P. J. (1977) *J. infect. Dis.*, **136**, 684.
18. Gonorrhea: CDC Recommended Treatment Schedules (1979) *Sex. transm. Dis.*, **6**, 38.
19. BROWN, S. T. and McMINN, T. (1974) *Br. J. vener. Dis.*, **50**, 298.
20. GRAY, R. C. F., PHILLIPS, I. and NICOL, C. S. (1970) *Br. J. vener. Dis.*, **46**, 401.
21. PANIKABUTRA, K. (1978) *J. med. Ass. Thai.*, **61**, 247.
22. ERIKSSON, G. (1970) *Acta derm.-vener. (Stockh.)*, **50**, 451.
23. ERIKSSON, G. (1971) *Acta. derm.-vener. (Stockh.)*, **51**, 305.
24. BRO-JØRGENSEN, A. and JENSEN, T. (1971) *Br. J. vener. Dis.*, **47**, 443.

25. KAUFMAN, R. E., JOHNSON, R. E., JAFFE, H. W., THORNSBERRY, C., REYNOLDS, G. H., WIESNER, P. J. and the Cooperative Study Group (1976) *New Engl. J. Med.*, **294**, 1.

26. MALMBORG, A-S., MOLIN, L. and NYSTRÖM, B. (1973) *Acta derm.-vener. (Stockh.)*, **53**, 501.

27. FORSTRÖM, L. (1974) *Br. J. vener. Dis.*, **50**, 61.

28. KRISTENSEN, J. K. and FROM, E. (1975) *Br. J. vener. Dis.*, **51**, 31.

29. FORSTRÖM, L. and LASSUS, A. (1972) *Br. J. vener. Dis.*, **48**, 510.

30. PRICE, J. D., FLUKER, J. L. and GILES, A. J. H. (1977) *Br. J. vener. Dis.*, **53**, 113.

31. WILLCOX, R. R. (1974) *Br. J. vener. Dis.*, **50**, 120.

32. PRICE, J. D. and FLUKER, J. L. (1975) *Br. J. vener. Dis.*, **51**, 398.

33. THIN, R. N., SYMONDS, M. A. E., SHAW, E. J., WONG, J., HOPPER, P. K. and SLOCOMBE, R. (1977) *Br. J. vener. Dis.*, **53**, 118.

34. KARNEY, W. W., TURCK, M. and HOLMES, K. K. (1974) *J. infect. Dis.*, **129**, suppl. 250.

35. GURWITH, M. J., McGINNIS, S., RONALD, A. R. and HENRY, R. (1974) *J. infect. Dis.*, **129**, suppl. 258.

36. KARNEY, W. W., PEDERSEN, A. H. B., NELSON, M., ADAMS, H., PFEIFER, R. T. and HOLMES, K. K. (1977) *New Engl. J. Med.*, **296**, 889.

37. JUDSON, F. N. and ROTHENBURG, R. (1976) *J. Am. vener. Dis. Ass.*, **3**, 56.

38. BAYTCH, H. and RANKIN, D. W. (1972) *Br. J. vener. Dis.*, **48**, 129.

39. SÖLTZ-SZÖTS, J. and KOKOSCHA, E. (1973) *Br. J. vener. Dis.*, **48**, 177.

40. WIESNER, P. J., HOLMES, K. K., SPARLING, P. F., MANESS, M. J., BEAR, T. M., GUTMAN, L. T. and KARNEY, W. W. (1973) *J. infect. Dis.*, **127**, 461.

41. ROBINSON, D. H. and SHEPHERD, D. A. (1974) *Curr. ther. Res.*, **16**, 214.

42. MASTERTON, G. and SCHOFIELD, C. B. S. (1972) *Br. J. vener. Dis.*, **48**, 121.

43. SCHOFIELD, C. B. S. and MASTERTON, G. (1974) *Br. J. vener. Dis.*, **50**, 303.

44. BROWN, S. T., PEDERSEN, A. H. B. and HOLMES, K. K. (1977) *J. Am. med. Ass.*, **238**, 1371.

45. MOSES, J. M., DESAI, M. S., BHOSLE, C. B. and TRASI, M. S. (1971) *Br. J. vener. Dis.*, **47**, 273.

46. HEINKE, E., SCHALLER, K. F. and SCHIRREN, H. (1969) *Dtsch. med. Wschr.*, **94**, 1182.

47. WILKINSON, A. E., RACE, J. W. and CURTIS, F. R. (1967) *Postgrad. med. J.*, suppl. May, 65.

48. HOOTON, W. F. and NICOL, C. S. (1967) *Postgrad. med. J.*, suppl. May, 68.

49. KEYS, T. F., HALVERSON, C. W. and CLARKE, E. J. (1969) *J. Am. med. Ass.*, **216**, 857.

50. FLUKER, J. L. and HEWITT, A. B. (1970) *Br. J. vener. Dis.*, **46**, 454.

51. PEDERSEN, A. H. B., WIESNER, P. J., HOLMES, K. K., JOHNSON, C. J. and TURCK, M. (1972) *J. Am. med. Ass.*, **220**, 205.

52. PANIKABUTRA, K. (1975) *Br. J. vener. Dis.*, **51**, 188.

53. REYN, A., SCHMIDT, H., TRIER, M. and BENTZON, M. W. (1973) *Br. J. vener. Dis.*, **49**, 54.

54. THORNSBERRY, C., JAFFE, H., BROWN, S. T., EDWARDS, T., BIDDLE, J. W. and THOMPSON, S. E. (1977) *J. Am. med. Ass.*, **237**, 2405.

55. MARSHALL, M. J. and CURTIS, F. R. (1967) *Postgrad. med. J.*, suppl. August, 121.

56. OLLER, L. Z. (1967) *Postgrad. med. J.*, suppl. August, 124.

57. NELSON, M. (1973) *J. infect. Dis.*, **128**, suppl., 404.

58. KARNEY, W. W., TURCK, M. and HOLMES, K. K. (1973) *J. infect. Dis.*, **128**, suppl., 399.
59. DUNCAN, W. C. (1974) *J. infect. Dis.*, **130**, 398.
60. THEODORIDIS, A., TSAMBAOS, D., SIVENAS, C. and CAPETENAKIS, J. (1976) *Curr. ther. Res.*, **19**, 20.
61. PRICE, T. D. and FLUKER, J. L. (1978) *Br. J. vener. Dis.*, **54**, 165.
62. ARYA, O. P., REES, E., PERCIVAL, A., ALERGANT, C. D., ANNELS, E. H. and TURNER, G. C. (1978) *Br. J. vener. Dis.*, **54**, 28.
63. WILLCOX, R. R. and WOODCOCK, K. S. (1970) *Postgrad. med. J.*, suppl. October, 103.
64. BROWNLOW, W. J., WATKO, L. P., AUCOIN, E. J. and IGLECIA-FERNANDEZ, R. (1974) *Br. J. vener. Dis.*, **50**, 113.
65. LANDES, R. R., MELNICK, I., HOFFMAN, A. A., FEHRENBAKER, L. G. and OAKES, A. L. (1972) *Clin. Med.*, **79**, 23.
66. MALMBORG, A. S., MOLIN, L. and NYSTRÖM, B. (1971) *Chemotherapy*, **16**, 319.
67. FELARCA, A. B., LAQUI, E. M. and IBARRA, L. M. (1971) *J. infect. Dis.*, **124**, suppl., 287.
68. HANTSCHKE, D., STRAUSS, P., LINZENMEIER, G., GAHLEN, D. and HELLER, W. (1973) *Br. J. vener. Dis.*, **49**, 62.
69. MORRISON, G. D. and REEVES, D. S. (1973) *Br. J. vener. Dis.*, **49**, 513.
70. BOWIE, W., RONALD, A. R., KAYWULAK, W., CATES, C. Y. and BOUTROS, A. (1974) *Br. J. vener. Dis.*, **50**, 208.
71. PERCIVAL, A., CORKILL, J. E., ARYA, O. P., ROWLANDS, J., ALERGANT, C. D., REES, E. and ANNELS, E. H. (1976) *Lancet*, **2**, 1379.
72. SPARLING, P. F., HOLMES, K. K., WIESNER, P. J. and PUZISS, M. (1977) *J. infect. Dis.*, **135**, 865.
73. PERINE, P. L., SCHALLA, W., SIEGEL, M. S., THORNSBERRY, C., BIDDLE, J., WONG, K-H. and THOMPSON, S. E. (1977) *Lancet*, **2**, 993.
74. SIEGAL, M. S., THOMPSON, S. E. and PERINE, P. L. (1977) *Sex. transm. Dis.*, **4**, 32.
75. HUTFIELD, D. C. (1965) *Br. J. vener. Dis.*, **41**, 137.

18

Chancroid

This condition is also called 'soft sore', 'soft chancre' and 'ulcus molle'. It is an acute, localized, auto-inoculable infection of the genitals caused by the streptobacillus of Ducrey (*Haemophilus ducreyi*), first isolated by Ducrey in 1889. It is characterized by ulceration at the sites of inoculation and is frequently accompanied by suppuration of the regional lymph nodes ('inflammatory bubo').[1]

INCIDENCE. It is not a common disease in the United Kingdom or in other Western countries, and seems to be becoming even more of a rarity. In Eastern countries and in tropical and subtropical regions the incidence is far higher and in some of these countries chancroid is the commonest cause of genital ulceration. There is a disproportionately low incidence in women, possibly due to difficulties in diagnosis, but it appears to be a particular hazard of prostitutes in certain parts of the world. It has been described as a disease of the 'socially unenlightened and economically unfortunate'. In Britain it is imported mainly by seamen, and, for the most part, is found only in the neighbourhood of dockland areas. In the year ending June 30, 1977, 43 cases were reported from the venereal disease clinics of England.[2]

CAUSATIVE ORGANISM. H. ducreyi is a short, slender, Gram-negative rod with rounded ends. Groups of organisms are often found in chains giving the appearance of a 'school of fish'. It may be difficult to find the organism in open lesions on the genitalia because of secondary bacterial infection; identification is usually easier if examination is made of pus aspirated from an inguinal abscess. The organism is fastidious and culture is difficult. Best results have been obtained with media containing whole human blood or defibrinated rabbits' blood.

EXPERIMENTAL INFECTIONS. Successful inoculations of recent strains of the cultured organism have been made in animals and in man.

CLINICAL CHARACTERISTICS

The incubation period is usually short, namely from one to five days, but it can occasionally be as long as 30 days. There may be only one lesion but often there are several. Extragenital chancroids are rare, and the initial lesion is almost always on the genitalia. It is a small, inflammatory papule, surrounded by a narrow zone of bright erythema; it soon becomes pustular and the pustule ruptures to form a painful, sharply circumscribed ulcer with ragged, undermined edges. On removing the pus, the floor of the ulcer is seen to be formed of unevenly distributed, very vascular granulation tissue. The lesions are shallow and vary in diameter from a few millimetres to one to two centimetres. They are tender to touch and bleed easily on gentle manipulation. Occasionally the ulcer spreads in linear fashion, forming a long, narrow and relatively superficial lesion. Palpation of the base of the sore shows it is usually free from induration, in contrast to the lesions of primary syphilis. Urine flowing over the ulcers causes a burning sensation, and this may be the main complaint of infected women.

There is a good deal of variation in the clinical appearance of chancroids and clinical types have been described as follows:

The follicular chancroid originates in the hair follicles and, at first, may simulate pus-coccal folliculitis, but the pustules soon ulcerate. Lesions of this type may be seen on the vulva and on the hairy surfaces round the genitalia. They are very superficial.

The dwarf chancroid is a very small lesion which may resemble the erosions of herpes genitalis, but the lesion has an irregular floor and sharply-cut haemorrhagic edges.

The transient chancroid ('chancre mou volant') is a small lesion of typical chancroidal type, which resolves rapidly in a few days but is apt to be followed within two to three weeks by the development of a typical inflammatory bubo in the groin. Because of the transitory nature of the initial lesion followed by involvement of inguinal lymphatic nodes, it has to be differentiated from the inguinal syndrome of lymphogranuloma venereum (see p. 259).

The papular chancroid ('ulcus molle elevatum') starts as an ulcer but later becomes raised, particularly around its edges. It may resemble the condylomata lata of secondary syphilis.

The giant chancroid may start as a small ulcer but extends rapidly and covers a considerable area. It is most likely to follow rupture of an inguinal abscess, when the ulcer forming at the point of rupture may spread to the suprapubic region and perhaps to the thigh by auto-inoculation (serpiginous chancroid).

The phagedenic chancroid may commence as a small lesion, but becomes large and destructive with widespread necrosis of tissue. The external

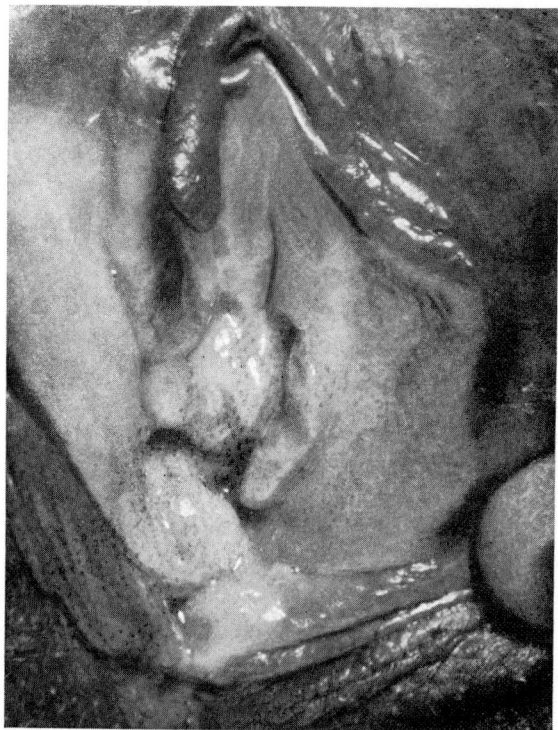

Fig. 119. Chancroid: multiple vulval ulcers.

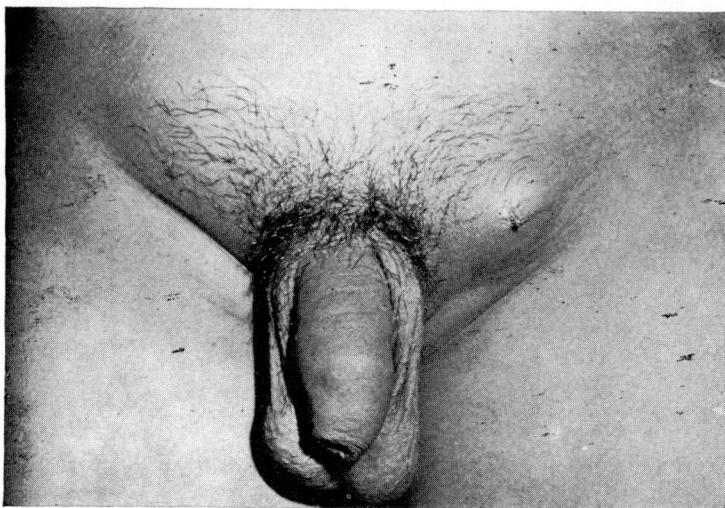

Fig. 120. Chancroid: bubo in the male, breaking down.

genitalia may be destroyed. In some cases superimposed infection with Vincent's organisms plays a part in the process.

Sites of Involvement (Plate V, i and Fig. 119)

Chancroidal lesions in males are usually found on the genital organs and the commonest sites are the preputial orifice, the mucous surface of the prepuce or the frenum of the prepuce, and the external urinary meatus. Intra-urethral chancroid can occur and present as non-gonococcal urethritis. Lesions may spread locally to the perineum and anus, to the scrotum, thighs or lower abdomen. In the female, ulceration is most likely to be found on the fourchette, in the vestibule, round the urinary meatus or on the inner surfaces of the labia minora. The perineum or anus may be involved and vaginal or cervical ulceration may occasionally be seen. Extragenital lesions, including lesions on the hands or breasts or in the mouth, have been described.

COMPLICATIONS

INGUINAL ADENITIS (*'inflammatory bubo'*) (Fig. 120). Adenitis of the inguinal lymph nodes is the commonest complication occurring in about half the cases; it follows the primary lesion within a few days to three weeks; it is usually unilateral. The nodes become enlarged and tender and then matted together. In about half the cases suppuration occurs with the formation of a unilocular abscess. There is erythema of the overlying skin and fluctuation may be felt. If untreated, the abscess ruptures through the skin forming a single sinus which breaks down to chancroidal ulceration. The ulceration may then enlarge to form a giant chancroid. Small, inaccessible lesions seem to be more liable to be complicated by bubo formation than large lesions which are readily accessible.

PHIMOSIS OR *PARAPHIMOSIS* may result from lesions affecting the prepuce.

URETHRAL FISTULA may occur as the result of a destructive ulceration of the glans penis. Involvement of the urethra is associated with severe pain on micturition. Urethral stricture may follow.

ASSOCIATED INFECTION with Vincent's organisms may enhance the severity and increase the destructive character of the lesion, as already mentioned. This complication may render the chancroids refractory to treatment unless this is adjusted to deal with the super-added infection.

Patients with chancroid may also have early syphilis ('mixed chancre', see Plate I, ii), lymphogranuloma venereum or granuloma inguinale.

DIAGNOSIS

Direct Smears

Direct smears taken from beneath the undermined edges of chancroidal ulcers may be stained with Gram's, Wright's or Pappenheim's stain, but most observers agree that it is not easy to recognize the typical morphological characteristics of *H. ducreyi* by this means. Estimations of the value of this method have varied considerably, but the probability is that useful information can be obtained from smears in no more than 30 per cent of cases, unless pus can be aspirated from an unruptured bubo.

Cultures

As already stated, the organism is fastidious, but good results have been obtained with cultures from chancroidal ulcers or pus from buboes, using media containing whole blood. A medium containing defibrinated rabbits' blood, cystine, dextrose and beef-infusion agar has proved particularly effective. The organism grows best at a temperature of 28 to 32°C, and shows optimum growth at 48 hours. A certain amount of moisture in the air surrounding the medium is essential. Success has been claimed by this and other specialized methods of culture in from 59 to 90 per cent of cases. However, the technique is difficult, and it is doubtful whether cultural methods can be developed to the point of giving really valuable information in areas where only occasional cases of chancroid are seen.

The Intradermal Test

The method of producing a cutaneous reaction by intradermal injection of a vaccine containing killed *H. ducreyi* in suspension was used for many years. It was employed by Ito and later by Reenstierna, and is therefore known as the Ito–Reenstierna test. The commercially produced vaccine (Dmelcos) contained 225 million organisms to the millilitre. The procedure was to inject intradermally one-tenth of a millilitre of the suspension and to inject a similar amount of the suspending fluid at another site. The minimum criterion for a positive result was the presence of an inflammatory papule 0·5 to 1 cm in diameter after 48 hours, with a negative control. The interval between appearance of the chancroidal ulcer and the likelihood of positive response to the test was from 6 to 15 days, and once present the reaction could still be obtained for a number of years, and perhaps for life. Opinions still vary on the diagnostic value of this test, but most observers regard it as unsatisfactory because of the considerable number of normal individuals who gave positive reactions. This diagnostic method is now generally considered to be obsolete and production of the commercial vaccine has ceased.

Biopsy

Some experienced workers in this field have regarded biopsy as the most efficient single method of diagnosis and as dependable in over 90 per cent of the cases. Sheldon and Heyman[3] described a combination of microscopical findings by which chancroidal ulceration could be differentiated from other genital lesions, as follows:

(*a*) The general architecture of the lesion consists of an ulcerated surface and one or two deeper layers.

(*b*) Marked endothelial proliferation of the blood vessels can be seen, predominantly in the mid-zone where the endothelium in various stages of overgrowth outnumbers all other cells.

(*c*) There is lack of appreciable fibroblastic proliferation in the mid-zone.

(*d*) There is palisading of blood vessels, with degeneration of their walls, and occasional thrombosis.

(*e*) In the deep zone there is dense infiltration by plasma cells and lymphocytes with a gradual transition into the surrounding tissue. In the superficial necrotic zone there is infiltration with polymorphonuclear leucocytes.

Auto-inoculation

The attempt to confirm a diagnosis by producing a typical lesion by inoculating material from a suspected sore into an incision made in a healthy area of skin of the affected patient is a very old method. It is said that the organism can be demonstrated more readily in lesions produced by auto-inoculation. However, the method is of restricted value because the inoculations do not 'take' with sufficient frequency, and it is now mainly of historical interest only.

TREATMENT

Prophylaxis

Suppressive treatment has been shown to be effective both for experimental chancroids and as a method of prevention in areas where the disease is very prevalent. Chancroid is a purely local disease, and the objections which were expressed to the suppressive treatment of syphilis are not valid. Nevertheless it is an infringement of a fundamental rule and it is not particularly satisfactory from the patient's point of view. The methods used include sulphonamide creams and ointments (which may give contact dermatitis), and sulphonamides by mouth, 1 to 4 g given within 12 hours of exposure. Good results have been claimed for local applications of chloramphenicol cream, but this has the disadvantage that it may mask the development of associated syphilitic infection.

Established Infection

Local Treatment

Local antiseptics are contraindicated because they may interfere with the early diagnosis of syphilis by dark-ground examination. Small, early lesions may heal after local cleansing with normal saline solution and the establishment of drainage. Larger and more established lesions require other methods.

Systemic Treatment

SULPHONAMIDES, such as sulphathiazole, sulphadiazine, and sulpha-dimidine, may be given by mouth, in dosage of 2 to 4 g at once and then 1 g every four hours until healing is well advanced or complete, which may take from 10 to 14 days. Co-trimoxazole tablets, a combination of sulpha-methoxazole 400 mg with trimethoprim 80 mg, may be used in a dosage of two tablets twice daily for 10 days. If any treatment is to be successful, local drainage must be established, and this may necessitate dorsal slitting of the prepuce. Suppurating buboes should not be incised but should be aspirated through healthy skin, repeatedly if necessary.

STREPTOMYCIN is also an effective remedy and, like the sulphonamides and co-trimoxazole, does not interfere with the diagnosis of syphilis. Daily injections of 1 g may be given for from 7 to 14 days, either alone or in association with a sulphonamide. The combination is especially useful if a bubo is present, or if the genital lesions are not healing with sulphonamides alone. Streptomycin has given good results in Singapore[4] where tetracycline is now less effective.

PENICILLIN has some effect in vitro on H. ducreyi, but is of little value in treatment unless associated infection with Vincent's organisms is present.

TETRACYCLINE AND OXYTETRACYCLINE are usually effective when given by mouth in dosage of 500 mg four times a day for 10 to 20 days. Tetracycline has, however, proved to be less effective in Singapore[4] and Vietnam.[5, 6] The tetracycline group of antibiotics have the disadvantage that they may mask the early signs of syphilis and, on that account, sulphon-amides and streptomycin are preferable.

KANAMYCIN was found to be effective in Vietnam by Marmar.[6] He used the drug to treat 62 patients who had not responded to sulphonamide and tetracycline. Each was given 500 mg intramuscularly twice daily for 6 to 14 days and all responded well. Kanamycin has no effect on T. pallidum and so will not mask syphilis.

CHLORAMPHENICOL by mouth is effective but should not be used because of its potentially severe toxic effects.

REFERENCES

1. GREENBLATT, R. B. (1953) Management of Chancroid, Granuloma Inguinale, Lympho-granuloma Venereum in General Practice, U.S. Publ. Hlth. Serv. Publ., Wash. No. 255.
2. A. R. med. Offr. Dept Hlth (Lond.) (1977) p. 58. H.M.S.O. 1978.
3. SHELDON, W. H. and HEYMAN, A. (1946) Am. J. Path., 22, 415.
4. TAN, T., RAJAN, V. S., KOE, S. L., TAN, N. J., TAN, B. H. and GOH, A. J. (1977) Asian J. infect. Dis., 1, 27.
5. KERBER, R. E., ROWE, C. E. and GILBERT, K. R. (1969) Archs Derm., 100, 604.
6. MARMAR, J. L. (1972) J. Urol., 107, 807.

19

Lymphogranuloma Venereum

In the past this disease has been known by many names, because most of the clinical manifestations were described separately and the condition was not fully recognized as a clinical entity until specific diagnostic tests became available.

INCIDENCE. Lymphogranuloma venereum is common in tropical and subtropical climates but uncommon in temperate countries. In the year ending June 30, 1977, 36 cases of the disease were diagnosed in the venereal disease clinics of England.[1] It is most often seen in immigrants who have come from areas where it is endemic, such as the West Indies.

THE CAUSATIVE AGENT, which was first isolated by Hellerström and Wassen in 1930, belongs to the *Chlamydia* group of agents, which includes the causative organisms of psittacosis, trachoma, and inclusion conjunctivitis. They were formerly described as large viruses but they resemble viruses only in the fact that they are obligatory intracellular parasites. Otherwise they are much more clearly related to bacteria: for example, in their structure, mode of reproduction, chemical constitution and susceptibility to chemotherapy.

The disease is usually transmitted sexually and commences with a transient, primary genital lesion followed by suppurative regional adenitis. After a latent phase which may last for years, there may be late manifestations due to rectal stricture or lymphatic obstruction.

EARLY MANIFESTATIONS

The incubation period is probably short in most cases, perhaps less than a week, but incubation periods of three to five weeks and longer have been reported.

Primary Genital Lesion (Fig. 121, p. 261)

This is usually a small herpetiform lesion but may be an ulcer, papule, vesicle or pustule, appearing on the glans penis, coronal sulcus, prepuce or shaft of the penis; although it is usually single, sometimes there are several lesions. It is small, painless and non-indurated and frequently the patient fails to notice it or describes it as a 'pimple'. It usually heals very quickly. It is rarely found in women. Occasionally, the lesion ulcerates more extensively and is more persistent.[2] Intraurethral lesions may give rise to urethral discharge, a rare form of non-gonococcal urethritis. Urethral stricture and fistula may follow.

Extragenital primary infection of the anus, mouth or hand has been described with involvement of the related lymph nodes.

Inguinal Adenitis ('Inguinal Syndrome')

This may follow the primary lesion after an interval of from a few days to several weeks. In males it may be associated with lymphangitis of the penis[2] and small abscesses along the course of the lymphatics (bubonuli). Involvement is limited to one groin in about two-thirds of the cases, but is bilateral in the remainder. This manifestation is considerably more common in men than in women, presumably because, in women, the initial lesion is likely to be deeply situated and to drain to the pelvic lymphatic nodes. Pain is usually the presenting symptom and the patient is aware of tender swelling in the groin. On examination, the superficial inguinal lymphatic nodes on the affected side are enlarged and tender. At first the swellings may be discrete, but they soon become matted together as the result of perinodal inflammation. They become attached to the skin and to the deep tissues. There may be palpable swelling and tenderness of iliac lymphatic nodes at the pelvic brim and also of the femoral nodes. Soon, suppuration occurs with the formation of multiple small abscesses. The skin overlying the abscesses is bluish-red in colour and fluctuation may be felt. The abscesses open on the skin surface to form multiple sinuses, discharging semi-caseous material, which may, however, be frankly purulent and bloodstained. The openings of the sinuses are not acutely inflamed and do not tend to ulcerate as in chancroid. The swelling is often an elongated sausage-shaped mass, and enlargement of nodes above and below the inguinal ligament may give the bubo a grooved appearance, called by Greenblatt[3] the 'sign of the groove' (Fig. 122). There are many variations in the clinical picture. The swelling may be painless and may resolve without suppuration; or it may break down to form a unilocular abscess resembling a chancroidal bubo. Involvement of iliac nodes may give the symptom of abdominal pain which, on the right side, has been mistaken for appendicitis. Rarely there is generalized enlargement of the lymphatic nodes.

Constitutional Symptoms

These are very variable. They may be absent, slight or severe. At the time of the inguinal syndrome, a patient may complain of chills, feverishness, headache, anorexia, nausea, arthralgia and loss of weight. The pulse rate is likely to be raised and there may be fever of up to 39·5°C or higher. Occasionally meningism occurs or a condition resembling a typhoid state. Splenomegaly, joint effusions and erythema nodosum can occur. Hepatic involvement has been described. Backache is not uncommon in women, and this may be due to involvement of pelvic lymphatic nodes.

Clinical recovery from the inguinal syndrome occurs in the course of weeks or months, but if there have been discharging sinuses, scars remain in the groin. Diagnosis at this stage of the disease depends on the results of intradermal and serological tests. Patients may become infected with this disease without experiencing symptoms or showing signs which attract attention. Signs of proctitis may be found on routine examination.

LATE MANIFESTATIONS

The interval between the early stage and the later manifestations may vary from a year or two to many years. In the later stage the patient may give the history of suppurative adenitis in the past, and there may be characteristic scarring in the groin.

Genital Elephantiasis (Esthiomene) (Fig. 123)

This is a swelling due to chronic lymphatic oedema of the vulva, a consequence of chronic inflammation involving the lymphatic vessels. The male genitalia may be affected by the same process, but less commonly. Vegetations and polypoid growths may develop on the skin surface; recto-vaginal or urinary fistulae may form and the area may break down to destructive ulceration. The oedema may extend from the clitoris to the anus. Elephantiasis in the male involves the penis and scrotum; warty growths, urinary fistulae and non-gonococcal urethritis have been described in these cases. Occasionally elephantiasis of one or both legs may occur. These changes are much more likely to occur in negroes than in white persons.

Anorectal Syndrome

This important late manifestation is commoner in women, probably as the result of direct spread of the infective process from the vagina to the rectum. Proctitis may be found early in the course of the disease but rectal stricture is a later development. Milder cases are frequently symptomless so that proctoscopy and digital examination of the rectum should be carried out in all cases of suspected lymphogranuloma venereum. The earliest symptoms are bleeding from the anus, and purulent anal discharge. Proctoscopy may reveal proctitis, rectal ulceration or rectal stricture, or a combination of these findings. In late neglected cases there may be severe proctocolitis resembling ulcerative colitis. Fistula-in-ano, perirectal

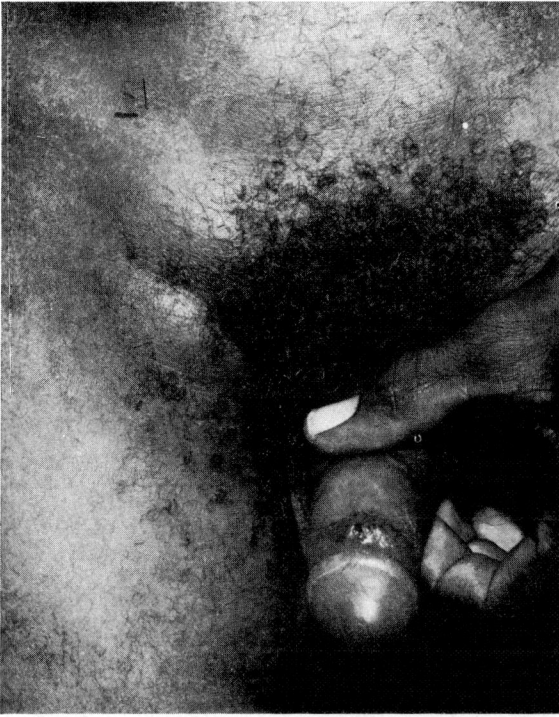

Fig. 121.
Lymphogranuloma
venereum: primary lesion
with right inguinal
adenopathy.

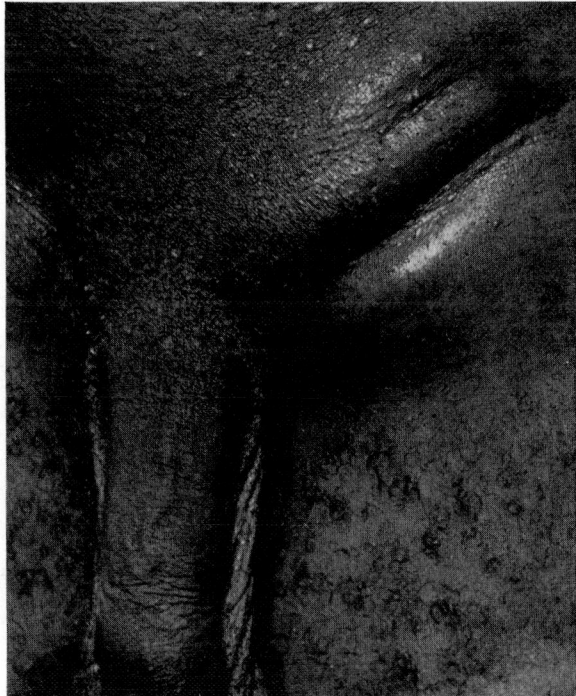

Fig. 122.
Lymphogranuloma
venereum: inguinal
syndrome with typical
'groove'.

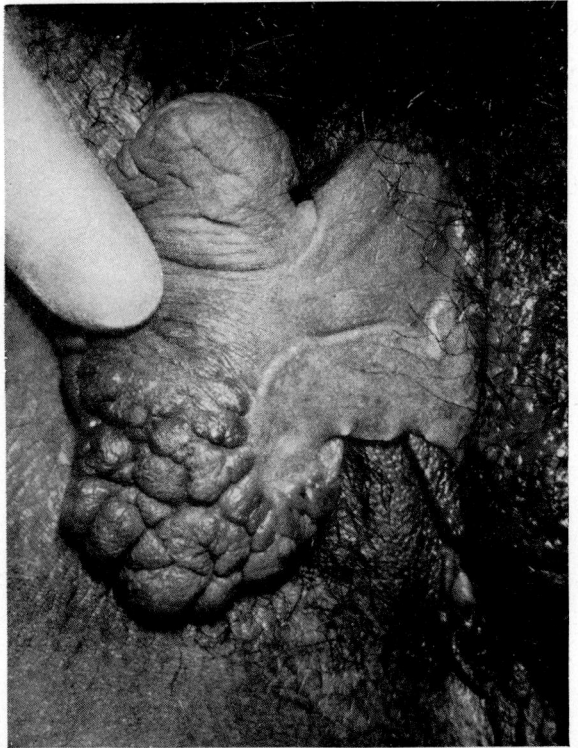

Fig. 123.
Lymphogranuloma
venereum: esthiomene
with ulceration of labium
minus.

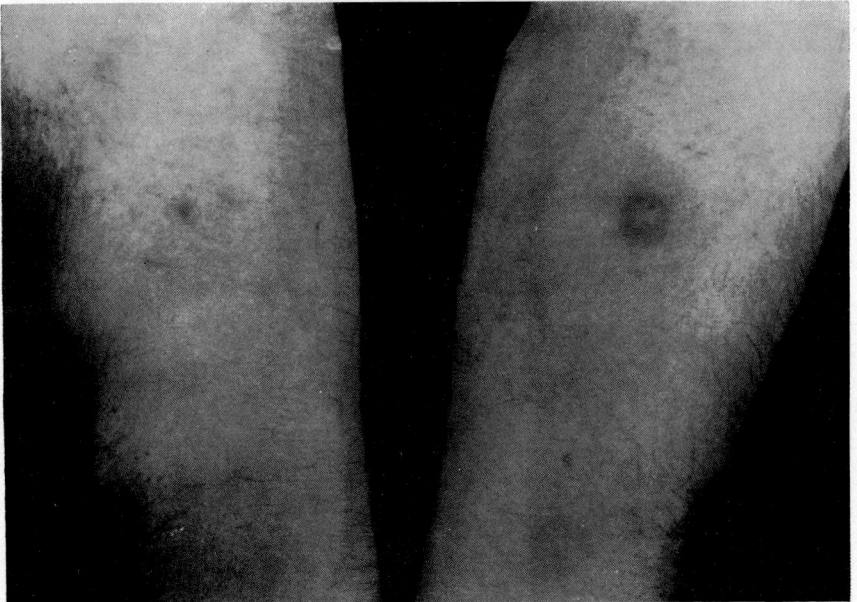

Fig. 124. Lymphogranuloma venereum: Frei test showing positive test left arm
with negative control right arm.

abscesses and rectovesical and rectovaginal fistulae may develop; lobulated tumour-like swellings may sometimes be seen at the anal orifice. Patients with progressive stricture formation are likely to complain of rectal discharge and bleeding, associated with constipation, colicky pain and the passage of 'ribbon stools'. Finally, complete obstruction may occur. The stricture is usually cylindrical and commonly about 5 cm long, although it can be diaphragmatic or as much as 20 cm in length with involvement of the sigmoid colon. The lowest part of stricture formation is generally 3 to 5 cm from the anal margin. When proctitis is found in the male, the infection has sometimes occurred as the result of homosexual practices.[4]

Malignant Changes

Malignant changes have been described as sequelae of genital elephantiasis and of the anorectal syndrome.[5]

DIAGNOSTIC TESTS

Culture

The most certain method of confirming the diagnosis is to obtain pus by aspiration of an unruptured inguinal abscess and to grow the organism in the yolk sacs of chick embryos or in cell culture. Even if the patient has received no treatment before this is undertaken, success in growing the organism is by no means certain.

The Frei Test (Fig. 124)

The original antigen, which was first introduced by Frei in 1925, was made from pus aspirated from unruptured buboes of patients suffering from the disease. This antigen was difficult to obtain in quantity; it varied considerably in potency and was sometimes contaminated by bacteria. Some of these difficulties were overcome by preparing antigen from the brains of infected mice. This preparation suffered from the fact that the concentration of the agent in the brains of diseased mice was not high and also many patients gave non-specific reactions to the control injection of normal mouse brain. A potent group-specific antigen became available in 1940 when Rake, McKee and Shaffer[6] succeeded in growing the agent in quantity in the yolk sacs of developing chick embryos. A reliable antigen of this kind is available commercially under the trade name of Lygranum. The test is performed by injecting 0·1 ml of such an antigen intradermally into the skin of one forearm, and 0·1 ml of control material, made from normal yolk, into the other forearm. The test is read at 48 and 72 hours; the control should give no reaction. If the test is positive, a raised, red papule, at least 6 mm across, surrounded by a variable area of erythema, appears at the site of injection of the antigen. The positive intradermal test is obtained at varying intervals after the time of infection. The limits of time are possibly from one week to six months, but usually the test is positive within two or three weeks. A negative test does not exclude the disease. Once reactivity is established it may persist for many years and perhaps for life. It is less likely to do so if the diagnosis is made early and adequate treatment is given. False-positive tests are frequent and many of these are probably due to infection by other chlamydial agents.

The Complement-fixation Test (CFT)

The same group-specific antigen is used for a complement-fixation test on blood serum, and it is generally agreed that this is a more sensitive and reliable test than the intradermal reaction. It is likely to give positive results earlier in the course of the disease. There is cross-reaction with the organism of psittacosis and an antigen made from that organism will give equally satisfactory results. The test is reported quantitatively, and a positive result in dilutions of the serum to 1 in 16 or above is usually taken to indicate the presence of active or recent infection with the organism. Positive results persisting in lower titre indicate the possibility that the patient has suffered from the disease but that it is probably inactive at the time of testing. They may also be due to infections with other organisms of the *Chlamydia* group. Both the intradermal test and the CFT should be done in cases in which this infection is suspected, and they may have to be repeated at intervals before the diagnosis of early infection can be established or excluded.

The Micro-immunofluorescence Test

The micro-immunofluorescence (Micro-IF) test has proved to be the best serological test for distinguishing the different chlamydial serotypes including the three serotypes of the agent of lymphogranuloma venereum.[7, 8] As well as being chlamydial type specific, it is much more sensitive than the group-specific complement-fixation test. It is likely to replace the CFT but is not yet widely available.

Other Tests

There is often an alteration in the serum proteins in cases of lymphogranuloma venereum. This usually takes the form of hyperproteinaemia with increase in the globulin fraction but normal or reduced albumin, giving reversal of the albumin–globulin ratio. Sonck[9] found an early rise in the level of immunoglobulins, especially IgA, in patients infected with the disease. This persisted with active infection and could be used to determine the efficacy of treatment over the longer term. The erythrocyte sedimentation rate is usually raised when active lesions of the disease are present.

TREATMENT

Chemotherapy

ANTIMONY. Preparations of antimony have been used in the past by both the intravenous and intramuscular routes. The efficacy of these drugs is doubtful and the toxic effects are not negligible. They should not now be used in the treatment of this disease.

SULPHONAMIDES. In early cases good results may follow the use of a sulphonamide, such as sulphathiazole, sulphadiazine or sulphadimidine. Dosage may be 5 g daily in divided doses for 10 to 20 days, but sometimes it may be necessary to give a second course of the same or another drug; toxic effects may follow. Co-trimoxazole, two tablets twice daily for 10 to 20 days may also be given. It has been claimed that cases of genital elephantiasis and the anorectal syndrome have shown clinical improvement as the result of treatment with sulphonamides, but the beneficial effect may well be due only to control of secondary infection. Sulphonamides are possibly the most effective remedies for this condition in which all treatment has been rather disappointing. It is customary to commence treatment with sulphonamides, unless there is some contraindication, and then to use an antibiotic if there is little response after five to seven days.

Antibiotics

PENICILLIN has some action against this organism in vitro and has been reported to be effective in animal experiments. Reports of its use in man are conflicting, but the consensus of opinion is that it is not a useful drug in the treatment of lymphogranuloma venereum. It is true to say, however, that it has never been given a systematic trial with a considerable number of cases and proper controls.

STREPTOMYCIN is believed to be ineffective and aminoglycosides in general have no action against *Chlamydia* in cell culture.

CHLORAMPHENICOL. Good results have been claimed from giving chloramphenicol by mouth in doses of 500 mg four times daily for 14 days or by intramuscular injections in doses of 4 g at intervals of two or three days, to a total of 12 g. The use of this drug is not recommended because of its potentially serious toxic effects.

TETRACYCLINES. Considerable claims have been made for these drugs in the treatment of lymphogranuloma venereum and they are the remedies of choice after sulphonamides. Nevertheless, they have sometimes proved disappointing. Tetracycline and oxytetracycline have slight preference over chlortetracycline because they are less likely to give minor toxic effects. The recommended dosage is 500 mg four times daily for 10 to 20 days.

If response is indifferent it may prove effective to repeat the course after an interval of seven days without treatment. Recently good results have been obtained with minocycline.[10] It was given in dosage of 300 mg initially followed by 200 mg twice daily for 10 days. Doxycycline 200 mg daily for 10 to 20 days should also be effective.

ERYTHROMYCIN. This is likely to give similar results to tetracycline when used in dosage of 500 mg four times daily for 10 to 20 days.

CORTICOSTEROIDS. Saad, De Gouveia and Da Silva[11] used corticosteroids (prednisolone, triamcinolone or dexamethasone) by mouth in the treatment of late cases of lymphogranuloma venereum, alone or in conjunction with sulphonamides or antibiotics. They noted improvement in some cases with diminution of rectal discharge, relief of rectal and intestinal pain and lessening of constipation. This treatment may help prevent further rectal fibrosis.

Surgical Treatment

Surgical intervention should only be undertaken after adequate antibiotic therapy has been given.

Fluctuant abscesses in the groins may need repeated aspiration, which is preferable to incision. Surgical removal of lymphatic nodes is inadvisable because of the danger that elephantiasis of the lower limbs may follow.

In cases of esthiomene, local vulvectomy may be indicated. Patients with the anorectal syndrome may need regular dilatation of rectal strictures with rectal bougies. Perianal and perirectal abscesses may need drainage. If the rectal obstruction is complete, colostomy may be necessary; in certain cases this may be followed by abdominoperineal excision of the rectum, particularly when multiple perianal fistulae are present.[12]

REFERENCES

1. A. R. med. Offr Dept Hlth (Lond.) (1977) p. 59. H.M.S.O. 1978.
2. HOPSU-HAVU, V. K. and SONCK, C. E. (1973) Br. J. vener. Dis., 49, 193.
3. GREENBLATT, R. B. (1953) Management of Chancroid, Granuloma Inguinale, Lymphogranuloma Venereum in General Practice. U.S. Publ. Hlth Serv. Publ., Wash., No. 255.
4. GREAVES, A. B. (1963) Bull. Wld Hlth Org., 29, 797.
5. LEVIN, I., ROMANO, S., STEINBERG, M. and WELSH, R. A. (1964) Dis. Colon Rectum, 7, 129.
6. RAKE, G., McKEE, C. M. and SHAFFER, M. F. (1940) Proc. Soc. exp. Biol. (N.Y.), 43, 332.
7. WANG, S-P. and GRAYSTON, J. T. (1971) Trachoma and Related Disorders, ed. R. L. Nichols, p. 305. Amsterdam and New York: Excerpta Medica.
8. PHILIP, R. N., CASPER, E. A., GORDON, F. B. and QUAN, A. L. (1974) J. Immunol., 112, 2126.

9. Sonck, C. E. (1972) *Hautarzt*, **23,** 280.

10. Sowmini, C. N., Gopalan, K. N. and Chandrasekhara, R. (1976) *J. Am. vener. Dis. Ass.*, **2,** 19.

11. Saad, E. A., De Gouveia, O. F. and Da Silva, J. R. (1962) *Am. J. trop. Med.*, **11,** 108.

12. Annamunthodo, H. (1961) *Ann. R. Coll. Surg.*, **29,** 141.

20

Granuloma Inguinale

This condition has been called 'ulcerating granuloma of the pudenda', 'sclerosing granuloma', and 'granulomatosis'. In Europe it used to be called 'granuloma venereum', but the name 'granuloma inguinale' is now accepted for the International Nomenclature of Diseases and helps to avoid confusion with lymphogranuloma venereum. Lal and Nicholas[1] have criticized this name on the grounds that the lesions of the disease are infrequently found in the inguinal region. They suggest the name 'granuloma donovani'. It is generally regarded as a venereal disease of low contagiousness, but doubts have been expressed as to the method of transmission because in most cases it is not communicated to the sexual partner.[2] Those who believe it to be a venereal disease point to the fact that the lesions are usually on the genitalia, and they are found in promiscuous individuals who often suffer from other venereal infections. Lal and Nicholas[1] examined the sexual partners (all marital) of 50 of their 165 patients and found the disease to be present in 26 (52 per cent) which is a much higher frequency than in most other reports. According to their data the incubation periods vary from three days to six months with periods of 7 to 30 days in the considerable majority. Of their 165 patients 45·5 per cent were also suffering from syphilis. Granuloma inguinale was probably first described by McLeod in India in 1882.[3]

INCIDENCE. Granuloma inguinale occurs almost exclusively in the coloured races. It is found in tropical and subtropical countries and is not uncommon in the southern states of the United States of America and in the West Indies. In the sub-continent of India before partition it was much more common in Hindus than in Muslims. Until recent years it was practically unknown in Great Britain, but it is now seen occasionally in recent immigrants. Where the condition has been common, it has been found twice as frequently in men as in women. Most patients are aged 20 to 40 years.

The causative organism, *Donovania granulomatis* (Donovan body), was probably discovered by Donovan in India in 1905 (see Fig. 127). He described bodies seen in epithelial cells of the skin. As now recognized, these bodies are encapsulated rods which are found within large mononuclear cells in material from the lesions, and measure 1·5 by 2·5 μm. With Wright's stain the capsule is pink and the body of the organism shows bipolar condensation of chromatin material. The nature of the organism is the subject of controversy, but many believe that it is bacterial and is perhaps related to the *Klebsiella* group. It is an extremely fastidious organism but has, nevertheless, been grown on various artificial media. Belief that the organism grown in culture is identical with that found in the lesions is based on morphological appearance, staining properties, failure to grow on ordinary media, susceptibility to streptomycin and antigenic relationship; it has not been confirmed by experimental reproduction of the typical disease in volunteers. The incubation period has not been determined accurately but in experimental infections in man using material from pseudobuboes the disease seems to be fully developed in about 50 days.

CLINICAL FINDINGS

The lesions may commence on the genitalia (Plate V, ii and Figs. 125 and 126), on the thigh, in the groins or in the perineum. They appear first as painless papules or vesicles which become ulcerated and slowly develop into rounded, elevated, velvety, ulcerating granulomatous masses, which bleed easily. There is little or no tendency to spontaneous healing as the condition spreads by continuity as friable, painless, 'beefy-red' ulcerogranulomatous lesions. Contact infection occurs between the skin of the scrotum and thigh. It may extend to the lower abdomen and buttocks. Inguinal swellings may be seen associated with the genital lesions, appearing as indurated masses or fluctuant abscesses which eventually break down to be replaced by the typical ulcers. They are called 'pseudobuboes', because they are, in fact, subcutaneous granulomata and not enlarged lymphatic nodes although the adjacent lymphatic nodes may show microscopical changes. The ulcers may become painful, but usually there is little constitutional disturbance. Discharge from the lesions is often serosanguineous. With extensive disease of some standing, in debilitated patients, there may be gross secondary infection, especially with Vincent's organisms, and phagedenic ulceration may follow, with much tissue destruction, foul-smelling discharge, and constitutional symptoms. Ultimately there may be much scarring, with distortion, and perhaps elephantiasis of the genitals The ulcerating process sometimes extends into the female genital tract and involves the cervix uteri.

The early lesions may closely resemble the early lesions of syphilis, especially condylomata lata. Later the ulcerating masses may resemble

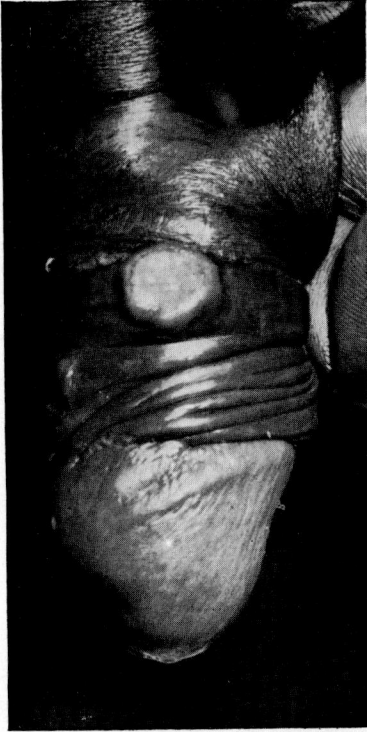

Fig. 125. Granuloma inguinale: early lesion of penis.

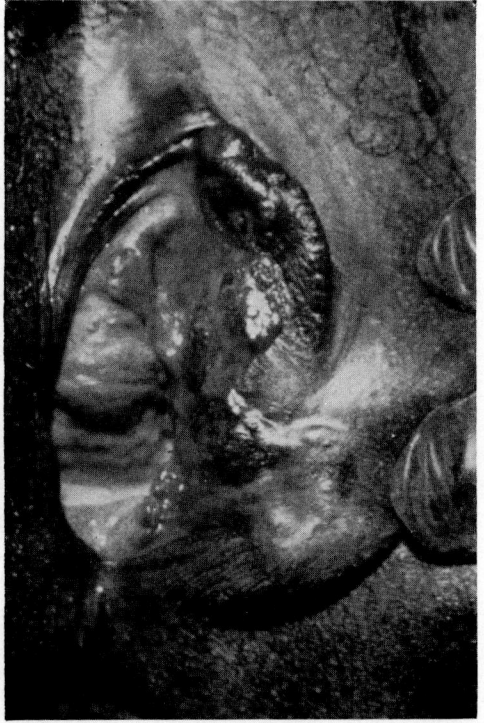

Fig. 126. Granuloma inguinale: later lesions with vulval oedema on left.

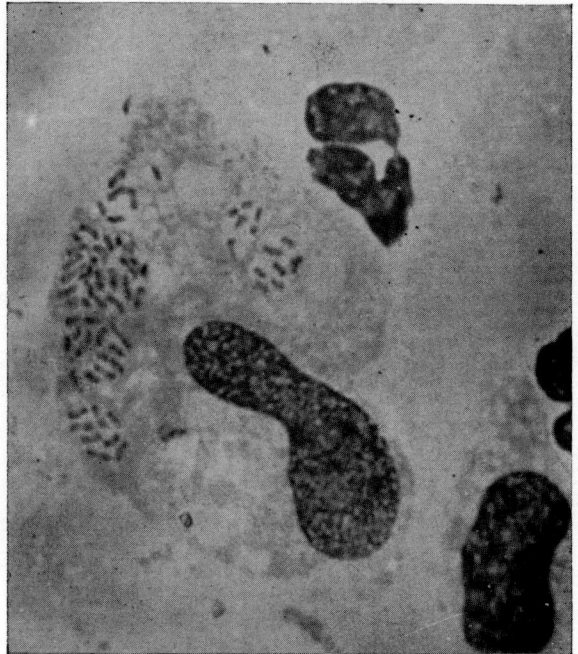

Fig. 127. Granuloma inguinale: Donovan bodies seen in mononuclear cell.

epitheliomatous lesions, and in the late stage they have to be differentiated from the genital syndrome of lymphogranuloma venereum.

EXTRAGENITAL LESIONS have been described on the face and neck, in the mouth and throat and occasionally at other sites on skin and mucous surfaces.

METASTATIC LESIONS, involving bones and joints and viscera, have been reported occasionally. They are more common in females.

MALIGNANT CHANGES have been reported as occurring in long-standing lesions of the genital or perianal regions. The disease itself produces a variable degree of pseudo-epitheliomatous hyperplasia and can at times be difficult to differentiate from carcinoma, both clinically and histologically.

DIAGNOSIS

STAINING METHODS. After thorough cleansing of the lesion a small piece of granulomatous tissue is removed from the edge of a lesion with a small scalpel or with a biopsy punch. The under surface of the tissue is smeared on to glass slides and the smears are allowed to dry. Smears may also be made by crushing the tissue between two slides. After drying they are then fixed with methyl alcohol for three minutes and stained with Wright's or Giemsa's stain. Donovan bodies must be searched for in the mononuclear cells, and they are usually recognized by their 'safety-pin' appearance, produced by the bipolar distribution of the chromatin material. Occasionally Donovan bodies may show no evidence of a capsule and may be extracellular.

BIOPSY. Donovan bodies may also be found in suitably stained sections.

INTRADERMAL AND SEROLOGICAL TESTS. Intradermal tests have been described but they have little value in diagnosis, because of frequent false-positive reactions. A complement-fixation test has proved more reliable but diagnosis should ordinarily rest on discovery of Donovan bodies.

TREATMENT

LOCAL TREATMENT, apart from saline washes to maintain cleanliness, is of no value in this condition.

ANTIMONY has been used in the past for early lesions, but now has no place in treatment.

SULPHONAMIDES AND PENICILLIN have no direct effect upon the lesions of granuloma inguinale. Benefit, which has been observed occasionally, is probably due to control of secondary infection.

CO-TRIMOXAZOLE, in contrast to sulphonamides alone, has recently proved effective in a small series of cases. Garg et al.,[4] in India, treated 10 patients with 2 tablets twice daily for 10 days with rapid healing in each case.

STREPTOMYCIN by intramuscular injection has usually been effective treatment for granuloma inguinale. Donovan bodies disappear and lesions heal. A total of 20 g is adequate dosage in most cases, and the most effective method of administration is to give 4 g in divided doses daily for five days. Smaller dosage for longer periods is also effective, but recovery is slower. Lal,[5] in India, has testified to the fact that this drug remains effective in that country. In the period 1966 to 1970 he treated 122 cases of the condition, giving 1 g intramuscularly twice daily, with good response in 91 per cent of the cases. The average amount required for successful treatment was 25 g. In New Guinea,[6] however, streptomycin has given poor results in recent years.

TETRACYCLINE, CHLORTETRACYCLINE AND OXYTETRACYCLINE are all effective in the treatment of granuloma inguinale. In a few days, Donovan bodies disappear from the lesions, which heal rapidly. Tetracycline or oxytetracycline is to be preferred, and either may be given in doses of 500 mg every six hours for 10 to 20 days, totalling 20 to 40 g. Poor results have, however, been reported from Vietnam.[7]

CHLORAMPHENICOL is effective by mouth and has been given successfully by intramuscular injection in single doses of 4 g, with intervals of two or three days, to a total of 12 to 16 g. Because of its potentially serious toxic effects this drug is not suitable for routine use and should be avoided if possible.

ERYTHROMYCIN is also said to be effective. It can be given in similar dosage to the tetracyclines.

AMPICILLIN was found to be effective by Thew et al.[8] in the treatment of 4 cases. They gave 1 g (in one case 2 g) by mouth daily for 3 to 12 weeks, the total dosage varying from 24 to 160 g. The biggest dosage was given to a patient whose condition relapsed after tetracycline. The lesions healed quickly and there were no recurrences after 4 to 6 weeks. On the other hand Davis[9] treated 2 of his 14 patients initially with ampicillin, without improvement. Excellent results were obtained in 31 cases in Vietnam[7] using 500 mg every six hours for 14 days.

GENTAMICIN has given good results in a small series of cases treated in New Guinea.[6] It was given intramuscularly in dosage of 1 mg per kg three times a day; the average total amount required was 2·4 g. Some of the patients had previously failed to respond to streptomycin.

LINCOMYCIN was found to be effective by Breschi et al.[7] in the treatment of six cases. They gave 500 mg by mouth every six hours for 14 days.

FOLLOW-UP

Clinical relapse occurs sometimes after apparently successful treatment, but repetition of the same treatment is usually successful.

Follow-up of cases should be prolonged, for relapse may occur several months or even years after apparently successful treatment.

REFERENCES

1. LAL, S. and NICHOLAS, C. (1970) *Br. J. vener. Dis.*, **46,** 461.
2. GREENBLATT, R. B. (1953) Management of Chancroid, Granuloma Inguinale, Lympho-granuloma Venereum in General Practice. *U.S. Publ. Hlth Serv. Publ., Wash.*, No. 255.
3. McLEOD, K. (1882) *Indian med. Gaz.*, **17,** 113.
4. GARG, B. R., LAL, S. and SIVAMANI, S. (1978) *Br. J. vener. Dis.*, **54,** 348.
5. LAL, S. (1971) *Br. J. vener. Dis.*, **47,** 454.
6. MADDOCKS, I., ANDERS, E. M. and DENNIS, E. (1976) *Br. J. vener. Dis.*, **52,** 190.
7. BRESCHI, L. C., GOLDMAN, G. and SHAPIRO, S. R. (1975) *J. Am. vener. Dis. Ass.*, **1,** 118.
8. THEW, M. A., SWIFT, J. T. and HEATON, C. L. (1969) *J. Am. med. Ass.*, **210,** 866.
9. DAVIS, C. M. (1970) *J. Am. med. Ass.*, **211,** 632.

21

'Non-specific' Urogenital Infection; Non-gonococcal Genital Infections in Children; Non-gonococcal Ophthalmia

The simplest classification of urethral inflammations is a broad division into gonococcal and non-gonococcal.* About 40 per cent of the non-gonococcal group are now known to be due to chlamydial infection. Of the remainder a definite cause can be identified in only a minority of cases; thus a specific organism may be identified as a pathogen or associated clinical findings may give a clue to the origin of the condition, as, for instance, in cases of disease higher in the urogenital tract (see Figs. 140 and 141, p. 318) or the presence of foreign bodies (see Figs. 142–145, pp. 318–9). In the rest, which is probably about half of the total, no cause can be found. For this reason this disease is often called 'non-specific' or 'abacterial' urethritis. The former name has only common usage to recommend it, because the strong probability is that there is a specific cause, or perhaps more than one, which has not yet been found. The proportional incidence of the causes of non-gonococcal urethritis in the male is shown in Table 4. If tests for *Chlamydia* are not done then over 90 per cent will be classed as 'non-specific'.

AETIOLOGY

Search for the cause of non-specific (abacterial) urethritis has proceeded along six main lines:

*Early work in this subject was very fully reviewed by Harkness[1] in his monograph.

TABLE 4
CAUSES OF NON-GONOCOCCAL URETHRITIS

Chlamydia trachomatis	40 per cent
Trichomonas vaginalis	2 to 5 per cent
Secondary to bacterial urinary infection	1 to 2 per cent
Herpes simplex virus	1 to 2 per cent
Other causes, for example, pre-existing urethral stricture, mycotic, bacterial, traumatic, chemical, neoplastic, and foreign bodies	1 to 2 per cent
'Non-specific'	50 per cent

Chlamydia

The finding of inclusion bodies in epithelial cells from the urethrae of patients suffering from non-gonococcal urethritis was described in 1910 and confirmed in later years. The organism of which these findings gave evidence is the cause of inclusion conjunctivitis (see p. 289) and the isolation of this organism in yolk-sac culture by Jones, Collier and Smith[2] gave the opportunity for further study of its significance in ocular and genital infections. It has been established that the organism responsible for inclusion conjunctivitis and related genital infection cannot be distinguished from the cause of trachoma and it is now believed that a single organism causes both of these clinical syndromes. It has been named by Gear et al.[3] 'TRIC agent', the TR standing for trachoma and -IC for inclusion conjunctivitis. The agent is a member of a group of organisms which includes the cause of lymphogranuloma venereum and for which the generic name *Chlamydia* is now used. There are two species of *Chlamydia*, *C. trachomatis* and *C. psittaci*. The inclusion bodies of *C. trachomatis* stain with iodine whereas those of *C. psittaci* do not. They are neither viruses nor bacteria. Although they can only grow in cells they divide by binary fission. They contain both RNA and DNA, have cell walls of bacterial type, ribosomes and enzyme systems. The technique of detection and isolation of this organism has been fully described by Gordon et al.,[4] and the technique has been simplified by Darougar et al.[5] The application of the micro-immunofluorescence technique has provided a practicable method of serotyping the different strains of *C. trachomatis*.[6,7] Hyperendemic trachoma is almost always associated with infection by serotypes A, B, Ba and C, whereas those involved in inclusion conjunctivitis and genital infection are generally types D, E, F, G, H, I, J and K. The lymphogranuloma venereum serotypes are LI, LII and LIII. The micro-immunofluorescence test can also be used to detect antichlamydial antibodies in serum and local antibodies in body secretions. There have now been numerous investigations employing the newer techniques for isolating *Chlamydia* and there is no doubt that it is a major cause of non-gonococcal urethritis, accounting for about 40 per cent of cases. Patients with gonorrhoea who also harbour *C. trachomatis* almost invariably have evidence of post-gonococcal urethritis on careful examination after treatment of their gonorrhoea. The subject was reviewed by Dunlop[8] in 1975 and more recently by Schachter.[9]

As will be evident later in this chapter, there is a wide spectrum of disease due to *C. trachomatis*. Disease of the eyes, non-gonococcal urethritis and lymphogranuloma venereum have already been mentioned. The organism has also been incriminated in cervical, rectal and pharyngeal infections, epididymitis, salpingitis, perihepatitis, endocarditis and neonatal pneumonia.

Mycoplasma

Cultural investigations have demonstrated the presence of *Mycoplasma hominis* in many cases of urethral and genital infection, although the results of such investigations have varied in different hands. The organisms have also been found, although less frequently, in subjects with no evidence of past or present infection of the urogenital tract. The frequency of recovery generally correlates with the degree of sexual activity of the individuals studied. The significance of strains of *M. hominis* found in cases of non-specific urethritis remains a matter for speculation. Whether they cause the condition, or are commensals or non-pathogenic organisms which become pathogenic under certain conditions, cannot be determined at the present time, but they are unlikely to be a significant cause of non-specific urethritis. The strongest point in favour of their pathogenicity is that on rare occasions they have been isolated in pure culture from the pus of tubo-ovarian abscesses in such profusion that they were probably the cause of the condition. Complement-fixing antibodies against *M. hominis* have been demonstrated in the serum of patients, the highest incidence being among patients attending VD clinics and the lowest in blood donors and children.

Considerable attention has also been directed to an organism described by Shepard,[10] who believed it to be a special variety of mycoplasma, the colonies of which were smaller than those of *Mycoplasma hominis* and which, from the tiny size of the colonies, he called 'T-strains'. T-mycoplasmas are indeed members of the genus *Mycoplasma* but, because they have the unique property of metabolizing urea, those of human origin are now termed *Ureaplasma urealyticum*.[11] Although they are found in the urethra in the majority of men with non-specific urethritis, they can also be found in healthy individuals, the rate of recovery correlating with the total number of sexual partners.[12] Nevertheless there is some evidence that they may be a cause of non-specific urethritis[13] and this has been supported recently by inoculation experiments in humans.[14]

Trichomonas vaginalis
(see Chapter 23)

This organism is found in the secretions of some men with non-gonococcal urethritis, although in proportions which have been found to vary greatly in the experience of different observers and in different groups of population. It is more common in Negroes than in white men, and in those with urethral stricture than those without. It is sometimes detected in the consorts of females suffering from trichomonal vaginitis, although in many of the cases it gives rise to neither symptoms nor signs and it may be very difficult to isolate. The belief that it is pathogenic is supported by the fact that treatment with the oral trichomonacide metronidazole cures most of the cases in which *Trichomonas vaginalis* appears to be the only cause of non-gonococcal urethritis. Metronidazole is, however, ineffective in cases of urethritis in which *Trichomonas vaginalis* is not present, and there is no support for the view that this organism, undetected by present laboratory methods, is a major cause of non-gonococcal urethritis.

Mycotic Infections

Candida albicans (see Chapter 24) and other fungi may be detected in the secretions of up to 5 per cent of cases of non-gonococcal urethritis, but true mycotic urethritis is a rare condition, associated in most cases with urethral trauma or pre-existing diabetes mellitus.

Bacteria

Organisms, particularly *Staphylococcus albus* and diphtheroid bacilli, are frequently grown from urethral secretions in these cases. The evidence points to the fact that these organisms are commensals. If they do cause urethritis, they do so in a minute proportion of the cases.

'Haemophilus vaginalis' (Corynebacterium vaginale)

This is a Gram-negative, non-motile, non-encapsulated, pleomorphic rod, alleged to be related to the genus *Haemophilus*. It was isolated from the genital tracts of men suffering from urethritis by Leopold in 1953[15] and from cases of vaginitis by Gardner and Dukes in 1954.[16] It has since been shown that this organism does not belong to the genus *Haemophilus* but is probably a *Corynebacterium*. Its significance has not been fully determined but present evidence suggests that in the urethra it is probably a commensal. Whether or not it is a vaginal pathogen still remains controversial. The matter has been reviewed recently by Dunkelberg.[17]

Corynebacterium genitalium

Another type of *Corynebacterium* called *Corynebacterium genitalium* has also been recovered from men with non-specific urethritis. Certain strains are thought to be pathogenic by Furness and Evangelista.[18] It has been recovered from the epididymis in cases of acute epididymitis, but its exact role in non-specific urethritis remains to be decided.

Allergy

This has been suggested as a cause of non-gonococcal urethritis as it has been suggested as a cause for many other conditions. The clinical behaviour of the disease, cellular content of the urethral discharge, and the response to antibiotics do not suggest that this form of urethritis is an allergic process. Treatment with antihistamines and corticosteroids neither cures nor relieves the condition.

NON-SPECIFIC UROGENITAL INFECTION IN THE MALE

The major problem is, therefore, a condition of unknown cause which, for want of a better name, must be called non-specific urogenital infection. When facilities for culture of *Chlamydia trachomatis* are not available, over 90 per cent of cases of non-gonococcal urethritis will fall into this category and the following account applies to both chlamydial and non-chlamydial cases.

METHOD OF SPREAD. There is little doubt that this condition is spread by sexual intercourse, but clearly, in the absence of a known cause, this opinion is based only on epidemiological experience. However, *Chlamydia trachomatis* is often recovered from women whose sexual partners have chlamydial urethritis, but seldom from those whose partners have *Chlamydia*-negative non-specific urethritis.[19,20]

INCIDENCE. It is a common condition and seems to be becoming more so. The number of cases in males reported as attending the venereal diseases clinics of England and Wales rose from 10,794 in 1951 to 59,023 (England only) in 1971 and 73,996 (England only) in the year ending June 30, 1977.[21] Of course these figures do not indicate the total incidence but they do show the trend of increase. However, this is a condition which is prone to relapse and some part of the increase may be due to attendance for relapses, which are difficult to distinguish from fresh infections. No figures are available for the United States, but the incidence is likely to be greater than that of gonorrhoea. It seems to be less common in homosexuals.

Clinical Course

The usual presentation is with low-grade urethritis with scanty or moderate mucoid or mucopurulent urethral discharge and variable dysuria; but in a minority of cases the appearance of the discharge and the severity of the condition make it clinically indistinguishable from gonorrhoea. In a small number of cases the discharge is accompanied by haematuria and symptoms of cystitis, when it is usually called 'acute abacterial haemorrhagic cystitis'. At the other end of the scale, subclinical urethritis seems to be common; the patient does not notice the condition but it may be found in the course of a routine examination or because the patient presents with a complication. Rodin,[22] using early morning tests, found 11 cases of non-specific urethritis among 88 asymptomatic men attending a venereal diseases clinic. It is this feature of the disease that has led to difficulty in determining the true *incubation period*. It is generally considered to be from one to three weeks, but shorter and considerably longer periods are described.

Diagnosis

If the patient gives the history of the onset of dysuria or urethral discharge after recent intercourse with someone other than the regular sexual partner, and if the gonococcus or other likely cause cannot be found microscopically or in culture, the diagnosis is seldom in doubt.

In the two-glass test of urine the first or both specimens may be hazy with pus, and 'threads' which usually sink to the bottom of the glass may be seen in the first specimen. Often the first portion of urine contains several 'threads' without any haziness. If both specimens of urine are hazy then bacterial cystitis should be excluded. If present, the centrifuged deposit will show numerous organisms as well as leucocytes and culture of the mid-stream urine will identify the organisms. With non-specific infection examination of the centrifuged deposit of urine shows an excess of leucocytes and few or no organisms. Conventional culture of the urethral secretion gives no growth or only that of urethral commensals, but if culture for *Chlamydia* is available the organism will be found in 40 per cent or so of cases.

Sometimes the patient notices discharge only first thing in the morning or the complaint is solely of dysuria, and there may be no symptoms and no signs if the urine has been held only for a short time. In such cases the surest method of diagnosis is to ask the patient to return in the early morning having held the urine overnight, for eight hours or so. This is usually not difficult if fluid intake is restricted. It may then be possible to find secretion for microscopical and cultural examination, and if there is infection, characteristic signs are generally present in the urine. It must be admitted, however, that in some cases the findings on microscopy are minimal and the diagnosis is uncertain. There are no generally accepted criteria in such cases but the finding of 10 or more pus cells in several fields of the urethral smear, using a $\times$ 1000 magnification, is likely to be significant. However, the area of the field also depends on the type of eyepiece used and significant parts of the smear may be missed if it is not first scanned under low power. These difficulties will remain until all the causal agents of non-specific urethritis are known and can be tested for as a routine.

Complications

Local

The local complications are similar to those which used to follow gonorrhoea but are now seldom seen; they are usually less severe. Some degree of *littritis* is probably inevitable in the course of any urethral infection. *Tysonitis*, *cowperitis* and infection of *paraurethral* ducts occur, but are uncommon.

Prostatitis, or perhaps more accurately *prostatovesiculitis*, is probably commonly present from the first. It is generally a symptomless condition and the signs of associated non-specific urethritis may be overlooked unless the patient is examined for urethral discharge and pyuria, after having held his urine all night. Some patients have discomfort on passing urine and vague aches in the perineum, groins, thighs, penis, suprapubic region or lower part of the back; painful ejaculation may occur. Sometimes there is urethral discharge on the passage of a motion but care should be taken not to confuse this with a physiological 'prostatorrhoea', occurring in men who have no regular sexual outlet. Occasionally the complaint is of general malaise and low grade fever. Acute prostatitis is very rare, and in most cases the process seems to be chronic from the first. In early cases of chronic prostatitis there is no distinctive feel to the prostate. In late cases, after the lapse of years, the prostate and seminal vesicles may be firm to palpation, and may show areas of induration. Calculi may develop in the prostate. A diagnosis can be made only by examining the fluid obtained by prostatic massage. The criteria on which the diagnosis of chronic prostatitis should be based is the subject of considerable divergence of opinion. Ten or more leucocytes in several × 1000 microscopic fields or clumping of leucocytes is accepted by many as evidence of prostatitis. On these criteria, however, about one in five apparently healthy men would be diagnosed as having chronic prostatitis.[23] Nevertheless, a strong association has been found between chronic prostatitis, as so defined, and Reiter's disease, ankylosing spondylitis and iritis, in each of which conditions about 80 per cent of male patients have chronic prostatitis. Prostatic fluid is obtained by digital massage of the prostate, and common practice is to fix and stain by Gram's method a single specimen for microscopical examination. A more accurate, although more complicated, method is to examine five consecutive portions of one specimen of freshly expressed prostatic fluid.[23] Experience shows that a single specimen may appear normal even though the prostate is infected. The '5-slide' method diminishes the possibility of this error and permits the recognition of 'clumping' of the leucocytes. Culture of the prostatic fluid either is sterile or shows only commensal organisms.

It should be remembered that infection of the *seminal vesicles* is often associated with prostatitis, and care should be taken to empty these organs in the course of prostatic massage. In the course of time the walls of one or both seminal vesicles may become thickened as the result of chronic inflammation and careful palpation will determine that fact.

Epididymitis is a less common complication, occurring in about one per cent of the cases. *Chlamydia trachomatis* has recently been recovered from aspirates of the epididymis in some of these cases.[24] The symptoms and signs tend to be less severe than with gonococcal infection. It has to be distinguished from other causes of non-gonococcal epididymitis, especially early tuberculous infection, mumps without parotitis, and epididymitis associated with infection higher in the urinary tract; the latter is particularly likely in older patients.[24] Torsion of the testis and testicular tumours must also be excluded.

Urethral stricture is not a common complication of non-specific urethritis but it occurs sometimes. It is identified by anterior urethroscopy, which should be performed as part of the tests for cure and in the investigation of chronic and relapsing cases. A urethrogram may be necessary in some cases. The presence of symptomless stricture due to previous urethral infection or trauma may cause failure of treatment and serious late results; the possibility of such a lesion should always be considered in cases of trichomonal urethritis because the latter is found in up to a third of patients with urethral stricture.

General

Reiter's disease is described in Chapter 22. Recently a case of endocarditis due to *Chlamydia trachomatis* in a female has been reported (see p. 286). Males will also presumably be at risk from this rare complication.

Treatment

If active treatment is withheld and the patient given a placebo, in 60 per cent of cases the symptoms and signs of the disease will gradually disappear in the course of 8 weeks.[25] This procedure causes considerable anxiety and discomfort to the patient, and may subject others to the risk of infection; also in 40 per cent of cases longer periods for spontaneous resolution will be required and recovery of chlamydial agent after a year has been reported.[26] The incidence of late complications in untreated cases of the disease is not known. Thus there are strong indications for treatment with modern remedies.

The patient should be instructed to abstain from alcohol until symptoms and signs have subsided. Sexual intercourse should be forbidden until tests for cure have been completed.

Many remedies have been used for the treatment of this condition, and claims have been made which have not been substantiated by further experience. In many of the studies the period of observation after treatment has been too short. Tests for cure have often been inadequate and, for that matter, there is no general agreement on what constitutes cure. In many cases it is impossible to distinguish between relapse and re-infection. As stated, relapse is common and there is reason to suppose that in some cases the organism which causes this condition may persist, although giving rise to no symptoms in between attacks. In some cases decrease of urethral discharge may be wrongly interpreted as recovery if the urine has been held for a comparatively short time and examination of asymptomatic patients after they have held urine overnight may reveal persistent urethritis.

On the whole, this disease responds only fairly well to treatment, but there is sound evidence that some remedies are effective in 70 to 80 per cent of cases. The drugs most active against *Chlamydia trachomatis* in cell culture are the tetracyclines, erythromycin and spiramycin. Sulphonamides show moderate activity and aminoglycosides none. Spectinomycin has only slight activity.[27]

Non-specific urethritis does not respond to penicillin, although, unfortunately, it seems to be common practice to try the effect of penicillin without undertaking microscopical diagnosis. If the symptoms are relieved it is possibly the result of spontaneous remission, which may occur in cases of mild degree, although the patient is probably still carrying infection.

The combination of *streptomycin and sulphonamides* has given good results in the past and was at one time the standard treatment in the United Kingdom.[28] Sulphonamides show activity against *Chlamydia* but not *U. urealyticum* and streptomycin has the reverse effects. Streptomycin 1 g is injected intramuscularly and this may be followed by sulphadimidine or other soluble sulphonamide, 5 to 6 g in divided doses by mouth daily for 7 to 14 days. The longer course is probably preferable but 10 days has been shown to be effective in eliminating *Chlamydia*.[29] Spectinomycin, 2 g by injection, may be given as an alternative to streptomycin.

Tetracycline and *oxytetracycline* by mouth seem to be the most effective remedies, although the combination of streptomycin and sulphonamides is probably only a little less effective. With the tetracyclines, effective dosage may be 1 to 2 g daily in divided doses for 7 to 14 days, but occasionally *Chlamydia* has been isolated again after 1 g daily for 14 days.[30] The optimum duration of therapy is uncertain but we recommend a dosage of 2 g daily, for at least seven days, and the effect should then be checked by an early morning smear and urine test. Symptomatic improvement is the rule but does not necessarily indicate cure. If the tests are not satisfactory the drug should be continued for another one to two weeks. In a double-blind trial using 500 mg of tetracycline four times daily for 7 days cases in which *Chlamydia* had been found responded better than those in which this agent was not found.[31] *Chlamydia* was not found in cases of persistent urethritis or recurrence within 6 weeks of treatment even when such cases were initially *Chlamydia*-positive. Oriel et al.,[30] however, obtained a similar response in those with and those without *Chlamydia*. Routine courses of treatment prolonged for three weeks irrespective of the initial response are often recommended, but so far there are no really convincing well-conducted trials which show any lasting benefit from this and a recent double-blind trial showed no benefit, recurrence being only delayed but not prevented.[13] Likewise, in the double-blind trial of Thambar et al.[32] the initial significant benefit of three weeks' treatment compared with one week was not maintained; furthermore, when the sexual partners were also treated there was no difference in the early outcome in relation to duration of treatment, but the groups concerned were small. Part of any apparent early benefit might be from temporary protection against re-infection provided by the longer course. Patients should be told not to take tetracycline with milk or dairy products, which reduce its absorption. *Doxycycline* is not affected in this way and 200 mg daily after food for 7 to 14 days should give good results, but it is far too expensive to be used as a routine. The absorption of doxycycline as well as tetracycline is affected by antacids containing polyvalent metallic cations and by iron preparations and these should not be given concurrently.

A popular method of giving tetracycline in the United Kingdom is a triple mixture consisting of 69 mg of demethylchlortetracycline hydro-chloride, 115·5 mg of chlortetracycline hydrochloride and 115·5 mg of tetracycline hydrochloride (Deteclo). One or preferably two tablets each containing 300 mg of the mixture can be given night and morning for one to three weeks with the likelihood of good response.

Some patients taking tetracyclines complain of troublesome nausea, for which it may be necessary to reduce the dose. The rare complication of severe enteritis believed to be due to a disturbance in the balance of the intestinal flora has already been mentioned (p. 150). Persistent anal irrita-tion may be due to the same cause from which an intestinal yeast flourishes unduly. All tetracyclines may cause photosensitivity and patients should be warned of this possibility, the incidence of which is related to the size of the dose as well as exposure to sunlight. Obviously the risk is greater in summer and in sunny climates. In winter it may affect skiing enthusiasts. The usual manifestation is a rash on exposed areas of skin. Of the tetra-cyclines demethylchlortetracycline (a component of Deteclo) is particularly prone to produce photosensitivity.

Erythromycin stearate given in dosage of 500 mg 12-hourly for 14 days has been found to be as effective as oxytetracycline 250 mg six-hourly for 14 days.[30] *Chlamydia* was occasionally recovered after this treatment, so that, as with tetracycline, 2 g daily for 7 to 14 days might be preferable. Absorption of erythromycin is said to be best if it is taken before a meal or with 250 ml of water on an empty stomach. If *U. urealyticum* does cause some cases of non-specific urethritis erythromycin may have advantages in that some strains of this organism are resistant to tetracycline but sensitive to erythromycin.[33] There is also no risk of photosensitivity from erythromycin. It may sometimes cause nausea and it may then be necessary to reduce the dose.

Spiramycin (Rovamycin) is also effective. The usual dosage is 500 mg every six hours for seven to 14 days.

Urethrovesical Irrigation

This is a time-honoured method of treatment which is now seldom required. It may be indicated in highly resistant cases of non-specific urethritis. The technique is described in the Appendix (p. 401).

Treatment of Chronic Non-specific Prostatitis (see p. 280)

Treatment of this condition is a difficult matter; the general experience is that it is often unsatisfactory. If there are no symptoms and no signs of urethral infection, there is a case for leaving these patients without treatment, because treatment may be prolonged and may provoke an anxiety neurosis. If the patient has symptoms, other than those resulting from active urethritis, they may be due to faulty drainage from the prostate, and treatment should be given.

In treatment, the broad-spectrum antibiotics used in cases of non-specific urethritis may help. Erythromycin and doxycycline are probably the most useful and may be given in the recommended dosage. Gentle systematic digital massage of the prostate is also likely to give relief. The massage should occupy one or two minutes and should be given not more than once a week as a rule. The course of prostatic massage may occupy six weeks and the patient should then rest from treatment for a month. The need for further courses of treatment must be decided in the individual case. The application of heat to the prostate is sometimes beneficial.

Tests for Cure

Tests after treatment should include early morning smear tests of the urethral secretion and examination for pus and threads in the urine on two or more occasions. Serological tests for syphilis should be carried out before treatment and at the end of three months (see p. 247). In some cases a poor response to treatment may be due to failure to take the tablets correctly, failure to abstain from sexual intercourse, a missed trichomonal infection or the presence of an underlying prostatitis or urethral stricture. In such cases the prostatic fluid may need to be examined and anterior urethroscopy carried out. In other unfortunate cases the patient responds poorly or suffers frequent relapses without any apparent reason. Such patients are likely to develop psychological disturbances (see p. 373).

NON-SPECIFIC UROGENITAL INFECTION IN THE FEMALE

INCIDENCE. The criteria of diagnosis of this condition in females are so uncertain that no true estimate of the incidence is possible; 20,156 such cases were reported from the clinics of England in 1977[21], but the number of women affected is undoubtedly much larger.

We are concerned here mainly with females who are known contacts of men with non-specific urethritis and if tests for *Chlamydia* are not taken the diagnosis often has to depend mainly on epidemiological evidence. Furthermore, as already mentioned, the partners of men with *Chlamydia*-negative non-specific urethritis are seldom found to harbour this organism. *Corynebacterium vaginale* is not considered to be of significance in this context.

In the United Kingdom and the United States of America *Chlamydia trachomatis* is found in 20 to 30 per cent of women attending venereal disease clinics. The highest rates of recovery are found in women with gonorrhoea and in contacts of men with non-specific urethritis; not surprisingly, it is found most often of all when the contact is known to harbour the organism. Among women attending a family planning clinic in Bristol[34] the isolation rate was 3 per cent and in Manchester it was found in 1 per cent of hospital staff.[35] In Seattle, U.S.A., it was isolated from 12·7 per cent of an unselected sample of pregnant women,[36] and in San Francisco in 5 per cent of pregnant women.[37] Infection can persist for many months.[26]

Clinical Course

The disease is often asymptomatic. If symptoms are present they are often of minor degree and may be disregarded or attributed to other causes. Acute or recurrent cystitis for which a causative organism cannot be demonstrated should always suggest the possibility of this diagnosis, but how often it causes the urethral syndrome or 'honeymoon cystitis' are open questions. Vaginal discharge of any degree is likely only if cervicitis is exceptionally severe or if there is associated trichomonal vaginitis. The signs may be of cervicitis, sometimes with an oedematous and congested erosion,[38] urethritis and proctitis. In many cases, however, the cervix appears normal or shows only a simple erosion although examination with a colposcope may sometimes reveal follicles in the marginal area. Follicles may also be seen in the rectum in cases of chlamydial infection. Evidence of urethritis may only be obtained if the urine has been held for some hours. Microscopical examination of smears of secretion is likely to show a considerable excess of leucocytes, especially in the cervical fluid, without specific organisms. However, normal cervical secretion contains variable numbers of leucocytes and this varies with the phase of the menstrual cycle, so that interpretation can be difficult. Conventional cultures are sterile or grow only commensals.

In a minority of cases, the condition presents with symptoms and signs of inflammation of the pelvic organs, without bacteriological evidence of gonorrhoea in the patient or her consort, or may come to light when a newborn baby develops chlamydial conjunctivitis.

Complications

Local

Non-specific *bartholinitis* is similar in symptoms and signs to bartholinitis caused by gonorrhoea. There are, of course, several causes of non-gonococcal bartholinitis and anaerobic organisms, especially *Bacteroides* species, are often recovered.[39] That *Chlamydia* may prove to be a cause in some cases is suggested by a recent study in which this organism was isolated from material obtained from Bartholin's duct[40] in 9 out of 30 of a selected group of women, 24 of whom had gonorrhoea.

Pelvic infection has to be distinguished on bacteriological grounds from that due to gonorrhoea. In a recent investigation by Mårdh et al.,[41] *Chlamydia trachomatis* was found in the cervix in 19 out of 53 women with acute salpingitis; it was recovered from 6 out of 20 specimens obtained at laparoscopy from the Fallopian tubes. Among the 20 were included six of the seven patients from whom *Chlamydia trachomatis* was isolated from the cervices. These workers believed that in some areas this organism was the commonest cause of salpingitis. They tested only for the gonococcus and *Chlamydia*, but a mixed infection, often involving anaerobic organisms, may be important in some cases of non-gonococcal salpingitis.[42] Very high levels of chlamydial antibody are often found in the serum and in fluid aspirated from the pouch of Douglas in women with severe salpingitis.[43] The rôle of mycoplasmas is uncertain. The use of an intrauterine device is associated with an increased risk of non-gonococcal salpingitis.[44] The non-specific variety of salpingitis seems to have a greater tendency to relapse. How important it is as a cause of sterility has not yet been determined, but Weström[45] found tubal occlusions to be more common after non-gonococcal than after gonococcal salpingitis and especially likely after multiple attacks.

Non-specific perihepatitis also occurs and there is serological evidence that some of these cases are due to chlamydial infection.[46]

General

Reiter's disease is described in Chapter 22. It is much less common in females than in males. Very recently a fatal case of endocarditis due to *Chlamydia trachomatis* has been reported.[47] The patient was 30 weeks pregnant and the affected aortic valve was previously normal.

Treatment

It has been the usual practice to give women with suspected non-specific urogenital infection treatment similar to that used for men. Even if a female patient is free from symptoms and signs, it may be wise to treat her in the hope of preventing complications in her case and re-infection of her consort.[32] If the consort has chlamydial urethritis, however, the need for treatment in her case could be decided on the results of cultural and serological tests for *Chlamydia*. Waugh and Nayyar[48] found that treatment for one week with the triple tetracycline Deteclo in dosage of 300 mg twice daily was effective in eliminating *Chlamydia* from the cervix. Erythromycin stearate or base would be the drug of choice for pregnant women and those who are breast feeding; the estolate should not be used for pregnant women because of the risk of jaundice. Abscesses of Bartholin's gland may require aspiration. In the event of recurrences excision or 'marsupialization' of the gland may be indicated (see p. 246). Women suffering from pelvic infection may be treated with oral tetracycline or oxytetracycline 2 g daily or doxycycline 200 mg daily, and the drug should be continued for at least fourteen days. For severely ill patients it might be advisable to give tetracycline intravenously until improvement occurs. Some add metronidazole to this regimen because of the possibility of infection with anaerobic organisms, some of which are resistant to tetracycline. This would certainly be worth doing in cases which are not responding well to the tetracycline. The suggested dosage is 400 mg three times daily for 10 to 14 days. In other respects, the general management of these patients is identical with that required for pelvic infection with the gonococcus (see p. 245).

Tests for Cure

Genital examinations and tests should be carried out after the course of treatment and again a week or two later. Serological tests for syphilis should be done before treatment and at the end of three months (see p. 232).

RECTAL, PHARYNGEAL AND PULMONARY INFECTION

The criteria for diagnosis of non-specific proctitis are controversial, but rectal involvement in women with genital chlamydial infection has been well described.[49,50] Rectal chlamydial infection has also been reported in newborn babies.[37] Although *Chlamydia* has been isolated from the urethra in 7 out of 22 (32 per cent) homosexual men with non-gonococcal urethritis[51] there is very little information on rectal infection in homosexuals apart from reports of two cases.[52]

Nasopharyngeal chlamydial infection in infants is usually associated with conjunctival infection but may occur without it. Some of these babies develop a distinctive, usually mild but chronic, pneumonia starting at the age of two or three weeks.[53-55] However, most cases are not diagnosed until the baby is aged six weeks or more. The infants are usually afebrile, have a staccato cough and rapid respiratory rate. There is often partial nasal obstruction with mucoid discharge. X-rays show diffuse infiltration and hyperinflation. Eosinophilia is common. High titres of both IgG and IgM antichlamydial antibodies are found in the serum.

Chlamydia may also be isolated from the throats of adults with chlamydial ocular disease, but there is as yet little information on pharyngeal disease in adults attending venereal diseases clinics. Schachter and Atwood[56] reported one case of cervical and pharyngeal involvement; the patient was a woman who complained of sore throat and who was having regular oral sexual intercourse with a man with recurrent non-gonococcal urethritis. Bowie et al.,[57] however, were unable to isolate *Chlamydia* from the throats of 11 women who had had oral intercourse with partners known to have chlamydial urethritis. Goldmeier and Darougar[52] grew *C. trachomatis* from the throat but not the urethra of a homosexual who complained only of urethral discharge.

NON-GONOCOCCAL GENITAL INFECTIONS IN CHILDREN

These occur most often in female children and they have to be distinguished from gonococcal vulvovaginitis, which is responsible for most highly contagious cases. Non-gonococcal vulvovaginitis is now much more common than the gonococcal variety,[58] which accounts for less than 5 per cent of cases. Faulty hygiene may be a contributory factor in some cases. The non-gonococcal causes may be classified as follows:

1. *Bacterial* – Numerous organisms have been recovered from the vaginae of children with vulvovaginitis.[58,59] These included coliform bacilli, *Staphylococcus aureus* and *S. albus*, diphtheroids, streptococci, *Neisseria* species other than the gonococcus, *Proteus* species and several others. Many of these organisms can also be found in the vaginae of healthy children, so that it is often difficult to be certain of their significance in cases of vulvovaginitis. Diphtheritic infection is now extremely rare.

2. *Mycotic* – Infection by *Candida albicans* accounts for a small number of cases of vulvovaginitis.

3. *Protozoal* – Infestation with *Trichomonas vaginalis* is seen only occasionally.

4. *Systemic disease* – Vulvovaginitis may present in the course of chickenpox, scarlet fever, measles and other exanthemata, or in association with coryza, pneumonia or other infections.

5. *Non-specific (abacterial)* – Vaginitis of this type seems to be a rare condition in children but cases have not been fully investigated with tests for *Chlamydia*.

6. *Other causes* – These include foreign bodies in the vagina and threadworms which have migrated from the anal canal. Irritation from 'bubblebaths', Dettol or other antiseptics used in the bath can also occur.

Non-gonococcal urethritis in young boys is very rare. It may be associated with bacterial urinary infection or may be seen in the rare cases of Reiter's disease in childhood, or in the Stevens–Johnson syndrome. However, some cases are unexplained.[60]

Treatment

Treatment is that of the causative condition. If pyogenic organisms are responsible, their sensitivity to antibiotics should indicate the appropriate remedies. Faulty hygiene should be corrected.

NON-GONOCOCCAL OPHTHALMIA

Adults

'Non-specific' infection may sometimes present in the form of acute follicular conjunctivitis affecting one or both eyes. The clinical and cytological findings are those of infection with TRIC agent. Characteristic inclusion forms may be found in the cytoplasm of conjunctival epithelial cells and *Chlamydia trachomatis* is grown in cell culture. The condition may present in men or women and most of the patients are unaware of genitourinary infection, which is found on routine investigation. There is a high rate of recovery of *Chlamydia* from genital specimens in these cases, especially from women.[50] It is uncommon to find this type of conjunctivitis in patients who are aware of genital symptoms, presumably because they promptly seek advice and are treated. The danger of transmission to eyes seems to be related to prolonged infection in asymptomatic cases.

Infants

As already mentioned (p. 229) most cases of ophthalmia neonatorum are due to causes other than the gonococcus, and a variety of organisms has been held to be responsible. Of these *Chlamydia trachomatis* is probably the commonest, accounting for a quarter or more of the cases. The organism is generally recovered from the genital tract of the mother who is also at high risk of developing salpingitis. Her sexual partner will commonly be found on careful examination to have non-specific urethritis and *Chlamydia trachomatis* will often be recovered in these cases.[61, 62] There is a 40 to 50 per cent chance of babies developing chlamydial ophthalmia in known cases of cervical infection in the mothers,[36, 37] and it has been estimated[37] that somewhere between 2 and 6 per cent of all newly borns in the United States will be affected. Prophylactic silver nitrate drops are ineffective.[36] The incubation period is 5 to 14 days but may be shorter. The condition is usually, but not always, milder than gonococcal ophthalmia neonatorum and the two conditions may co-exist. The clinical differences between the infant and adult forms of the disease appear to be related to the inability of the infant's conjunctiva to react by follicle formation in the first few weeks of life. Scarring and pannus can occur in apparently mild cases. This is especially likely if treatment is delayed and it is essential that the condition should never be taken lightly.

Babies with chlamydial ophthalmia often have associated nasopharyngeal infection and there is a risk that they may develop chlamydial pneumonia (see p. 287). Harrison et al.,[55] in Seattle, U.S.A., found that *Chlamydia trachomatis* was the cause of 30 per cent of all cases of pneumonia in infants less than six months of age which required admission to hospital from September, 1976, to February, 1977. It was responsible for 13 out of 21 (62 per cent) cases seen between 3 and 11 weeks of age.

Treatment
Adults

Chlamydial conjunctivitis responds reasonably well to local applications of eye ointment containing 1 per cent of chlortetracycline four times daily. Improvement is prompt but full recovery may take six weeks or more. Response is usually more rapid if tetracycline is also given systemically and, in any case, this is generally required because of associated genital infection; 2 g daily for three weeks should be given. If there is corneal haze or ulceration, the pupil should be dilated with 1 per cent atropine sulphate.

Infants

Gonorrhoea must be excluded by culture as well as by examination of smears. If the conjunctival smear shows pus cells and organisms other than Gram-negative diplococci, neomycin eye ointment 0·5 per cent should be applied four times daily (after each feed) until the condition has resolved. Neomycin has a broad antibacterial spectrum but does not affect *Chlamydia*. If the smear is abacterial or there is no response to neomycin, then tests for *Chlamydia* should be taken. Babies with chlamydial ophthalmia are usually treated with chlortetracycline eye ointment, 1 per cent, four times daily after feeds for six weeks. It is very important to make sure that the mother is able to apply the ointment correctly. Local treatment, however, does not always give satisfactory results;[62,63] for this reason, and because of the high frequency of associated nasopharyngeal infection which can lead to pneumonia, systemic treatment also is advisable. Systemic tetracycline should not be given to babies. Ridgway and Oriel[63] obtained excellent results using erythromycin, 30 mg per kg daily for 21 days, together with chlortetracycline eye ointment locally for the same period. Others advise 40 mg per kg of erythromycin, especially when pneumonia is suspected. The medicine is divided into four doses during the day and given before feeds. Examination of the mother and her sexual partner should not be neglected.

The management of all these cases should be conducted in consultation with an ophthalmologist.

REFERENCES

1. HARKNESS, A. H. (1950) *Non-Gonococcal Urethritis*. Edinburgh: Livingstone.
2. JONES, B. R., COLLIER, L. H. and SMITH, C. H. (1959) *Lancet*, **1**, 902.
3. GEAR, J. H. S., GORDON, F. B., JONES, B. R. and BELL, S. D. (1963) *Nature (Lond.)*, **197**, 26.
4. GORDON, F. B., HARPER, I. A., QUAN, A. L., TREHARNE, J. D., DWYER, R. ST. C. and GARLAND, J. A. (1969). *J. infect. Dis.*, **120**, 451.
5. DAROUGAR, S., KINNISON, J. R. and JONES, B. R. (1971) In: *Trachoma and Related Disorders*, ed. R. L. Nichols, pp. 63 and 501. Amsterdam and New York: Excerpta Medica.
6. WANG, S-P. and GRAYSTON, J. T. (1971) In: *Trachoma and Related Disorders*, ed. R. L. Nichols, p. 305. Amsterdam and New York: Excerpta Medica.
7. JONES, B. R. (1972) *Br. J. vener. Dis.*, **48**, 13.
8. DUNLOP, E. M. C. (1975) In: *Recent Advances in Sexually Transmitted Diseases*, ed. R. S. Morton and J. R. W. Harris, p. 280. London: Churchill Livingston.
9. SCHACHTER, J. (1978) *New Engl. J. Med.*, **298**, 428.
10. SHEPARD, M. C. (1956) *J. Bact.*, **71**, 362.
11. SHEPARD, M. C., LUNCEFORD, C. D., FORD, D. K., PURCELL, R. H., TAYLOR-ROBINSON, D., RAZIN, S. and BLACK, F. T. (1974) *Int. J. syst. Bact.*, **24**, 160.
12. McCORMACK, W. M., LEE, Y-H. and ZINNER, S. H. (1973) *Ann. intern. Med.*, **78**, 696.
13. BOWIE, W. R. (1978) *Sex. transm. Dis.*, **5**, 27.
14. TAYLOR-ROBINSON, D., CSONKA, G. W. and PRENTICE, M. J. (1977) *Quart. J. Med.*, **46**, 309.
15. LEOPOLD, S. (1953) *U.S. arm. Forces med. J.*, **4**, 263.
16. GARDNER, H. L. and DUKES, C. D. (1954) *Science*, **120**, 853.
17. DUNKELBERG, W. E. (1977) *Sex. transm. Dis.*, **4**, 69.
18. FURNESS, G. and EVANGELISTA, A. T. (1978) *Invest. Urol.*, **16**, 1.
19. ORIEL, J. D., REEVE, P., POWIS, P., MILLER, A. and NICOL, C. S. (1972) *Br. J. vener. Dis.*, **48**, 429.
20. HOLMES, K. K., HANDSFIELD, H. H., WANG, S-P., WENTWORTH, B. B., TURCK, M., ANDERSON, J. B. and ALEXANDER, E. R. (1975) *New Engl. J. Med.*, **292**, 1199.
21. A. R. Chief med. Offr Dept Hlth (Lond.) (1951–77) H.M.S.O. 1952–78.
22. RODIN, P. (1971) *Br. J. vener. Dis.*, **47**, 452.
23. OATES, J. K. (1957) *Acta derm.-vener. (Stockh.)*, Proc. Internat. Congr. Derm., 1957, vol. III, p. 994.
24. BERGER, R. E., ALEXANDER, E. R., MONDA, G. D., ANSELL, J., McCORMICK, G. and HOLMES, K. K. (1978) *New Engl. J. Med.*, **298**, 301.
25. GARTMAN, E. and LEIBOVITZ, A. (1955) *Br. J. vener. Dis.*, **31**, 92.
26. SCHACHTER, J., HANNA, L., HILL, E. C., MASSAD, S., SHEPPARD, C. W., CONTE, J. E., COHEN, S. N. and MEYER, K. F. (1975) *J. Am. med. Ass.*, **231**, 1252.
27. RIDGWAY, G. L., OWEN, J. M. and ORIEL, J. D. (1978) *Br. J. vener. Dis.*, **54**, 103.
28. KING, A. J. (1964) *Recent Advances in Venereology*, p. 384. London: J. & A. Churchill.
29. BOWIE, W. R., FLOYD, J. F., MILLER, Y., ALEXANDER, E. R., HOLMES, J. and HOLMES, K. K. (1976) *Lancet*, **2**, 1276.
30. ORIEL, J. D., RIDGWAY, G. L. and TCHAMOUROFF, S. (1977) *Scot. med. J.*, **22**, 375.
31. HANDSFIELD, H. H., ALEXANDER, E. R., WANG, S-P., PEDERSEN, A. H. B. and HOLMES, K. K. (1975) *J. Am. vener. Dis. Ass.*, **2**, 5.

32. THAMBAR, I. V., SIMMONS, P. D., THIN, R. N., DAROUGAR, S. and YEARSLEY, P. (1979) Br. J. vener. Dis., 55, 284.

33. PRENTICE, M. J., TAYLOR-ROBINSON, D. and CSONKA, G. W. (1976) Br. J. vener. Dis., 52, 269.

34. HILTON, A. L., RICHMOND, S. J., MILNE, J. D., HINDLEY, F. and CLARKE, S. K. R. (1974) Br. J. vener. Dis., 50, 1.

35. WOOLFITT, J. M. G. and WATT, L. (1977) Br. J. vener. Dis., 53, 93.

36. CHANDLER, J. W., ALEXANDER, E. R., PHEIFFER, T. A., WANG, S-P., HOLMES, K. K. and ENGLISH, M. (1977) Trans. Am. Acad. Ophthal. Otolar., 83, 302.

37. SCHACHTER, J. (1978) New Engl. J. Med., 298, 540.

38. REES, E., TAIT, I. A., HOBSON, D. and JOHNSON, F. W. A. (1977) In: Non-gonococcal Urethritis and Related Conditions, ed. D. Hobson and K. K. Holmes, p. 67. Washington D.C.: American Society for Microbiology.

39. WREN, M. W. D. (1977) J. clin. Path., 30, 1025.

40. DAVIES, J. A., REES, E., HOBSON, D. and KARAYIANNIS, P. (1978) Br. J. vener. Dis., 54, 409.

41. MÅRDH, P-A., RIPA, T., SVENSSON, L. and WESTRÖM, L. (1977) New Engl. J. Med., 296, 1377.

42. ESCHENBACH, D. A., BUCHANAN, T. M., POLLOCK, H. M., FORSYTH, P. S., ALEXANDER, E. R., LIN, T-S., WANG, S-P., WENTWORTH, B. B., McCORMACK, W. M. and HOLMES, K. K. (1975) New Engl. J. Med., 293, 166.

43. TREHARNE, J. D., RIPA, K. T., MÅRDH, P-A., SVENSSON, L., WESTRÖM, L. and DAROUGAR, S. (1979) Br. J. vener. Dis., 55, 26.

44. ESCHENBACH, D. A., HARNISCH, J. P. and HOLMES, K. K. (1977) Am. J. Obstet. Gynec., 128, 838.

45. WESTRÖM, L. (1975) Am. J. Obstet. Gynec., 121, 707.

46. MÜLLER-SCHOOP, J. W., WANG, S-P., MUNZINGER, J., SCHLÄPFER, H. U., KNOBLAUCH, M. and AMMANN, R. W. (1978) Br. med. J., 1, 1022.

47. VAN DER BEL-KAHN, J. M., WATANAKUNAKORN, C., MENEFEE, M. G., LONG, H. D. and DICTER, R. (1978) Am. Heart J., 95, 627.

48. WAUGH, M. A. and NAYYAR, K. C. (1977) Br. J. vener. Dis., 53, 96.

49. DUNLOP, E. M. C., VAUGHAN-JACKSON, J. D. and DAROUGAR, S. (1972) Br. J. vener. Dis., 48, 425.

50. VAUGHAN-JACKSON, J. D., DUNLOP, E. M. C., DAROUGAR, S., DWYER, R. ST. C. and JONES, B. R. (1972) Br. J. vener. Dis., 48, 445.

51. ORIEL, J. D., REEVE, P., WRIGHT, J. T. and OWEN, J. (1976) Br. J. vener. Dis., 52, 46.

52. GOLDMEIER, D. and DAROUGAR, S. (1977) Br. J. vener. Dis., 53, 184.

53. BEEM, M. O. and SAXON, E. M. (1977) New Engl. J. Med., 296, 306.

54. SCHACHTER, J., GROSSMAN, M., HOLT, J., SWEET, R., GOODNER, E. and MILLS, J. (1979) Lancet, 2, 377.

55. HARRISON, H. R., ENGLISH, M. G., LEE, C. K. and ALEXANDER, E. R. (1978) New Engl. J. Med., 298, 702.

56. SCHACHTER, J. and ATWOOD, G. (1975) J. Am. vener. Dis. Ass., 2, 12.

57. BOWIE, W. R., ALEXANDER, E. R. and HOLMES, K. K. (1977) Sex. transm. Dis., 4, 140.

58. SERSIRON, D. and ROIRON, V. (1967) Br. J. vener. Dis., 43, 33.

59. HELLER, R. H., JOSEPH, J. M. and DAVIS, H. J. (1969) J. Pediat., 74, 370.

60. WILLIAMS, D. I. and MIKHAEL, B. R. (1971) Proc. R. Soc. Med., 64, 133.

61. DUNLOP, E. M. C., GOLDMEIER, D., DAROUGAR, S. and JONES, B. R. (1976) In: *Sexually Transmitted Diseases*, ed. R. D. Catterall and C. S. Nicol, p. 83. London: Academic Press.
62. REES, E., TAIT, I. A., HOBSON, D., BYNG, R. E. and JOHNSON, F. W. A. (1977) *Br. J. vener. Dis.*, **53,** 173.
63. RIDGWAY, G. L. and ORIEL, J. D. (1977) *New Engl. J. Med.*, **297,** 512.

22

Reiter's Disease*

The syndrome of non-gonococcal urethritis, polyarthritis, and conjunctivitis or iritis was described in some detail by Benjamin Brodie in 1818 and 1836,[3] by Fournier in 1868 and by Launois in 1899. In 1916 Hans Reiter[4] published details of a case in which he mistakenly believed he had isolated a causative spirochaete. The condition was thereafter termed 'Reiter's disease'.

In Great Britain and in North America the disease is found in association with venereally transmitted urethritis. On the continent of Europe, in Asia, and in North Africa, it is more commonly reported in association with bacillary or amoebic dysentery, *Salmonella* and *Yersinia* infections and non-specific diarrhoea. In both epidemiological varieties, an early indication of the presence of the syndrome is likely to be a non-gonococcal urethritis, and the subsequent behaviour of the fully-developed condition appears to be constant irrespective of the nature of the antecedent illness.

In a minority of cases of the venereally-acquired disease, there may be a recent history or signs of gonorrhoea. These patients are generally found to have residual non-specific urethritis after successful treatment of gonorrhoea and the Reiter's disease is probably precipitated by this rather than by gonococcal infection.

INCIDENCE. It has been suggested that from 0·8 to 3·0 per cent of patients suffering from non-gonococcal venereal urethritis subsequently develop Reiter's disease, but these figures are probably unreliable. It is likely that many more cases of Reiter's disease exist than are diagnosed but the same can be said of non-gonococcal venereal urethritis, so that it is impossible to determine the true incidence. Returns from the clinics of England for the year ending June 30, 1977,[5] report 593 cases of non-specific genital infection with arthritis, 551 in men and 42 in women. The total number of cases of non-specific genital infection reported in that year was 94,152 (73,996 in men and 20,156 in women).

*The literature on this subject is massive and complicated. It was reviewed in detail by J. A. H. Hancock[1] and in part by King and Mason.[2]

CLINICAL FEATURES

The condition affects males predominantly, at an estimated ratio of 15 males to 1 female. The majority of patients develop their first attack between the ages of 21 and 40, though onset in late life also occurs. The very rare cases occurring in children are generally of the post-dysenteric type.

The full syndrome consists of non-specific urogenital infection in the form of urethritis, prostatitis or cystitis, in that order of frequency; non-suppurative arthritis which is usually polyarticular; conjunctivitis or iritis; and distinctive lesions of the mucous membrane and skin, the latter being called by the traditional misnomer 'keratoderma blennorrhagica'. The presenting symptoms, in order of frequency, are usually those of urethral discharge or dysuria, arthritis and conjunctivitis (see Figs. 128–137). Even when the condition is venereally acquired there may sometimes be short-lived mild non-specific diarrhoea.

Arthritis

The onset of the arthritis may be acute or subacute. It is associated with pyrexia and tachycardia of varying degrees. In severe cases, particularly those with generalized keratoderma, the patient appears very ill and may rapidly become cachectic. The blood picture shows a moderate normocytic anaemia, and a slight neutrophil leucocytosis. The erythrocyte sedimentation rate is raised, being more than 100 mm per hour in the more severe cases; and the plasma proteins show a non-specific pattern of elevation of the alpha-2-globulins. Results of serological tests for rheumatoid factor are almost invariably negative; lupus erythematosus cells are not found and serum uric-acid levels are within normal limits in most cases. In less severe cases constitutional changes may be slight and changes in the blood picture and erythrocyte sedimentation rate are proportionally diminished. The attack of arthritis is usually self-limiting, the course lasting from one to four months in most cases, although it can last as long as eighteen months. Many patients are prone to recurrent attacks. The joints usually involved are those of the lower limbs, especially the knees, ankles, metatarsophalangeal joints and other small joints of the feet (Figs. 128–130). Backache is fairly common in the acute attacks and there may be tenderness over one or both sacro-iliac joints; although conventional X-rays of the sacro-iliac joints are usually normal in the early phase of the disease, sacro-iliitis can often be demonstrated by a bone scan technique.[6]

Sometimes there is widespread involvement of joints which may include those of the hands, elbows and shoulders, and temporomandibular and costochondral joints. If only one joint is involved it is most likely to be the knee. Rupture of the synovium of a swollen knee joint has been described.[7] Suppuration does not occur in the joints. Aspirated joint fluid is yellow

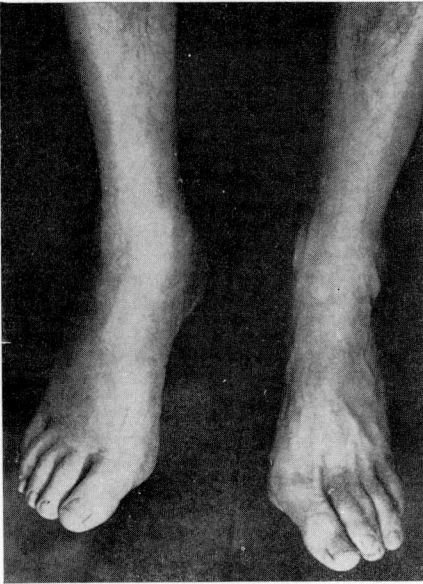

Fig. 128. Reiter's disease (acute):
arthritis of right ankle and foot.

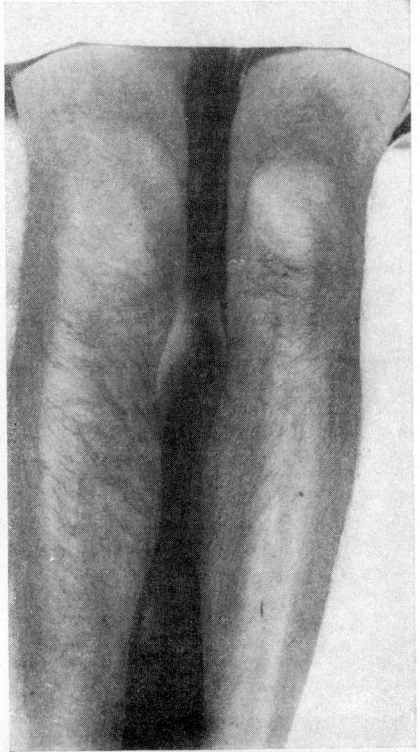

Fig. 129 (right). Reiter's disease
(acute): arthritis of right knee.

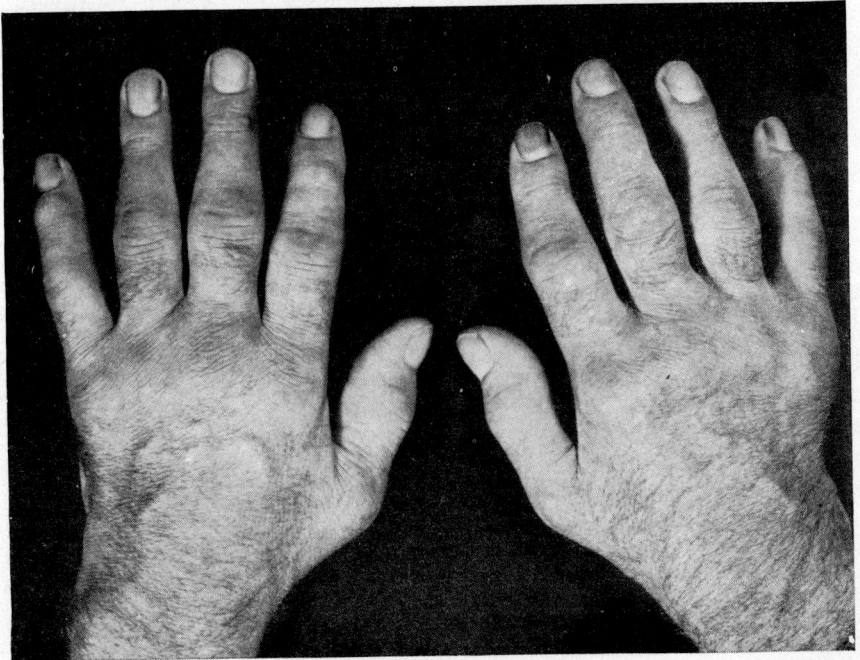

Fig. 130. Reiter's disease (acute): arthritis of hands simulating rheumatoid arthritis.

and turbid and clots readily on standing. At first it contains a predominance of polymorphonuclear leucocytes but the proportion of lymphocytes later increases. The number of leucocytes is usually less than 20,000 per ml but can be as high as 50,000 and the synovial fluid sugar content normal (80 mg/100 ml), or reduced; levels of complement are increased. The fluid is sterile on culture. Histopathological examination of the synovium gives no characteristic diagnostic features. In the early stage of the disease, radiographs of the joints show little or no change. The acute process may also involve soft tissues such as the plantar fasciae and the Achilles tendons. Occasionally only soft tissues are involved.

Lesions of the Eyes

Conjunctivitis (see Plate V, iii)

This occurs in about one-half of the cases. It is usually bilateral and, characteristically, is most severe in the tarsal conjunctivae of the lower lids at the lateral angles. In most cases it is mild and transient, but occasionally there may be severe purulent conjunctivitis with chemosis.

Anterior Uveitis

This sometimes occurs late in the course of a first attack of arthritis, and may be preceded by an attack of conjunctivitis, but most commonly it appears months or years from the time of the original infection, by which time other manifestations of the disease may have become relatively symptomless. Some patients suffer as many as 20 or 30 attacks, and blindness may result. There is evidence of a close correlation between the presence of chronic sacro-iliitis and the development of anterior uveitis. Posterior uveitis is very rare.

Keratitis and Corneal Ulceration

These occur infrequently.

Optic Neuritis

This is very rare. Two cases were described by Zewi[8] and one by Oates and Hancock.[9]

Parotitis

Parotitis is known to occur, as a rarity, with the dysenteric syndrome. Reckless[10] has described a case associated with the venereal syndrome in a woman of 27 years. Very rarely, there may be swelling of the lachrymal as well as salivary glands.

Lesions of the Skin

Keratoderma blennorrhagica is found in about 10 per cent[11] of patients with the venereal syndrome but seems to be much less common in post-

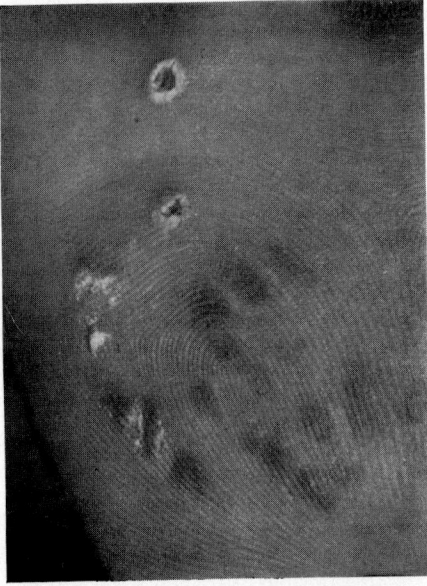

Fig. 131. Reiter's disease (acute): close-up view of keratoderma of sole of foot.

Fig. 132 (*right*). Reiter's disease (acute): circinate balanitis.

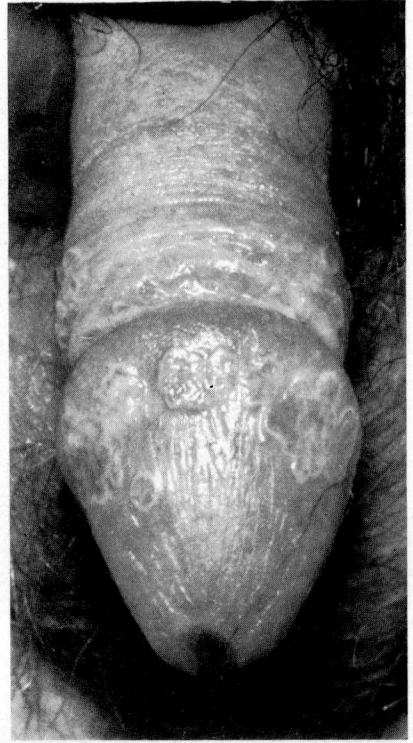

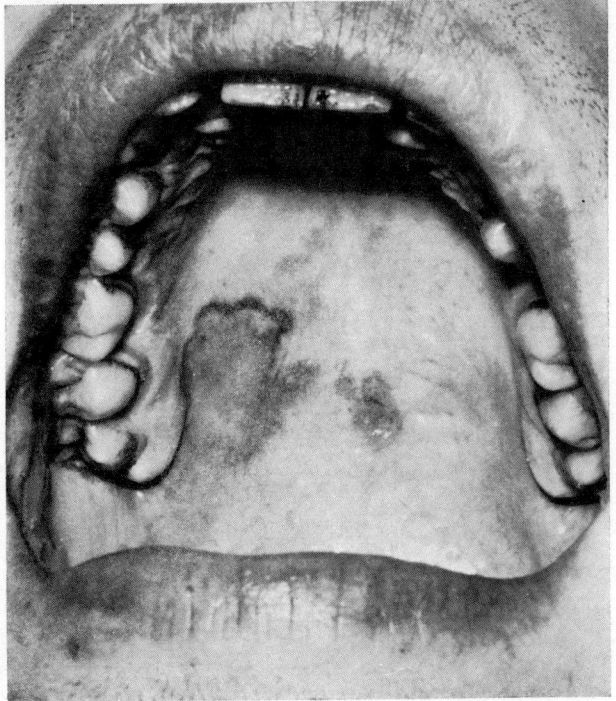

Fig. 133. Reiter's disease (acute): lesions of palate.

dysenteric cases. The lesions nearly always commence in the skin of the soles of the feet, first as dull-red macules, then as vesicles becoming pustular, and then keratotic. Keratotic patches may be hard and nodular, or may form grotesque, limpet-like, soft masses of scale. Though more commonly confined to the feet, the rash may, in severe cases, spread to involve the limbs, trunk and scalp (see Plate V, iv and Fig. 131). The lesions may appear at sites of trauma (Koebner's phenomenon). In severe cases the nails and nail beds of the toes and sometimes of the fingers may be involved. The nails become thickened and opaque and separation of the nail plate occurs.

Lesions of the Tongue and Buccal Mucosa

These occur in about 10 per cent of patients[11] and are usually painless, superficial erosions sometimes surmounted by greyish patches of necrotic epithelium. They are often found on the mucosa covering the hard palate (Fig. 133) and sometimes on the soft palate, uvula, tongue and mucosa of the cheek and lip. Occasionally vesicular lesions may be seen, representing an earlier stage of the condition.

Lesions of the Penis and Vulva

Lesions of the penis are found in about a quarter[11] of the cases. They usually affect the mucosa of the glans penis and of the preputial sac, appearing as rounded, shallow, red erosions, with slightly raised edges, which assume a circinate outline as adjacent lesions coalesce. On this account this manifestation is often called 'circinate balanitis' (Fig. 132). In circumcised patients keratodermic crusts may form at the sites of the lesions. Occasionally patients develop circinate balanitis without arthritis; this can persist for several months. Recently circinate vulvitis has been described in two cases of Reiter's disease in women.[12]

Other Systemic Manifestations

Involvement of the nervous system has been reported in both the venereally acquired and the dysenteric varieties of the disease. It is rare, but peripheral neuritis, 'shoulder-girdle' neuritis and meningoencephalitis have been described.[9,13,14] Pericarditis, myocarditis, partial or complete heart block, aortic incompetence[15-21] and lesions of the lung have all been described as occurring in the course of the disease. Csonka[22] described thrombosis of deep veins of the legs in 3 per cent of his patients. Recovery was rapid and uneventful. However, it is possible that some of these were cases of acute synovial rupture of the knee rather than deep vein thrombosis. There have been two case reports of amyloidosis associated with Reiter's disease.[23,24]

Late Course of the Disease

It is probable that few patients who suffer from arthritis due to this cause make a complete and permanent recovery. Csonka[25] estimated that the annual risk of a first recurrence was in the region of 15 per cent. There were recurrences in 62 per cent of 144 cases which he had followed for two or more years. The later effects fall into five groups: (1) multiple attacks without residual damage to joints; (2) painful deformities of the feet; (3) painful feet without obvious deformity; (4) the syndrome of spondylitis; and (5) recurrent attacks of uveitis.

Multiple Attacks without Residual Damage to the Joints

The later episodes of arthritis are sometimes related to sexual intercourse and to fresh attacks (or relapses) of urethritis; sometimes they occur without evident precipitating cause. The intervals between recurrences vary greatly, from a few weeks or months to a number of years. In recurrent attacks, as with first attacks, the distribution of the arthritis follows no set pattern, for although the knees and feet are usually affected, some patients show more generalized polyarthritis with involvement of the hands and wrists.

Painful Deformities of the Feet

Pes planus is sometimes a residual deformity. In other cases pes cavus occurs, and may be associated with fixed dorsiflexion of all the toes at the metatarsophalangeal joints, and hyperflexion at the proximal interphalangeal joints, giving multiple hammer-toe deformities. The hammer-toe deformities and also lateral deviation of the toes at the metatarsophalangeal joints (Fig. 135) may also occur without pes cavus.

Painful Feet without Obvious Deformity

The most usual effect of this kind is tenderness of the heel on walking, localized in the region of the posterior attachment of the plantar fascia to the os calcis. This is generally associated with the presence of a spur of the inferior surface of the calcaneum of fluffy appearance on X-ray (Fig. 136). Gross examples of this are highly characteristic of Reiter's disease. The posterior surface of the calcaneum may be involved and a spur may also develop at the site of attachment of the Achilles tendon. Calcaneal spurs, even of florid type, may be asymptomatic for long periods, hence the need for X-ray examination of the heels as a routine procedure in suspected cases of Reiter's disease.

The Syndrome of Spondylitis

In the course of years a few of these patients develop a condition resembling ankylosing spondylitis (Fig. 137). This does not conform to the pattern of classical ankylosing spondylitis, in which progressive spinal stiffness is the predominant symptom. The condition presents with polyarthritis, affecting chiefly the ankles and feet; spinal stiffness with comparatively little pain

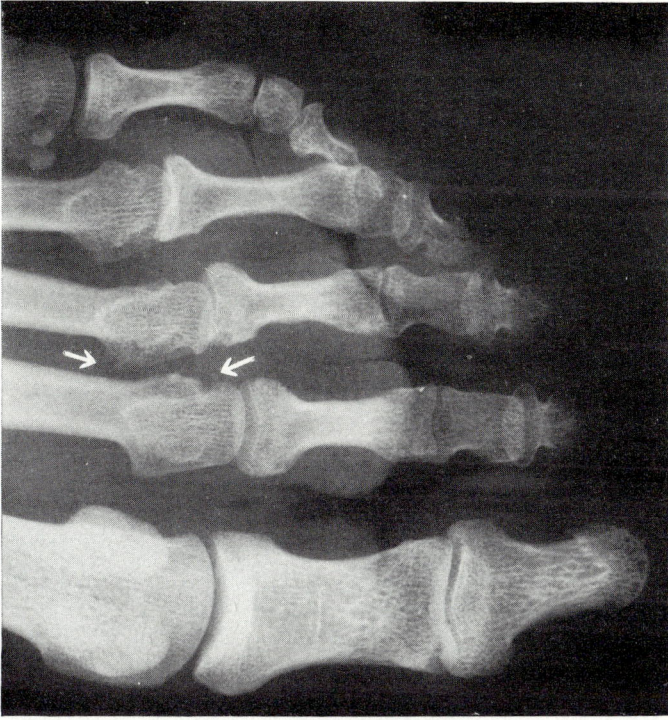

Fig. 134. Reiter's disease (acute): osteoporosis with small erosions on second and third metatarsal heads.

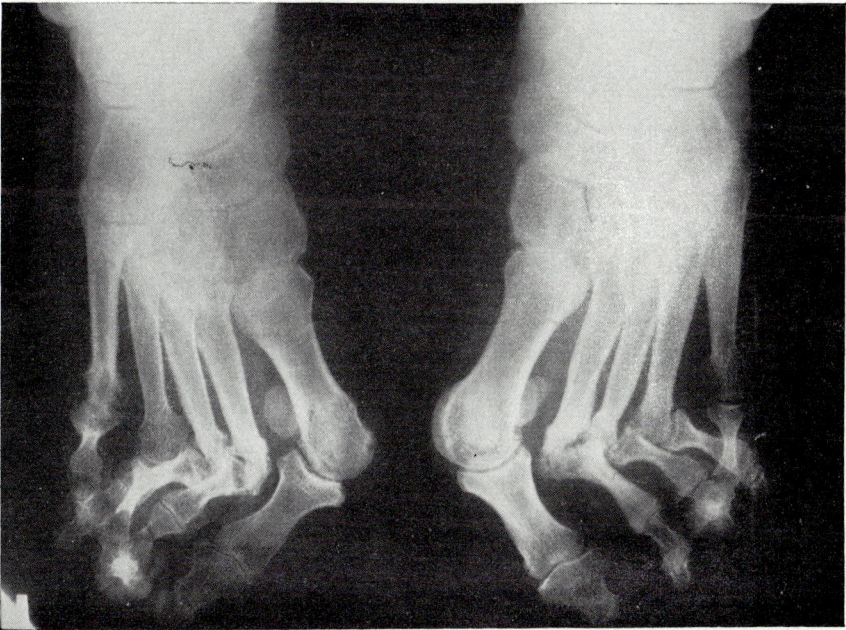

Fig. 135. Reiter's disease (chronic): X-ray showing destructive lesions of metatarso-phalangeal joints and lateral deviation of the toes.

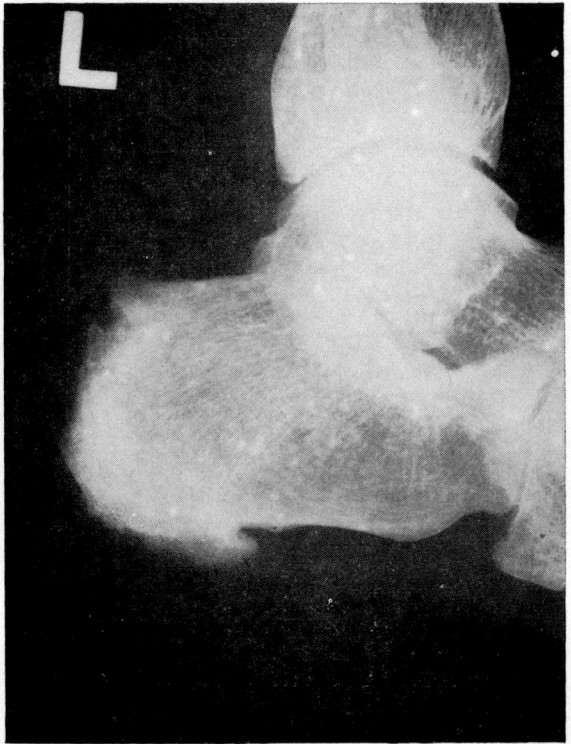

Fig. 136. Reiter's disease (chronic): X-ray showing calcanean spurs.

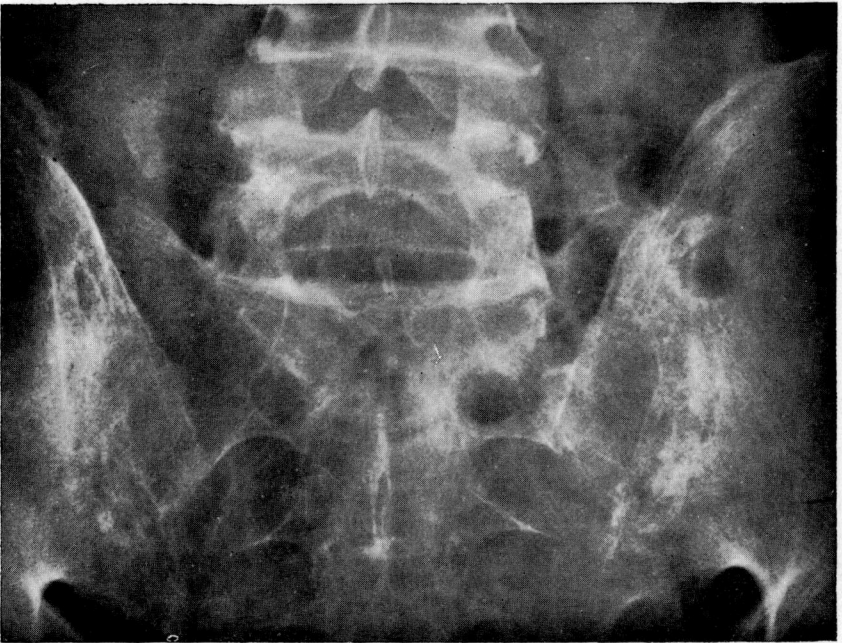

Fig. 137. Reiter's disease (chronic): X-ray showing obliteration of the sacro-iliac joints.

follows later. Routine X-rays in relapsing cases of Reiter's disease have shown evidence of chronic sacro-iliitis in 45 per cent of cases,[26] and in many of them there have been few symptoms of the involvement. Changes in the sacro-iliac joints tend to be progressive and the end result may well be complete obliteration of the joints. Many patients with classical ankylosing spondylitis have evidence of chronic inflammation of the seminal vesicles and prostate gland; some of them suffer from anterior uveitis. Although the significance of this is speculative, it seems likely that there is some relationship between the two conditions which has recently been supported by studies of histocompatibility antigens.

Sholkoff and Glickman[27] reviewed the radiological changes found in 55 cases of Reiter's disease, of which only 2 were in females. The sacro-iliac joints were involved in 42 per cent but, unlike ankylosing spondylitis, the changes were usually asymmetrical and rarely associated with spinal lesions. The knees were involved in 15 (34 per cent) of 44 cases for which films were available and ankles in 12 (28 per cent) of 43. Lesions of the heels were present in 27 (59 per cent) of 46 cases, but none of these showed large and fluffy spurs. The toes were involved in 20 (44 per cent) of 45 cases, particularly the interphalangeal joint of the great toe. The hands were less often affected and the hips and shoulders not at all. The main changes which occur are those of erosions of bone and periosteal new bone formation.

Recurrent Attacks of Uveitis

Reference has been made to the occurrence of anterior uveitis as a manifestation of Reiter's disease. Patients with chronic sacro-iliitis seem to be particularly prone to recurrent anterior uveitis.[26] Investigation of patients with anterior uveitis of unknown cause has shown that 72 per cent of them have chronic prostatovesiculitis, as compared with 29 per cent of patients of the same age groups with no history of uveitis or of genital infection.[28] Some of the patients with uveitis have been found to be suffering from undiagnosed Reiter's disease and others from ankylosing spondylitis or plantar fasciitis. This association suggested that the common factor in this condition was genital infection, in the form of urethritis or chronic prostatovesiculitis.

DIFFERENTIAL DIAGNOSIS

In straightforward cases observed in the early stages this presents no difficulty, but there are many less typical cases in which the diagnosis from other rheumatic diseases presents considerable difficulty. Reiter's disease may have to be distinguished from rheumatoid arthritis, ankylosing spondylitis, gout, psoriatic arthritis, gonococcal and other infective arthritis, acute rheumatic fever, the arthritic manifestations of serum sickness, systemic lupus erythematosus, Behçet's disease, the Stevens–Johnson syndrome and chronic inflammatory bowel disease.

AETIOLOGY

The cause of Reiter's disease is unknown. The constant association with sexually acquired urethritis in Western countries has led to the belief that it is a complication of the form of non-gonococcal urethritis usually called 'non-specific', of which about 40 per cent of cases are now known to be due to *Chlamydia trachomatis*. The matter has been discussed on pages 274 to 278. This relationship has led to attempts to isolate *Chlamydia* from joint fluid and conjunctival exudate in cases of Reiter's disease, so far with unconvincing results. Vaughan-Jackson et al.[29] tested 29 men suffering from acute Reiter's disease. Nineteen had received recent treatment with anti-chlamydial preparations and no isolate was obtained from them. Of the remaining 10, *Chlamydia* was isolated in cell culture from urethral material in three. No isolates were obtained from conjunctival material collected from 12 patients of whom four were untreated, or from synovial fluid from knees in nine of whom three were untreated. Fourteen contacts were examined and isolates were obtained from the contact of one man with positive urethral tests. Sera of 10 patients with Reiter's disease were tested with the microimmunofluorescence test with positive results showing titres of 1 : 16 or more in eight of them. Gordon et al.,[30] employing cell culture, isolated *Chlamydia* from both conjunctival and urethral material from a patient with Reiter's disease, but 54 specimens from 15 other patients gave negative results. These specimens included 12 of synovial fluid, 6 of synovial tissue, 12 of conjunctival material and 9 of urethral material; most of the patients were believed to have been untreated. Thus the evidence is that *Chlamydia* is not to be found in the joints of patients with Reiter's disease and it is found in the urethra no more often in those cases of non-specific urethritis which develop arthritis than in those which do not. This has recently been confirmed[31] in a prospective study of 531 men with non-specific urethritis, 16 of whom developed arthritis. *Chlamydia* was recovered from the urethra in 36 per cent of those with arthritis and in the same proportion of those without arthritis. However, patients with *Chlamydia*-positive urethritis who develop arthritis tend to have higher titres of IgG antibodies to *Chlamydia* than those with uncomplicated chlamydial urethritis.

In recent years much work has been done on the association of histo-compatibility (HLA) antigens with various diseases. As regards Reiter's disease it has been shown[32] that 76 per cent of these patients possess B27 antigen compared with 9 per cent of patients with non-specific urethritis and 6 per cent of age-matched male blood donors. Of those with only urethritis and peripheral arthritis B27 is possessed by 65 per cent but when there is sacro-iliitis, uveitis or circinate balanitis it is almost always present.[33] Those lacking B27 tend to pursue a milder course. The frequency of B27 is also high in Reiter's disease following dysentery.[34] There is an even stronger association of B27 and ankylosing spondylitis, the antigen being present in about 90 per cent of cases. Not unexpectedly patients with anterior uveitis are also likely to possess B27, particularly when there is evidence of associated disease.

The mechanism by which the HLA antigen influences susceptibility to the disease is unknown, but it may be an effect on the patient's immune response to various agents which could lead to autoimmunity.

Other evidence of a genetic influence is that psoriasis has been found in 13 per cent of the male relatives of patients with Reiter's disease compared with one per cent of a control population.[35] Clinical ankylosing spondylitis and radiological bilateral sacro-iliitis were also more common in male relatives of those with Reiter's disease but the difference was not statistically significant.

TREATMENT

The patient should be admitted to hospital until the active phase of the attack has passed. The course of the arthritis is not influenced by antibiotics, but some of them have a favourable effect on the urogenital infection associated with the venereal form of the disease. It is advisable, therefore, to give tetracycline by mouth, 500 mg four times daily, or doxycycline, 200 mg daily, for fourteen days (see p. 282). Strict bed rest, good nursing and good feeding are important, and these measures, combined with calcium aspirin or paracetamol for the relief of pain, may suffice for the mild case.

In more severe cases, phenylbutazone (Butazolidin), 200 mg given by mouth twice daily, is usually strikingly effective in relieving pain. Oxyphenbutazone (Tanderil), a derivative of phenylbutazone, has given similar results and is less likely to produce gastric side-effects. The dose is in the region of 200 mg two or three times daily, but whichever drug is used, the dose should be reduced progressively as the pain remits. Because of the risk, albeit small, of blood dyscrasia and hepatic necrosis, we prefer to use another drug before resorting to phenylbutazone. Other drugs which sometimes prove effective in giving relief are indomethacin (Indocid) 25 to 50 mg two or three times daily and mefenamic acid (Ponstan) 500 mg three times daily. Any of the propionic acid derivatives such as ibuprofen, ketoprofen and naproxen should also be suitable but there is little experience of their use in Reiter's disease. The use of cytotoxic or immunosuppressive drugs in other forms of inflammatory arthropathy has led to their consideration in severe or intractable cases of Reiter's disease. Methotrexate has been used in a few cases.[36-38] In one case 25 mg of this drug was given on one day of each week by mouth for three months, and in another up to 50 mg weekly intramuscularly with apparent benefit. This treatment is, however, purely experimental and carries with it the major hazard of marrow suppression.

There can be no hard and fast rules in the decision as to which patient should receive steroid hormones. This treatment is probably better reserved for the patient with florid disease, severe pain, wasting, fever and an increasing erythrocyte sedimentation rate, who is failing to respond to the measures already outlined. The initial dose may be in the region of 60 mg daily of prednisone or its equivalent, slowly reduced to a daily maintenance dose in the region of 15 to 20 mg. The patient whose disease is mainly confined to the knee joints has sometimes benefited from aspiration of synovial fluid and injections of hydrocortisone into the joint cavity, but this procedure may result in destructive changes if repeated too frequently. In general we do not advocate aspiration except to provide symptomatic relief in cases of gross effusion.

In cases of severe, prolonged, painful arthritis, the patient will benefit from the use of light splints at night, but immobilization must not be constant or prolonged, or ankylosis may result. By day the patient should be encouraged to move the affected joints.

As soon as the more active phase of the arthritis has subsided, the patient should be mobilized and more active physiotherapy should be given.

If keratoderma blennorrhagica and circinate balanitis are present, the most that is usually required is the institution of simple hygienic measures to prevent secondary infection from occurring in moist areas. If necessary, 1 per cent hydrocortisone cream may be used to suppress circinate balanitis and this may be combined with an antibiotic if there is secondary infection. The more widespread attacks of keratoderma blennorrhagica are usually found in patients with severe general illness which requires the use of steroid hormones, and these agents in sufficient dosage will partially suppress the skin lesions. Conjunctivitis is usually mild and does not generally require treatment, but in more severe cases chloramphenicol eye-drops (0·5 per cent) may be used to control secondary infection. Anterior uveitis, which may recur long after other manifestations of the disease have subsided, requires skilled management by an ophthalmologist. The principles of treatment are dilatation of the pupil with atropine drops (gutt. atrop. 1 per cent N.F.) and the frequent topical use of soluble prednisolone (Predsol = prednisolone disodium phosphate 0·5 per cent in aqueous solution). In very severe cases it may be necessary to give systemic prednisone. This treatment is usually remarkably effective in controlling any one attack but even so iridectomy may be required in very severe relapsing cases.

It should not be forgotten that Reiter's disease, as it is seen in Western countries, is commonly associated with communicable genital infection and the correct management of cases must include investigation of sexual partners. As recurrent attacks are sometimes precipitated by freshly acquired non-specific urethritis, patients should be warned of this risk. They should also be told to report for treatment promptly if they do acquire non-specific urethritis, but whether very early treatment of the condition lessens the risk of developing Reiter's disease remains an open question; it certainly does not abolish it.

REFERENCES

1.   KING, AMBROSE (1964) *Recent Advances in Venereology*, pp. 395–471. London: J. & A. Churchill.

2.   KING, A. J. and MASON, R. M. (1969) In: *Textbook of Rheumatic Diseases*, 4th ed., ed. W. S. C. Copeman, pp. 366 et seq. Edinburgh: Livingstone.

3.   BRODIE, B. C. (a) (1818) *Pathological and Surgical Observations on Diseases of the Joints*, p. 55. London: Longman, Hurst, Rees, Orme and Brown. (b) *ibid.* (1836) 4th ed., p. 57.

4.   REITER, H. (1916) *Dtsch. med. Wschr.*, **42**, 1535.

5.   *A.R. med. Offr Dept Hlth (Lond.)* (1977) p. 59. H.M.S.O. 1978.

6.   RUSSELL, A. S., DAVIS, P., PERCY, J. S. and LENTLE, B. C. (1977) *J. Rheum.*, **4**, 293.

7.   WEESE, W. C. and McCARTY, D. J. (1969) *J. Am. med. Ass.*, **208**, 825.

8.   ZEWI, M. (1947) *Acta ophthal.*, **25**, 47.

9.   OATES, J. K. and HANCOCK, J. A. H. (1959) *Am. J. med. Sci.*, **238**, 79.

10.   RECKLESS, J. P. D. (1972) *Br. J. vener. Dis.*, **48**, 207.

11.   HANCOCK, J. A. H. (1960) *Br. J. vener. Dis.*, **36**, 36.

12.   THAMBAR, I. V., DUNLOP, R., THIN, R. N. and HUSKISSON, E. C. (1977) *Br. J. vener. Dis.*, **53**, 260.

13.   LAFON, R., PAGES, P., ROUX, J., TEMPLE, J. P. and MINVIELLE, J. (1955) *Rev. neurol.*, **92**, 611.

14.   CSONKA, G. W. (1958) *Ann. rheum. Dis.*, **17**, 334.

15.   CSONKA, G. W. and OATES, J. K. (1957) *Br. med. J.*, **1**, 866.

16.   CSONKA, G. W., LITCHFIELD, J. W., OATES, J. K. and WILLCOX, R. R. (1961) *Br. med. J.*, **1**, 243.

17.   RODNAN, G. P., BENEDEK, T. G., SHAVER, J. A. and FENNELL, R. H. (1964) *J. Am. med. Ass.*, **89**, 889.

18.   CLIFF, J. M. (1971) *Ann. rheum. Dis.*, **30**, 171.

19.   COLLINS, P. (1972) *Br. J. vener. Dis.*, **48**, 300.

20.   PAULUS, M. E., PEARSON, C. M. and PITTS, W. (1972) *Am. J. Med.*, **53**, 464.

21.   BLOCK, S. R. (1972) *Arthritis Rheum.*, **15**, 218.

22.   CSONKA, G. W. (1966) *Br. J. vener. Dis.*, **42**, 93.

23.   BLEEHEN, S. S., EVERALL, J. D. and TIGHE, J. R. (1966) *Br. J. vener. Dis.*, **42**, 88.

24.   CAUGHEY, D. E. and WAKEM, J. (1973) *Arthritis Rheum.*, **16**, 695.

25.   CSONKA, G. W. (1960) *Arthritis Rheum.*, **3**, 164.

26.   OATES, J. K. and YOUNG, A. C. (1959) *Br. med. J.*, **1**, 1013.

27.   SHOLKOFF, S. D., GLICKMAN, M. G. and STEINBACH, H. L. (1970) *Radiology*, **97**, 497.

28.   CATTERALL, R. D. (1960) *Br. J. vener. Dis.*, **36**, 27.

29.   VAUGHAN-JACKSON, J. D., DUNLOP, E. M. C., DAROUGAR, S., DWYER, R. ST. C. and JONES, B. R. (1972) *Br. J. vener. Dis.*, **48**, 445.

30. GORDON, F. B., QUAN, A. L., STEINMAN, T. I. and PHILIP, R. N. (1973) *Br. J. vener. Dis.*, **49,** 376.

31. KEAT, A. C., MAINI, R. N., NKWAZI, G. C., PEGRUM, G. D., RIDGWAY, G. L. and SCOTT, J. T. (1978) *Br. med. J.*, **1,** 605.

32. BREWERTON, D. A., CAFFREY, M., NICHOLLS, A., WALTERS, D., OATES, J. K. and JAMES, D. C. O. (1973) *Lancet*, **2,** 996.

33. BREWERTON, D. A. (1978) *J. R. Soc. Med.*, **71,** 331.

34. AHO, K., AHVONEN, P., ALKIO, P., LASSUS, R., SAIRENEN, E., SIEVERS, K. and TIILIKAINEN, A. (1975) *Ann. rheum. Dis.*, **34,** Suppl. I, p. 29.

35. LAWRENCE, J. S. (1974) *Br. J. vener. Dis.*, **50,** 140.

36. MULLINS, J. F., MABERRY, J. D. and STONE, O. J. (1966) *Arch. Derm.*, **94,** 335.

37. FARBER, G. A., FORSHNER, J. G. and O'QUINN, S. E. (1967) *J. Am. med. Ass.*, **200,** 171.

38. TOPP, J. R., FAM, A. G. and HART, G. D. (1971) *Can. med. Ass. J.*, **105,** 1168.

23

Trichomonal Infestation of the Genital Tract

The protozoal organism *Trichomonas vaginalis* was first described by Donné in 1836,[1] who observed it in purulent genital secretions from both women and men; the name is misleading because the organism is frequently found in the female urethra, and is by no means uncommon in the male urethra. The organism varies considerably in size, from that of a pus cell up to two and a half times that size. It may be oval or pear-shaped. It has a nucleus which is situated anteriorly, and between the nucleus and the surface of the broader end of the organism lie one or more rounded structures called blepharoplasts. From these arise four flagella, which by their rapid, jerky activity give the organism its characteristic movement by which it is easily identified in a fresh specimen of secretion observed microscopically. Also springing from one of the blepharoplasts is an undulating membrane, which may often be seen extending down the margin of one side of the body of the organism for about two-thirds of its length. It has a characteristic, undulating movement. Extending posteriorly from the nucleus and projecting beyond the margin of the cytoplasm is a long, narrow axostyle. Bacteria can usually be seen lying on or within the cytoplasm of the organism.

T. vaginalis can be identified in most cases by direct microscopical examination, using freshly obtained secretion on a slide with coverslip or a hanging-drop preparation (Fig. 139). It can be recognized, with the 4 mm or 2 mm objective, by its characteristic jerky movements. It can be well seen with ordinary illumination after elimination of peripheral rays of light by partial closure of the sub-stage diaphragm of the microscope, or with dark-ground or phase-contrast illumination. It can also be grown satisfactorily in various artificial media (see the Appendix, p. 401); the combination of smear and culture tests is more effective in diagnosis than either test alone. Various methods of staining to show the organism have been recommended. Opinions vary as to their value, but in general stained

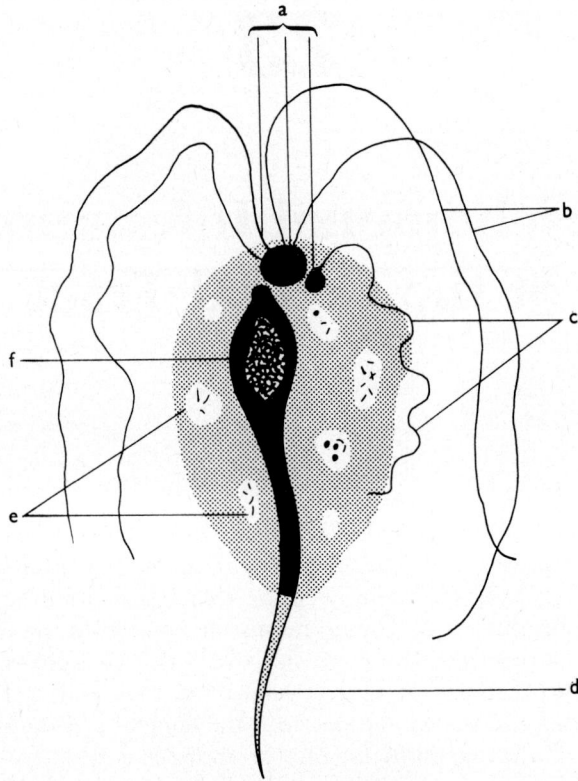

Trichomonas vaginalis

(*After Burke.*)

a. Blepharoplasts	*d.* Axostyle
b. Flagella	*e.* Vacuoles containing bacteria
c. Undulating membrane	*f.* Nucleus

preparations have proved less reliable than fresh preparations. However, good results have been claimed with Papanicolaou stain[2] and with brilliant cresyl blue.[3] *Trichomonas tenax (buccalis)*, found in the mouth, and *Trichomonas hominis*, found in the intestine, do not infest the genito-urinary tract.

TRICHOMONIASIS IN THE MALE

Infestation with *T. vaginalis* in the male often gives rise to no symptoms and the signs may be very slight or absent. In other cases, however, it presents as low-grade, non-gonococcal urethritis which cannot be distinguished from 'non-specific' urethritis on clinical grounds (see p. 277).

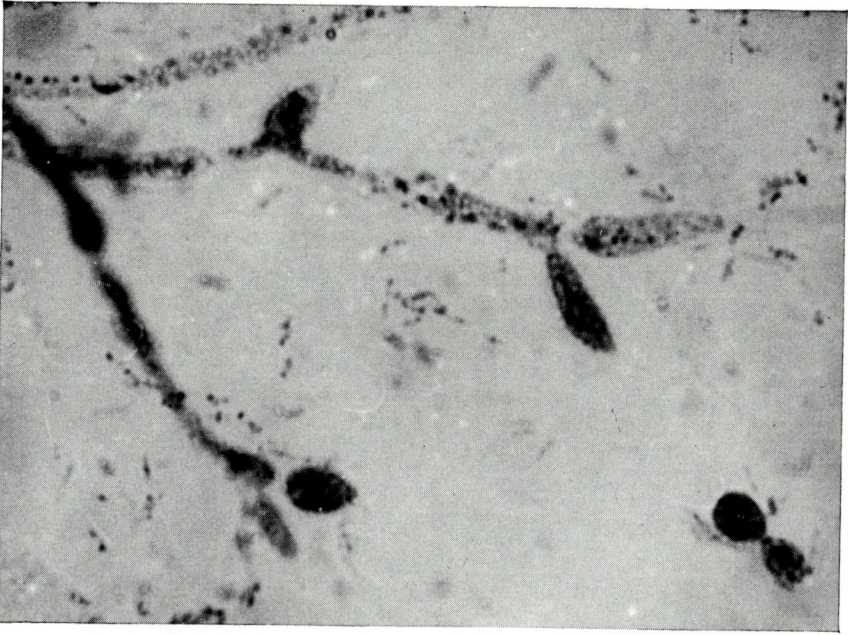

Fig. 138. Candidosis (*Candida albicans*): yeast-like spores and mycelium in vaginal secretion.

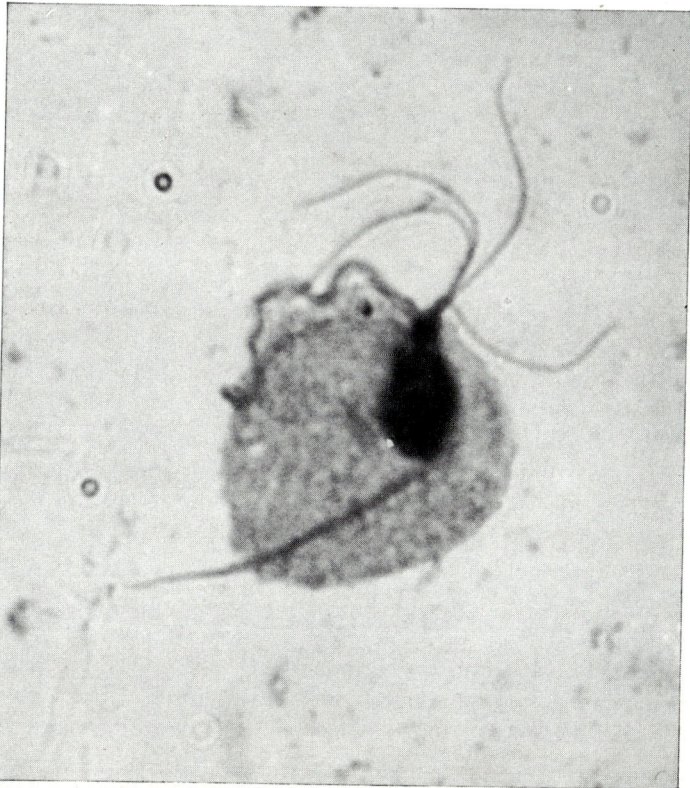

Fig. 139. *Trichomonas vaginalis* in moist slide of vaginal secretion. (*Photograph by courtesy of May and Baker Ltd.*)

The diagnosis is made by finding the organism in urethral secretion by smear or culture, or both. It may appear less active in specimens from the urethra than in those from the vagina, the body becoming spherical with sluggish flagella lying alongside. The proportion of cases of non-gonococcal urethritis in which this organism can be found has varied in different series, but 5 per cent is probably a representative figure. The organism has also been isolated from the subpreputial sac, prostatic secretion, seminal fluid and urine; but there is very little evidence as to whether any of these sites can be regarded as its regular habitat. Experimental evidence suggests that the infestation may be self-limiting in some cases in the male; this may apply to some naturally acquired infestations, but others can persist for years. The longer the infestation has been present the more difficult it may be to identify the organism. Urethrogenital trichomoniasis seems to be two to five times more common in coloured than white patients.[4,5]

THE INCUBATION PERIOD is generally from four days to three weeks.

SYMPTOMS are often absent or minimal. The patient may notice slight urethral discharge, which is mucoid or mucopurulent in appearance, and may complain of a tickling sensation in the urethra. Frankly purulent discharge and dysuria are uncommon.

SIGNS are often absent or those of low-grade non-gonococcal urethritis, but it may be necessary to examine for urethral secretion and the presence in the urine of small comma-like threads when the patient has held urine all night. There is a greater chance of finding the organism in specimens obtained by scraping the urethral wall with a firm platinum loop and mixing the material with a small drop of saline rather than taking a specimen from free discharge. Repeated examination may be required to demonstrate the organism. Sometimes it can be found in smear and culture of urinary deposit after light centrifugation. Some of these patients have pre-existing urethral strictures or stenosis of the external urinary meatus. Occasionally there is evidence of a purulent balanoposthitis.

COMPLICATIONS. Little is known about the complications of this condition. Evidence of littritis, prostatitis and occasionally epididymitis may be found, but it is difficult to know whether these are due to trichomonal infestation or to associated 'non-specific' infection. The organism has been found in specimens of semen[6] but whether it originates in the prostate, seminal vesicle, urethra or elsewhere has not been determined. Haemospermia has been reported. There is no evidence that metastatic complications occur. T. vaginalis is not found in the rectum.

TRICHOMONIASIS IN THE FEMALE

Infestation in females usually occurs during the years of greatest sexual activity, but it is found not infrequently during or after the menopause.[7] It is occasionally found in female infants shortly after birth and there have been very rare reports of finding the organism in the conjunctivas of babies with conjunctivitis.[8] Trichomoniasis is nearly always transmitted during sexual intercourse but it may very occasionally result from contamination by moist secretions recently deposited on a lavatory seat, from splashing in water closets,[4, 9, 10] or from borrowed towels or clothing. Other possible sources of infestation are douche nozzles, rubber gloves or improperly sterilized instruments used for examination. Trichomonal vaginitis is sometimes found in girls or women with intact hymens, but the probability is that transmission has occurred by sexual contact without penetration. Trichomoniasis is often of long standing when the diagnosis is made and there may be no history of recent sexual contact. Trichomonal vaginitis may be associated with gonococcal infection.[11] In several series a third to a half of female patients with gonorrhoea have been found to have trichomoniasis in addition. As in the male, the incubation period is generally from four days to three weeks.

Vaginitis

In the great majority of cases the vagina is involved. Fairly often there are no or only insignificant symptoms but most patients complain of vaginal discharge which is characteristically yellow, thin and offensive. It may be very profuse and cause marked vulvitis with intertrigo and excoriation of the inner aspects of the thighs. The patient may complain of dyspareunia, and the passage of a speculum may be very painful. The vagina is seen to contain thin, yellow, frothy secretion with an offensive smell; the vaginal wall is reddened and in acute cases there may be punctate red spots on the vagina and vaginal portion of the cervix, the so-called strawberry cervix. In some cases the type of discharge does not suggest a trichomonal infestation and in patients without symptoms the appearances may be normal. The vaginal pH usually varies from 5 to 8, as compared with the normal of between 4 and 5.

Before the advent of successful systemic remedies the condition would often become chronic with exacerbations, particularly after menstrual periods.

Urethritis

Approximately half the cases of trichomonal vaginitis also have infestation of the urethra. The condition may be asymptomatic or may cause dysuria and perhaps frequency if spread has occurred to the trigone of the bladder.

Endocervicitis

Endocervicitis may be associated with vaginitis of this kind, but it is doubtful whether *T. vaginalis* does penetrate the cervical mucus to reach the cervical glands, the uterine cavity or Fallopian tubes. The endocervicitis is probably due to associated 'non-specific' infection, and so also is pelvic infection which sometimes occurs in the presence of trichomoniasis.

Skenitis and Bartholinitis

Skenitis and bartholinitis with abscess formation may be associated with trichomoniasis, and occasionally *T. vaginalis* can be isolated from the secretions of these organs. As far as is known, metastatic spread does not occur. The anorectal region is generally believed not to be susceptible to this organism, although in the past there have been occasional case reports of proctitis from this organism in women with severe trichomonal vaginitis.

Diagnosis

The diagnosis must depend upon finding *T. vaginalis*, but it is also important to look for evidence of associated infection. It is essential to exclude gonorrhoea in all cases, bearing in mind that both conditions are often present especially in patients attending venereal disease clinics. Smears and cultures for the gonococcus should be taken on at least two occasions. Trichomoniasis is often present with 'non-specific' genital infection but vaginal candidosis seems to occur less often in patients with trichomonal infestations.[7,12] Vulval warts may be associated. The evidence of 'non-specific' genital infection can only be determined after successful treatment of the trichomoniasis; chlamydial infection should be diagnosed by appropriate culture tests if these are available. Vaginitis may also be caused by chemical and physical agents; by foreign bodies such as a retained tampon; by fungi, such as *Candida albicans* (vaginal thrush) (see Fig. 138); and possibly other organisms such as *Corynebacterium vaginale*. After the menopause women may have atrophic vaginitis. It may or may not be possible to find *T. vaginalis* in the male partner, and he may or may not have evidence of urethrogenital infection.

PREVALENCE

IN MALES

It is a reasonable assumption that the sexual partner of a woman with trichomonal vaginitis is likely to be harbouring the organism but the fact may be difficult to establish and the organism may be carried only transiently. In various studies on male consorts of infected women the presence of trichomonads has been demonstrated in from 19 to 76 per cent of cases. The number of male patients with trichomoniasis reported as attending the venereal disease clinics of England in the year ending June 30, 1977, was 1703.[13] In the large industrial city of Lódz in Poland,[14] urinary deposits were examined by phase-contrast microscopy in the cases of 7844 unselected men aged 18 to 60 years and *T. vaginalis* was found in 1·74 per cent. Among 3864 males aged less than 18 years or more than 60 years the

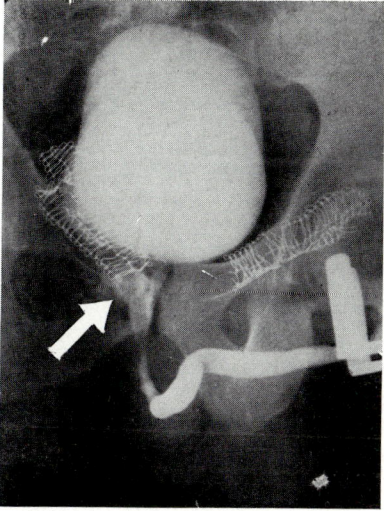

Fig. 140. Urethrogram showing urethral stricture and urethral calculus (*see arrow*); urethritis was secondary.

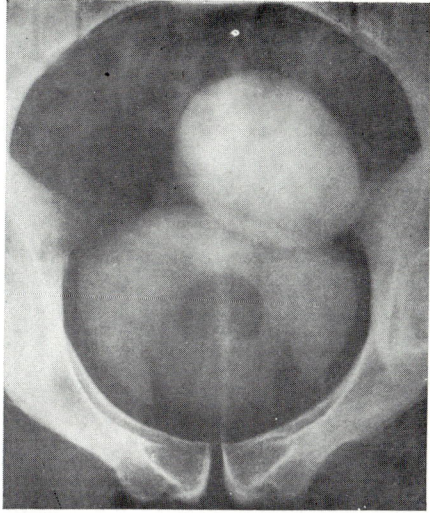

Fig. 141. IVP showing diverticulum of the bladder; urethritis was secondary to bacterial urinary infection.

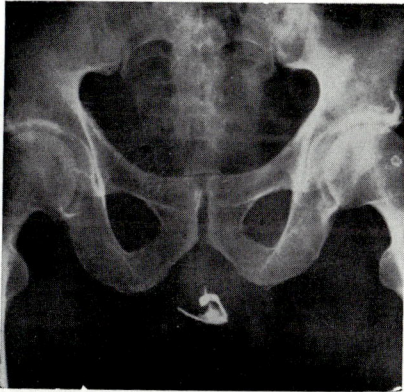

Fig. 142. Foreign body (safety-pin) in the urethra; urethritis was secondary.

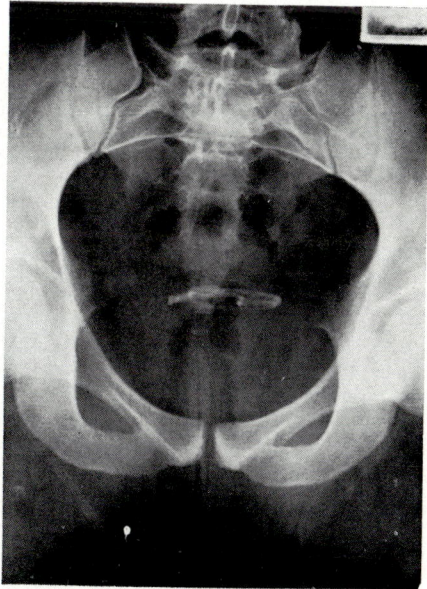

Fig. 143. Foreign body (flex) in the bladder; urethritis was secondary to bacterial urinary infection.

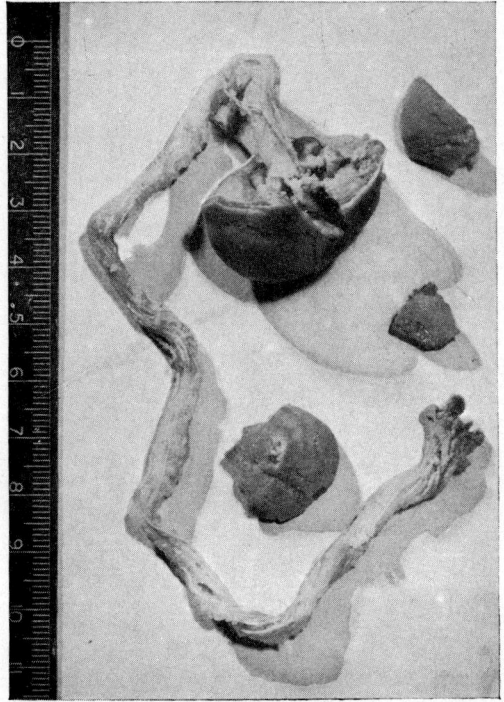

Fig. 144. Foreign body (wax
taper) as nucleus of vesical
calculus; urethritis was
secondary to bacterial urinary
infection. (*Scale in inches*; 1 in
= 2·54 cm)

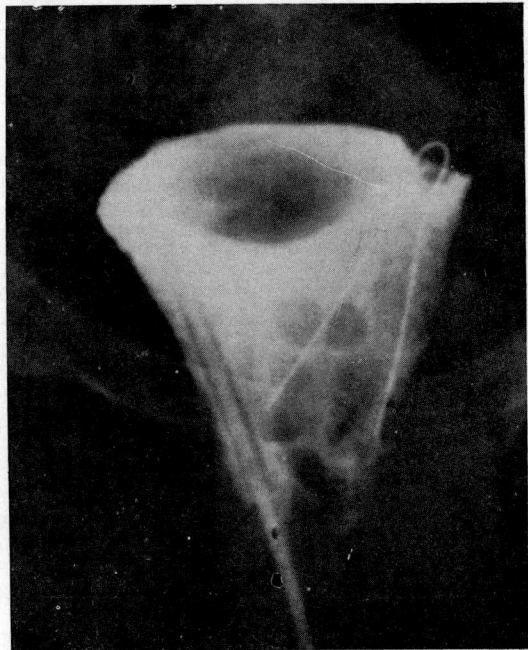

Fig. 145. Foreign body (hair-
pin) in vagina, which has been
filled with radio-opaque fluid;
vaginitis was secondary.

prevalence was 0·85 per cent, with none of the positive cases occurring in those under 18 years.

IN FEMALES

It is difficult to estimate the likely prevalence in the general population because almost all the available studies relate to special groups. The disease is at least twice as common in negro women as in whites. Of 562 women attending a birth control clinic in Western England, 5·3 per cent were found to be infected.[15] At the London Hospital,[4] 12·8 per cent of 400 women attending the gynaecological department and 21·3 per cent of 400 attending the venereal disease department were harbouring the organism. In Cardiff,[16] T. vaginalis was found in 4·7 per cent of 625 antenatal patients attending consecutively. The number of cases in women attending the venereal disease clinics of England in the year ending June 30, 1977, was 18,285.[13] In the survey in Lódz[14] mentioned above, urinary deposits from a large number of women were also examined. T. vaginalis was found in 10·67 per cent of 7432 unselected women aged 18 to 60 years and 3·76 per cent of 3795 aged less than 18 years or more than 60 years. The prevalence in those under 18 years was only 0·32 per cent. If vaginal specimens had also been examined these figures would almost certainly have been higher. Gallagher[17] examined 716 delinquent girls aged from 14 to 17 years, admitted to a Remand Home in London, and found the condition in 28 per cent. A study in the United States of America[18] of 465 employees of an insurance company showed a frequency of 6·3 per cent in married women and 1·4 per cent in single women. Among 715 inmates of mental institutions the frequency was 15 per cent, and of 221 women prisoners, most of whom had been prostitutes or drug addicts, 70 per cent had trichomoniasis. On the other hand, of 157 undergraduates of a women's college, aged 20 to 22 years, none had trichomonal infestation. Female partners of men known to have trichomonal infestation will almost invariably be found to harbour the organism.[19]

TREATMENT

The oral trichomonacide metronidazole (Flagyl)[20, 21] has proved very effective in the treatment of trichomoniasis in both sexes and is still the treatment of choice. Standard dosage is 200 mg by mouth three times daily for seven days. It may also be given effectively as 400 mg twice daily for five days,[22] and in a single dose of 2 g of metronidazole by mouth.[23-25] Other regimens which have given good results include 800 mg in the morning and 1200 mg in the evening for two days, and 500 mg twice daily for three days. The toxic effects are negligible, but occasionally there is gastrointestinal disturbance which is usually mild. The patient should avoid alcohol during treatment because of reports of Antabuse-like effects, but these have not been confirmed in double-blind trials in alcoholics.[26] This regimen gives over 80 per cent of successes and no local therapy is required. The sexual partners should receive the same treatment, after proper investigation, even if it proves impossible to find the organism. In cases of recurrence, the possibility of re-infestation should always be considered. Keighley,[27] who treated 496 women in the closed community of a prison in London giving 400 mg of metronidazole twice daily for seven days, claimed success in 98·3 per cent of the cases. Treatment failure is only very rarely associated with reduced sensitivity of the organism to this remedy. There is no evidence to suggest damage to the fetus when metronidazole has been administered to pregnant women, but until this point has been finally determined many clinicians have preferred to withhold the drug during the first three months of pregnancy.[28] The manufacturers advise against short treatments with high doses during pregnancy or breast-feeding.

More recently a preparation called nimorazole (Naxogin), also a nitro-imidazole compound, has been claimed to be equally as effective as metronidazole.[29, 30] The recommended dosage was initially 250 mg twice daily by mouth for six days. Modifications of this dosage have been used by Jones[31] and Ross,[32] who gave single doses of 2 g by mouth, and by Campbell,[33] who gave either two doses of 1 g or three doses of 1 g within 24 hours. The results claimed with these methods were all good with success in from 80 to more than 90 per cent of cases. Best results have been obtained with single doses of 2 g and three doses of 1 g within 24 hours. There is no doubt that nimorazole is a useful remedy but there seems no reason why it should replace metronidazole for routine treatment.

Various other nitroimidazole derivatives have recently undergone trials. These include tinidazole,[34] ornidazole,[35,36] carnidazole[37] and secnidazole.[38] All have given excellent results when used in single doses of 2 g by mouth, and ornidazole was also effective in single doses of 1·5 g.[36] Whether any of these offer any particular advantages over metronidazole remains to be seen. They are not yet marketed in the United Kingdom.

Before the introduction of metronidazole, local treatment was employed in the form of antiseptic urethrovesical irrigations in the male and vaginal pessaries in the female. The most successful vaginal preparation consisted of a pentavalent arsenical, acetarsol, which was inserted regularly each night for a considerable period. Results were poor, owing mainly to re-infestation from the urinary tract or from male partners. Occasional cases of sensitivity reactions to the arsenical were reported.

REFERENCES

1. DONNÉ, A. (1836) C.R. Acad. Sci. (Paris), **3**, 385.
2. SUMMERS, J. L. and FORD, M. L. (1972) J. Urol., **107**, 840.
3. BARTUNEK, J. and SCHULTZE, M. (1972) Hautarzt, **23**, 368.

4. WHITTINGTON, M. J. (1957) *Br. J. vener. Dis.*, **33**, 80.
5. NICOL, C. S. (1958) *Br. J. vener. Dis.*, **34**, 192.
6. WHITTINGTON, M. J. (1951) *J. Obstet. Gynaec. Br. Emp.*, **58**, 616.
7. NIELSEN, R. (1973) *Br. J. vener. Dis.*, **49**, 531.
8. NOVOTŇÝ, L. (1973) *Cs. Oftal.*, **29**, 292.
9. KESSEL, J. F. and THOMPSON, C. F. (1950) *Proc. Soc. exp. Biol. (N.Y.)*, **74**, 755.
10. BURGESS, J. A. (1963) *Br. J. vener. Dis.*, **39**, 248.
11. KING, A. J., MASCALL, W. N. and PRICE, I. N. O. (1936) *Lancet*, **2**, 18.
12. ORIEL, J. D., PARTRIDGE, B. M., DENNY, M. J. and COLEMAN, J. C. (1972) *Br. med. J.*, **4**, 761.
13. *A.R. med. Offr Dept Hlth (Lond.)* (1977) p. 59. H.M.S.O., 1978.
14. GLEBSKI, J. (1965) *Przegl. derm.*, **52**, 617.
15. WHITTINGTON, M. J. (1951) *J. Obstet. Gynaec. Br. Emp.*, **58**, 399.
16. SPARKS, R. A., WILLIAMS, G. L., BOYCE, J. M. H., FITZGERALD, T. C. and SHELLEY, G. (1975) *Br. J. vener. Dis.*, **51**, 110.
17. GALLAGHER, E. (1970) *Br. J. vener. Dis.*, **46**, 129.
18. BUXTON, C. L., WEINMAN, D. M. and JOHNSON, C. (1958) *Obstet. Gynec.*, **12**, 699.
19. CATTERALL, R. D. and NICOL, C. S. (1960) *Br. med. J.*, **1**, 1177.
20. COSAR, C. and JULOU, L. (1959) *Annls Inst. Pasteur*, **96**, 238.
21. DUREL, P., ROIRON, V., SIBOULET, A. and BOREL, L. J. (1960) *Br. J. vener. Dis.*, **36**, 21.
22. McCLEAN, A. N. (1971) *Br. J. vener. Dis.*, **47**, 36.
23. CSONKA, G. W. (1971) *Br. J. vener. Dis.*, **47**, 456.
24. WOODCOCK, K. R. (1972) *Br. J. vener. Dis.*, **48**, 65.
25. MORTON, R. S. (1972) *Br. J. vener. Dis.*, **48**, 525.
26. PLATZ, A., PANEPINTO, W. C., KISSIN, B. and CHARNOFF, S. M. (1970) *Dis. nerv. Syst.*, **31**, 631.
27. KEIGHLEY, E. E. (1971) *Br. med. J.*, **1**, 207.
28. RODIN, P. and HASS, G. (1966) *Br. J. vener. Dis.*, **42**, 210.
29. CANTONE, A., DECARNERI, I., EMANUELI, A., GIRALDI, P., LOGEMANN, W., LONGO, R., MEINARDI, G., MONTE, G., NANNINI, G., TOSOLINI, G. and VITA, G. (1969) *G. Mal. infett.*, **21**, 954.
30. McCLEAN, A. N. (1972) *Br. J. vener. Dis.*, **48**, 69.
31. JONES, J. P. (1972) *Br. J. vener. Dis.*, **48**, 528.
32. ROSS, S. M. (1973) *Br. J. vener. Dis.*, **49**, 310.
33. CAMPBELL, A. C. H. (1972) *Br. J. vener. Dis.*, **48**, 531.
34. WALLIN, J. and FORSGREN, A. (1974) *Br. J. vener. Dis.*, **50**, 148.
35. SKÖLD, M., GNARPE, H. and HILLSTRÖM, L. (1977) *Br. J. vener. Dis.*, **53**, 44.
36. HILLSTRÖM, L., PETTERSSON, L., PÁLSSON, E. and SANDSTRÖM, S. O. (1977) *Br. J. vener. Dis.*, **53**, 193.
37. NOTOWICZ, A., STOLZ, E. and DE KONING, G. A. J. (1977) *Br. J. vener. Dis.*, **53**, 129.
38. VIDEAU, D., NIEL, G., SIBOULET, A. and CATALAN, F. (1978) *Br. J. vener. Dis.*, **54**, 77.

24

Candidosis of the Genital Tract

The 'thrush' fungus—*Candida albicans*—was first discovered by Langenbeck in 1839. The various clinical conditions caused by this organism on the skin, in the mouth, lungs, gut and vagina, have been termed candidosis (candidiasis) in preference to the older term moniliasis, according to Winner.[1] The condition may rarely become systemic and involve the endocardium and other sites; this is only likely to occur in cases of severe illness, for which treatment with immunosuppressive drugs, corticosteroids or broad-spectrum antibiotics is required. Frank in 1792 first observed candidal involvement of the vagina without causing symptoms. It is now established that candidosis can also involve the vulva in the female and the male genitalia, in particular the subpreputial sac (balanoposthitis). Certain factors appear to favour the presence of the organism and to produce a clinical condition where previously it had been carried as a commensal; these include the state of pregnancy, glycosuria and the administration of broad-spectrum antibiotics and steroid and immunosuppressive drugs. Various workers, including Jensen et al.,[2] have found an association with the taking of a combined oral contraceptive but some, including Morris,[3] have not.

    Candida albicans is commonly identified by stained smear and culture, but yeast-forms or mycelium may be seen in the moist saline preparations used in the identification of *T. vaginalis*. Gram-stained slides show the yeast spores, which may have buds, and the mycelium, both of which are Gram-positive (see Fig. 138); culture is more sensitive and may be taken on to a maltose-peptone agar (Sabouraud's medium) plate which is then incubated at 36°C for two to five days. Specimens may be taken from the vagina or vulva in women and from the subpreputial sac, urethra or genital skin in men. Certain other yeasts are sometimes isolated from the genital tract. Oriel et al.[4] studied 533 women attending a venereal diseases clinic and found yeasts in culture in 138 (26 per cent). *Candida albicans* accounted for 112 (81 per cent), *Torulopsis glabrata* for 22 (16 per cent) and other yeasts for only 4 (3 per cent).

In the year ending June 30, 1977,[5] there were 6756 males and 29,995 females attending the venereal diseases clinics of England and Wales who were diagnosed as having candidosis. This was a considerably higher figure than for trichomoniasis. The disease in men is generally acquired through sexual contact. This applies to some cases in females, but the proportion is uncertain and certainly many vaginal infections are acquired in other ways, perhaps most often from the gut.

CANDIDOSIS IN THE MALE

Yeasts are carried on the penis just as often by circumcised as by uncircumcised men,[6, 7] although the latter are more likely to have symptoms.[7] Rodin and Kolator[6] found that 10 per cent of 175 men attending a venereal diseases clinic with no evidence of balanitis carried *Candida* species on the penis and the majority were *C. albicans*. Approximately half of male contacts of women with *Candida* infections have been found to harbour the organism,[8] and most female contacts of men with *Candida* infection will be affected. The patient may complain of intense irritation or burning and there may be a white or slightly purulent discharge; the prepuce may be difficult to retract and fissured. If retraction is possible, the inner surface of the prepuce and glans penis may be seen to be red and inflamed, with dispersed white patches and sometimes vesicles and erosions. The condition often extends into the fossa navicularis. The involvement of the latter site makes it difficult to assess urethral infection with *Candida*, which is probably rare but can occasionally occur even in the absence of balanitis.[9] Itchy and scaling lesions may also be present on the penile and scrotal skin, or even occasionally in the groins due to candidosis. However, it is most important to realize that many males will present no symptoms or signs but nevertheless be a potential source of infection or reinfection of females. In a number of these cases, *Candida* will be found by smear and culture taken with a sterile swab in saline applied to the coronal sulcus.

Sometimes a male contact of a woman with *Candida* infection will complain of itching and burning and the appearance of small vesicles and ulcers soon after intercourse and lasting a day or two; *Candida* is not found and these cases are believed to be the result of an allergic reaction to the organism carried by the female.[9]

CANDIDOSIS IN THE FEMALE

In many cases women with candidosis are symptomless or have only slight symptoms, but a considerable number complain of intense vulval and vaginal irritation with or without vaginal discharge. The latter is characteristically white and thick, but often it is scanty and watery and sometimes purulent. There may also be a history of dyspareunia and dysuria. On examination of the vulva, the mucosa is reddened and sometimes oedematous, and white patches, fissures or erosions may be present; there may be discomfort on passing a vaginal speculum which will reveal a similar picture on the vaginal mucosa with additional white 'cheese-like' secretion covering the vaginal portion of the cervix. The typical white vaginal plaques that occur are difficult to remove and after removal bleeding points are seen. As already mentioned the vaginal secretion may be watery and sometimes purulent. Generally the pH of the discharge is below 5.

In every case the diagnosis must be confirmed by smear or culture and tests to exclude other genital infections should be taken. The difficult problem is to assess the significance of asymptomatic candidosis in women; if hyphae (mycelium) are observed in the Gram-stained smear, then the fungal infection is probably due to *Candida albicans* and should be treated, but even if yeast forms only are identified, or evidence of *Candida* is only obtained by culture, the organism may still have to be considered a pathogen and the patient in need of treatment, particularly if she is pregnant. Certain species of *Candida* other than *C. albicans* may be pathogenic as well as other yeasts such as *Torulopsis glabrata*.

There is an association between vaginal candidosis and rectal infection with *Candida*.[10, 11] This is particularly strong in cases of recurrent *Candida* vaginitis, reaching 100 per cent in one study in the United States of America.[12] However, in another study[13] the association was less obvious and it has not been proved that the vaginal infection is a consequence of the rectal infection, although there is suggestive evidence that this might sometimes be so.[14]

TREATMENT

As long as the treatment of candidosis depends on local rather than systemic antifungal drugs, the results are likely to remain relatively poor and relapse common. It is also difficult to assess which of the locally acting antifungal preparations are more effective than others.

The principle of local treatment is to apply the preparations to all skin and mucosal surfaces involved for a sufficient length of time to eliminate the fungus, while preventing autoinfection from the gut and reinfection from the sex partner. Any causative factor such as glycosuria should be investigated, and if the patient is diabetic, suitable treatment given. The use of cotton rather than synthetic underwear may facilitate recovery.

Nystatin is an antifungal antibiotic which can be prescribed as an ointment or cream for male genital candidosis; it should be applied twice daily to the areas involved for at least two weeks. Females with candidosis can be given nystatin ointment or cream for vulvitis plus nystatin vaginal pessaries, which may be incorporated into an effervescent matrix for better dispersal. The pessaries should be used once or twice daily and the cream twice daily for at least two weeks, regardless of any intervening menstrual period. The cream should be applied to the perineum and perianal area as well as the vulva. In addition women with genital candidosis may need oral nystatin tablets (500,000 units), one to be taken four times daily for at least two weeks to prevent autoinfection from the gut. The nystatin in these tablets is not absorbed and thus there is no systemic effect. However, the value of oral nystatin is doubtful as faecal recolonization soon occurs after it is stopped.[13,15] In the rare cases of male urethral candidosis, 3 per cent amphotericin (Fungilin) lotion may be instilled into the urethra over two weeks, but a simpler and equally effective technique is to give 1/8000 oxycyanide of mercury urethral irrigations for the same period of time.

Miconazole (Gyno-Daktarin and Monistat), clotrimazole (Canesten) and econazole (Ecostatin and Gyno-Pevaryl) are relatively new antifungal preparations which are claimed to be effective in shorter courses. Dosages recommended by the manufacturers are one pessary twice daily for seven days or one nightly for 14 days for miconazole, two nightly for three days or one nightly for six days for clotrimazole, and one nightly for three days for econazole. Some patients find these preparations more acceptable than nystatin which tends to stain clothing. Other local preparations on the market include candicidin (Candeptin), amphotericin (Fungilin), nata-mycin (Pimafucin), hydragraphen (Penotrane) and chlordantoin (Sporosta-cin). Several vaginal preparations can be used in the form of a cream which can be inserted with an applicator over a period of two weeks. If treatment fails, reinfection and autoreinfection should be excluded. The sex contacts should be examined and, if infected, treated concurrently. The regularity of administration of treatment should be checked. Retreatment regimens may employ a different antifungal preparation and some advocate longer courses of treatment although there is little evidence that they are more effective. Short courses of treatment after each menstrual period have proved effective in preventing symptomatic recurrences even though they did not affect the rate of recovery of yeasts in specimens taken just before the next period.[13]

If all else fails in the case of a female patient on a combined oral contra-ceptive she may have to be advised to use some other form of contraception in which case routine retreatment may then be successful. However, this should rarely be necessary; in two studies[16,17] there were no significant differences in results of treatment between those who were taking oral contraceptives and those who were not. Traditional forms of local applica-tion such as 1 per cent gentian violet are now rarely indicated. Gentian violet can sometimes cause a severe local reaction; if it is used at all the strength of the solution should be 0·5 per cent.

REFERENCES

1. WINNER, H. I. and HURLEY, R. (1964) *Candida Albicans*. London: J. & A. Churchill.
2. JENSEN, H. K., HANSEN, P. Å. and BLOM, J. (1970) *Acta obstet. gynec. scand.*, **49**, 293.
3. MORRIS, C. A. (1969) *J. clin. Path.*, **22**, 488.
4. ORIEL, J. D., PARTRIDGE, B. M., DENNY, M. K. and COLEMAN, J. C. (1972) *Br. med. J.*, **4**, 761.
5. A. R. med. Offr Dept Hlth (Lond.) (1977) p. 59. H.M.S.O., 1978.
6. RODIN, P. and KOLATOR, B. (1976) *Br. med. J.*, **1**, 1123.
7. DAVIDSON, F. (1977) *Br. J. vener. Dis.*, **53**, 121.
8. WILLMOTT, F. E. (1975) *Br. J. vener. Dis.*, **51**, 119.
9. CATTERALL, R. D. (1966) In: *Symposium on Candida Infections*, ed. H. I. Winner and R. Hurley, p. 113 et seq. Edinburgh: Livingstone.
10. DE SOUSA, H. M. and VAN UDEN, N. (1960) *Am. J. Obstet. Gynec.*, **80**, 1096.
11. HILTON, A. L. and WARNOCK, D. W. (1975) *Br. J. Obstet. Gynaec.*, **82**, 922.
12. MILES, M. R., OLSEN, C. and ROGERS, A. (1977) *J. Am. med. Ass.*, **238**, 1836.
13. DAVIDSON, F. and MOULD, R. F. (1978) *Br. J. vener. Dis.*, **54**, 176.
14. WARNOCK, D. W., SPELLER, D. C. E., MILNE, J. D., HILTON, A. L. and KERSHAW, P. I. (1979) *Br. J. vener. Dis.*, **55**, 357.
15. MILNE, J. D. and WARNOCK, D. W. (1979) *Br. J. vener. Dis.*, **55**, 362.
16. JUSTIN, R. G. (1973) *J. Am. med. Wom. Ass.*, **28**, 198.
17. PASQUALE, S. A., YULIANO, S. E., LAWSON, J., McLEOD, M. and McNELLIS, D. (1977) *Contraception*, **15**, 355.

25

Herpes Genitalis and Hepatitis B Infection

HERPES GENITALIS

This condition has become so common in venereological practice and is often so troublesome to patients that it requires special consideration.

The virus of herpes simplex (*Herpesvirus hominis*) may cause lesions on and in the mouth, on the face, cornea, perianal region, buttocks, genitalia (see Fig. 164, p. 351) and elsewhere on the body surface, in both sexes.

The virus isolated from the genital tract can be distinguished antigenically and biologically from that which affects other sites.[1,2] Hence it is classified as herpesvirus Type 2, as opposed to Type 1 which is ordinarily found in other areas, especially round the mouth. However, Smith et al.,[3] in Scotland, found Type 1 virus in 16·9 per cent of their cases of genital herpes and Nahmias et al.,[4] in the United States of America, in 8 per cent. In both surveys Type 1 strain was involved more commonly in females than in males. Experience indicates that the genital infection is sexually transmitted and there is other evidence which seems to confirm this view, namely that in developed countries Type 2 antibodies are not found in the blood of an individual before sexual activity begins. Moreover, women who are members of religious orders are virtually free from these antibodies which are found most often in promiscuous women. Isolation of the virus from female sexual partners of men with genital herpes is said to be over 10 times more frequent than from controls, and genital herpes occurs more often among women attending venereal disease clinics than among those who attend gynaecological departments.[5-7] However, there is some evidence that non-venereal transmission of Type 2 virus may occur in humid environments, particularly when children often sleep with older relatives and share clothing and towels. In a recent study in Nigeria[8] Type 2 antibody was present in 10·9 per cent of children aged 3 to 5 years with only a slight increase up to the age of 20 years.

In the year ending June 30, 1977[9], there were 4692 males and 2635 females attending the venereal diseases clinics of England who were diagnosed as having genital herpes, but the number with virological confirmation is unknown.

THE INCUBATION PERIOD is usually four to five days, but longer and shorter incubation periods are known.

Clinical Findings

Most cases of genital infection with Type 2 virus occur in persons with previous Type I infections. Genital infections in patients without such prior experience tend to be more severe, but in either instance the genital infection may be asymptomatic, particularly in cases of cervical involvement. The patient usually complains of some burning and itching at the sites of lesions, often beginning a few hours before they appear. In the first attack there may be malaise, fever and muscular pains. The lesions do not differ in appearance from those caused by Type 1 virus. They present as small grouped rounded vesicles on skin but a vesicular stage is not often observed on mucous membranes; each is surrounded by a narrow zone of bright red erythema. In men, the lesions may be found on the prepuce, glans penis and shaft of the penis and there is sometimes evidence of urethritis; anal lesions and proctitis may occur in homosexuals. In females, lesions may be found on the labia majora, the labia minora, the clitoris, the perineum, at the introitus and sometimes on the cervix uteri; less common sites are the perianal area, the thighs, the buttocks and the mons pubis. Occasionally the throat or a finger is affected by Type 2 virus. The vesicles soon break down, leaving multiple superficial erosions which may become infected by secondary organisms. The erosions may become confluent and then show a typical arciform outline. The inguinal lymphatic nodes may be slightly to moderately enlarged and tender. Sometimes there is more widespread tissue destruction and then the patient may suffer severe pain and tenderness of the area involved. This development is usually limited to first attacks. Infection of the cervix uteri may produce varied changes including diffuse inflammation, multiple small ulcers, a larger single ulcer and occasionally severe necrotic ulceration. On the other hand, there is evidence that a carrier state exists in women, and isolation of herpesvirus Type 2 from the cervix has most often been made in the absence of signs.[10] In a first attack the tissues are slow to heal and may take from two to four weeks or more. In later attacks healing is quicker but may take up to 10 days. Scarring is unusual but may occur when there has been secondary infection. Recurrences are common and may occur at long or short intervals over the years. The virus probably persists in sacral ganglia and has, in fact, been isolated from these.[11]

Dysuria is common, especially with primary infection in females. This may be due to lesions involving the urethra itself and the periurethral region or to urine coming into contact with other lesions. Sometimes the pain is so severe that retention of urine occurs. Retention of urine may also result from involvement of the sacral region of the spinal cord and it has been stated that anogenital herpes with sacral meningomyelitis and radiculitis is probably the commonest cause of acute retention of urine in young sexually active persons.[12] Intestinal obstruction, as well as retention of urine, complicating anorectal herpes in a homosexual has also been described.[13]

Diagnosis

The diagnosis may be confirmed by finding inclusion bodies in a smear of the contents of a vesicle, stained with Giemsa's stain, or, better still, by growing the virus in cell culture. Rodin et al.[14] have shown that Stuart's transport medium may be used satisfactorily for the preservation of specimens for culture when delay in transfer to a virus laboratory is unavoidable.

The presence of antibodies to herpesvirus Type 2 may be a useful pointer to the nature of a genital lesion, but the antibody response varies considerably in individuals and, except when seroconversion occurs, the presence of antibodies is no more than suggestive evidence.

DIFFERENTIAL DIAGNOSIS is from all other inflammatory lesions of the genitalia including, and especially, the early lesions of syphilis.

Complications

The most dangerous complications are those which affect newborn infants. Nahmias et al.[4,10] showed that the cervix uteri was the main source of neonatal infection with herpes and that the risk of infection of infants of mothers carrying the virus late in pregnancy was 60 per cent. They also showed that the risk is much reduced, although not eliminated, if the baby is delivered by Caesarean section before or within 4 hours of rupture of the membranes. Many of the affected infants died or had visceral infection with serious sequelae in some cases. Apart from infection late in pregnancy, infection early in pregnancy may be associated with abortion[15] and there have been occasional reports of an association with congenital malformations, particularly microencephaly.[16]

Hepatitis due to *Herpesvirus hominis* has been described as a rarity in adults[17] and meningitis, myelitis and encephalitis are known to occur. In adults herpetic meningitis is generally caused by the Type 2 virus[18] and encephalitis by Type 1.[4] These are usually, but not always, primary infections.

Sequelae

There is evidence suggesting the possibility of an association between infection with herpesvirus Type 2 and the later development of neoplasia of the cervix uteri. Most of the evidence is based on the finding of a higher prevalence of antibody to herpesvirus Type 2 among women with cervical dysplasia, carcinoma-in-situ and invasive cervical carcinoma than in control groups. This was the case in studies done in the United States of America and others in Belgium and Denmark, but not in studies in Taiwan, New Zealand and Colombia. The matter is reviewed by Rawls et al.,[19] who believed that the different results might be explained, in part, by the different types of tests used. Naib et al.[20] found cervical anaplasia in 23·7 per cent of 245 women with cytological evidence of genital herpes, as compared with 1·6 per cent in 245 women, matched for age and social background, in whom there was no evidence of such infection. Nahmias et al.[21] found that the rate of development of cervical dysplasia was greater than twofold and that of carcinoma-in-situ eightfold higher in a group of women with serological, cytological or virological evidence of Type 2 herpes infection, compared with a control group of women in whom Type 2 antibody could not be detected. Further evidence of an association has been the finding of fragments of DNA of herpes simplex virus in cervical cancer cells.[22] The evidence at present is insufficient to say that the association between genital herpes and cancer of the cervix is causal. Nevertheless, even if herpes is only a covariable of cervical cancer, women with known genital herpes should have regular cervical cytological tests.

There is, at present, no evidence of any association between carcinoma of the prostate and Type 2 herpes infection; in a recent study[23] there was no significant difference in the frequencies of occurrence of Type 2 antibody in patients with cancer of the prostate and in those with benign hypertrophy.

Treatment

Local applications to the lesions of herpes genitalis have given disappointing results. However, if the lesions are mild all that is necessary is simple hygiene by cleansing the area with normal saline. It was hoped that the antiviral agent, idoxuridine, would promote healing of the lesions. At first it was used as 0·5 per cent idoxuridine ointment but initial claims of success with this have not been confirmed.[24, 25] Idoxuridine is very insoluble in water but can be dissolved easily in dimethylsulphoxide. The latter substance also increases skin penetration. A 5 per cent solution of idoxuridine in 100 per cent dimethylsulphoxide is available commercially (Herpid) and is painted on the lesions four times daily for four days. Again results with this in the treatment of genital herpes have been variable and a recent double-blind trial comparing 40 per cent idoxuridine in dimethylsulphoxide with dimethylsulphoxide alone showed no benefit from idoxuridine (Morgan, quoted by Belsey and Adler[26]). Nevertheless, it is possible that idoxuridine in concentrations of 5 per cent or higher in dimethylsulphoxide may sometimes abort recurrences of herpes if applied as soon as the patient notices the itching sensation which commonly precedes the eruption. However, these preparations are very expensive and their use in this way would seldom be justified. They should not be used for pregnant women.

Local applications of the antiviral agents cytosine arabinoside[27] and adenine arabinoside[28] have both proved ineffective. Herpes simplex virus is sensitive to ether but the application of ether is painful and a recent double-blind trial[29] showed that it was of no benefit.

Certain heterocyclic dyes, such as neutral red and proflavine, can be bound irreversibly to herpesvirus and subsequent brief exposure to fluorescent light causes inactivation of the virus. Again initial trials employing such photodynamic inactivation showed promise, but later several carefully designed trials[25,30,31] did not demonstrate any benefit from this form of treatment.

Acycloguanosine is a new antiviral agent which is highly specific for the herpes group of viruses. It has given impressive results in animals[32] and a preliminary report from Moorfields Eye Hospital[33] showed it to be highly effective as a local application for dendritic corneal ulcers. As it has low toxicity, it is hoped that it will be safe for systemic administration, which will be necessary if persisting virus in nerve ganglia is to be eliminated and thus recurrences prevented.

Vaccines employing inactivated herpes simplex virus have been used for several years in some European countries in an attempt to reduce the frequency of recurrences. Lupidon H (Type 1 virus) and Lupidon G (Type 2 virus) are produced by Hermal-Chemie of Hamburg. Treatment consists of multiple injections over several months. It is notoriously difficult to assess the effect of any treatment in the prevention of recurrences which are naturally so variable, but there has been a recent double-blind trial[34] in which the vaccine gave significantly better results when compared with a placebo. Further controlled trials are needed before the treatment can be recommended, and there are also objections to its use because of the theoretical possibility of tumour enhancement by blocking antibodies. Another approach to the prevention of recurrence is the stimulation of cellular immunity by levamisole. There have been few controlled trials[35] and these have not been encouraging; the drug can also have serious toxic effects. At one time it was also claimed that vaccination with BCG could reduce the frequency of recurrences, but this was not confirmed in a recent trial.[36]

If there is considerable secondary infection patients might require a local antibiotic and occasionally a systemic antibiotic is required. In the latter case co-trimoxazole would be the most suitable choice because it would not mask syphilis. If there are painful lesions in or near the urethra or at the anus then the application of 1 or 2 per cent lignocaine gel prior to micturition or defaecation will give relief. Analgesics should also be given. Catheterization may be required in patients with retention of urine. Difficulties are most likely to occur in primary rather than recurrent attacks, but the psychological effects of frequent recurrences should not be ignored.

HEPATITIS B INFECTION

In 1973 there were reports from venereal diseases clinics in London that laboratory evidence of hepatitis B infection was ten times as common in patients attending these clinics as in blood donors.[37,38] The highest rates were found among homosexual men. In the same year there were also reports of a high proportion of homosexuals among men with acute hepatitis B infections admitted to two London hospitals; Vahrman[39] found that 20 out of 32 men with non-parenterally transmitted hepatitis B were homosexual and Heathcote and Sherlock[40] described the same finding in 15 out of 31. Subsequent work in the United States of America[41,42] and in London[43-45] has confirmed this strong association with homosexual practice. Only about a quarter of those affected give a history of jaundice. There is some correlation with duration of homosexual activity and the number of partners and those practising frequent anorectal intercourse seem to be at greater risk.[41,43] As might be expected those affected are also more likely to have had gonorrhoea or syphilis. The frequency of hepatitis B infection among female homosexuals is not increased.[41] Two studies of prostitutes did not show any significant increase of hepatitis B surface antigen (HB$_s$Ag),[46,47] but in one of these[46] anti-HB$_s$ was found more commonly than in a control group.

Those HB$_s$Ag carriers who also possess the e antigen (HB$_e$Ag) or the antibody to hepatitis B core antigen (anti-HB$_c$) are particularly likely to be infectious. HB$_s$Ag has been demonstrated in many of the body secretions including saliva, vaginal secretions, menstrual blood, semen, sweat, urine and faeces. However, the precise way that infection is transmitted between sexual partners is uncertain although there does seem to be some correlation with anorectal intercourse and this might partly explain the difference in the findings between homosexuals and prostitutes. Ellis et al.[45] found that 5 per cent of 2612 homosexual men were asymptomatic carriers of HB$_s$Ag and two-thirds of these had abnormal liver function tests. Over half of the latter had evidence of chronic active hepatitis or active cirrhosis in liver biopsies. There is also some evidence,[48] albeit circumstantial, that in some areas of New York City hepatitis non-B as well as hepatitis B may be more common in homosexuals.

As well as hepatitis B infection enteric infections, particularly protozoal infections with *Entamoeba histolytica* and *Giardia lamblia*, may be frequent in certain homosexual populations.[49]

REFERENCES

1. PARKER, J. D. J. and BANATVALA, J. E. (1967) *Br. J. vener. Dis.*, **43**, 212.
2. DOWDLE, W. R., NAHMIAS, A. J., HARWELL, R. W. and PAULS, F. P. (1967) *J. Immunol.*, **99**, 974.

3. SMITH, I. W., PEUTHERER, J. F. and ROBERTSON, D. H. H. (1973) Br. J. vener. Dis., 49, 385.
4. NAHMIAS, A. J., JOSEY, W. E., NAIB, Z. M. and VISINTINE, A. M. (1976) In: Sexually Transmitted Diseases, ed. R. D. Catterall and C. S. Nicol, p. 135. London: Academic Press.
5. NAHMIAS, A. J., DOWDLE, W. R., NAIB, Z. M., JOSEY, W. E., McLONE, D. and DOMESCIK, G. (1969) Br. J. vener. Dis., 45, 294.
6. RAWLS, W. E., TOMPKINS, W. A. F. and MELNICK, J. L. (1969) Am. J. Epidemiol., 89, 547.
7. RAWLS, W. E., GARDNER, H. L., FLANDERS, R. W., LOWRY, S. P., KAUFMAN, R. H. and MELNICK, J. L. (1971) Am. J. Obstet. Gynec., 110, 682.
8. SOGBETUN, A. O., MONTEFIORE, D. and ANONG, C. N. (1979) Br. J. vener. Dis., 55, 44.
9. A.R. med. Offr Dept Hlth (Lond.) (1977) p. 59. H.M.S.O., 1978.
10. NAHMIAS, A. J., JOSEY, W. E., NAIB, Z. M., FREEMAN, M. G., FERNANDEZ, R. J. and WHEELER, J. H. (1971) Am. J. Obstet. Gynec., 110, 825.
11. BARINGER, J. R. (1974) New Engl. J. Med., 291, 828.
12. OATES, J. K. and GREENHOUSE, P. R. D. H. (1978) Lancet, 1, 691.
13. GOLDMEIER, D., BATEMAN, J. R. M. and RODIN, P. (1975) Br. med. J., 2, 425.
14. RODIN, P., HARE, M. J., BARWELL, C. F. and WITHERS, M. J. (1971) Br. J. vener. Dis., 47, 198.
15. NAIB, Z. M., NAHMIAS, A. J., JOSEY, W. E. and WHEELER, J. H. (1970) Obstet. Gynec., 35, 260.
16. KOMOROUS, J. M., WHEELER, C. E., BRIGGAMAN, R. A. and CARO, I. (1977) Archs Derm., 113, 918.
17. Br. med. J. (1973). 1, 248.
18. SKÖLDENBERG, B., JEANSSON, S. and WOLONTIS, S. (1973) Br. med. J., 1, 611.
19. RAWLS, W. E., ADAM, E. and MELNICK, J. L. (1973) Cancer Res., 33, 1477.
20. NAIB, Z. M., NAHMIAS, A. J., JOSEY, W. E. and KRAMER, J. H. (1969) Cancer, 23, 940.
21. NAHMIAS, A. J., NAIB, Z. M., JOSEY, W. E., FRANKLIN, E. and JENKINS, R. (1973) Cancer Res., 33, 1491.
22. FRENKEL, N., ROIZMAN, B., CASSAI, E. and NAHMIAS, A. J. (1972) Proc. nat. Acad. Sci., U.S.A., 69, 3784.
23. HERBERT, J. T., BIRKHOFF, J. D., FEORINO, P. M. and CALDWELL, G. G. (1976) J. Urol., 116, 611.
24. NG, A. B. P., REAGAN, J. W. and YEN, S. S. C. (1970) Obstet. Gynec., 36, 645.
25. TAYLOR, P. K. and DOHERTY, N. R. (1975) Br. J. vener. Dis., 51, 125.
26. BELSEY, E. M. and ADLER, M. W. (1978) Br. J. vener. Dis., 54, 115.
27. MARKS, R. and KOUTTS, J. (1975) Med. J. Aust., 1, 479.
28. GOODMAN, E. L., LUBY, J. P. and JOHNSON, M. T. (1975) Antimicrob. Chemother., 8, 693.
29. COREY, L., REEVES, W. C., CHIANG, W. T., VONTŇER, L. A., REMINGTON, M., WINTER, C. and HOLMES, K. K. (1978) New Engl. J. Med., 299, 237.
30. ROOME, A. P. C. H., TINKLER, A. E., HILTON, A. L., MONTEFIORE, D. G. and WALLER, D. (1975) Br. J. vener. Dis., 51, 130.
31. MYERS, M. G., OXMAN, M. N., CLARK, J. E. and ARNDT, K. A. (1975) New Engl. J. Med., 293, 945.

32. Schaeffer, H. J., De Miranda, P., Elion, G. B., Bauer, J. D. and Collins, P. (1978) Nature, **272**, 583.

33. Jones, B. R., Fison, P. N., Cobo, L. M., Coster, D. J., Thompson, G. M. and Falcon, M. G. (1979) Lancet, **1**, 243.

34. Weitgasser, H. (1977) Z. Hautkr., **52**, 625.

35. Chang, T-W. and Fiumara, N. (1978) Antimicrob. Chemother., **13**, 809.

36. Bierman, S. M. (1976) Archs Derm., **112**, 1410.

37. Jeffries, D. J., James, W. H., Jefferiss, F. J. G., Macleod, K. G. and Willcox, R. R. (1973) Br. med. J., **2**, 455.

38. Fulford, K. W. M., Dane, D. S., Catterall, R. D., Woof, R. and Denning, J. V. (1973) Lancet, **1**, 1470.

39. Vahrman, J. (1973) Lancet, **2**, 157.

40. Heathcote, J. and Sherlock, S. (1973) Lancet, **1**, 1468.

41. Szmuness, W., Much, M. I., Prince, A. M., Hoofnagle, J. H., Cherubin, C. E., Harley, E. J. and Block, G. H. (1975) Ann. intern. Med., **83**, 489.

42. Dietzman, D. E., Harnisch, J. P., Ray, C. G., Alexander, E. R. and Holmes, K. K. (1977) J. Am. med. Ass., **238**, 2625.

43. Lim, K. S., Wong, V. T., Fulford, K. W. M., Catterall, R. D., Briggs, M. and Dane, D. S. (1977) Br. J. vener. Dis., **53**, 190.

44. Coleman, J. C., Waugh, M. and Dayton, R. (1977) Br. J. vener. Dis., **53**, 132.

45. Ellis, W. R., Coleman, J. C., Fluker, J. L., Keeling, P. W. N., Banatvala, J. E., Murray-Lyon, I. M., Evans, B. A., Bull, J., Simmons, P. D., Willcox, J. R. and Thompson, R. P. H. (1979) Lancet, **1**, 903.

46. Papaevangelou, G., Trichopoulos, D., Kremastinou, T. and Papoutsakis, G. (1974) Br. med. J., **2**, 256.

47. Adam, E., Hollinger, F. B., Melnick, J. L., Dueñas, A. and Rawls, W. E. (1974) J. infect. Dis., **129**, 317.

48. William, D. C., Felman, Y. M., Marr, J. S. and Shookhoff, H. B. (1977) N.Y. St. J. Med., **77**, 2050.

49. Keen, B. H., William, D. C. and Luminais, S. K. (1979) Br. J. vener. Dis., **55**, 375.

26

Yaws; Endemic Syphilis; Bejel; Pinta

Throughout the world there occur various diseases due to treponemata that are closely related to venereal syphilis, although not themselves transmitted sexually. The causative organisms are morphologically indistinguishable from *Treponema pallidum*, and the diseases give positive results to serological tests, both specific and non-specific, which are indistinguishable from those given by venereal syphilis. Members of this group of 'treponematoses' may be distinguished on clinical and epidemiological grounds, but there are similarities in the clinical manifestations and in the courses of the diseases.

Hudson[1] has maintained the view that all these conditions are really differing manifestations of the same infection, but most observers believe them to be separate clinical entities. In certain parts of the world syphilis occurs in some communities as a non-venereal, endemic disease; elsewhere, venereal syphilis, yaws and other treponematoses may be found in adjacent districts. Treponemal diseases are widespread in the Middle East, Africa, the Pacific area, and South America; in the past, owing to lack of economic and social development, efforts to control them were few and sporadic. Since the Second World War, the World Health Organization has introduced schemes for mass treatment with penicillin of the populations of some of these areas, in an attempt to eradicate the infections.

YAWS[2]

Yaws is a chronic, infectious disease occurring in the tropical belt and particularly related to tropical heat, considerable rainfall and humidity. It mainly affects rural peoples, especially the poor living in overcrowded conditions and lacking clothing and footwear. It is due to *Treponema pertenue*, which was discovered by Castellani in 1905, and is morphologically indistinguishable from *Treponema pallidum*. A study of *T. pertenue* with the electron microscope by Ovčinnikov and Delektorskij[3] showed minor structural differences between the two organisms but failed to establish reliable criteria for distinguishing them. It is not a venereal disease and is usually contracted in infancy or childhood through surface contact with infected children or adults. It is probable that flies and other insects also transfer infection. Entry of the organisms often occurs at sites of minor trauma, especially on the legs. The lesions of yaws may be divided into 'early' and 'late' lesions; those which are early develop, in general, within five years of infection.

Early Yaws

The Initial Lesion

The initial lesion develops at the point of entry of the organism after an incubation period of usually three to five weeks, with limits of two to eight weeks. It commences as a large, rounded papule, usually on a limb and most often on a leg (Fig. 146). It may also be found in the mouth of the suckling infant or on the breasts of nursing women. The lesion varies in diameter from 1 to 6 centimetres. It tends to ulcerate on the surface. Thus the first or initial yaw may be *papillomatous* or *ulceropapillomatous*. The lesion is relatively painless unless it becomes secondarily infected. Sometimes more than one lesion is present. If ulceration occurs the surface becomes crusted; if the crust is removed, a raspberry-like (framboesiform) granuloma is seen. If such a lesion occurs on the sole of the foot, it is often called a 'crab yaw'; this is because walking is painful and the patient is apt to move with a 'crab-like' gait. There is usually enlargement of the regional lymphatic nodes. If the condition remains untreated it may take weeks or months to heal and sometimes leaves considerable scarring. Serological tests become positive within the first few weeks of infection.

Secondary Lesions (Figs. 147–151)

Generalized eruptions appear on the skin from three to six or more weeks after the appearance of the initial lesion. The most characteristic lesion of this, the secondary stage of the disease, is the yaws *papilloma*, which is composed of hypertrophic papillae and is from 5 to 25 mm or more in diameter. The papillomata may be moist or dry. Constitutional symptoms are generally mild or absent.

Classification of Lesions

The eruptions of early yaws have been classified as follows:

1. *Erythematous macular rash* corresponds to the roseolar rash of syphilis. It is apt to be inconspicuous and transient and is particularly difficult to see on a pigmented skin.

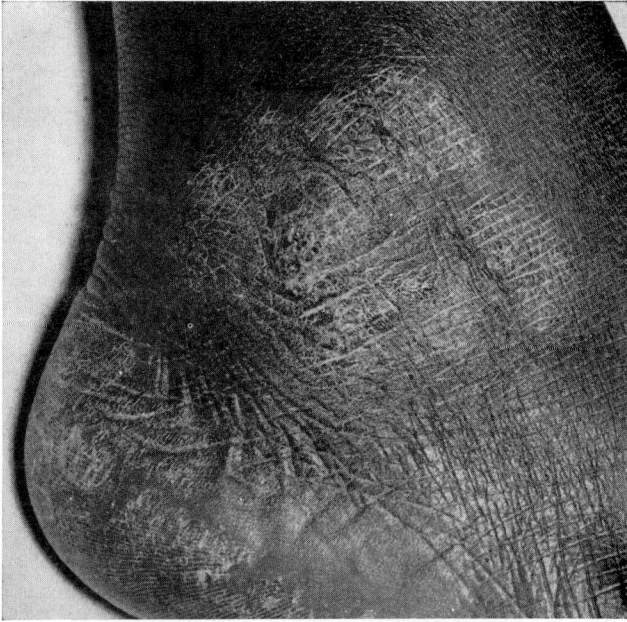

Fig. 146. Early yaws (occurring in the U.K.): initial lesion on the ankle.

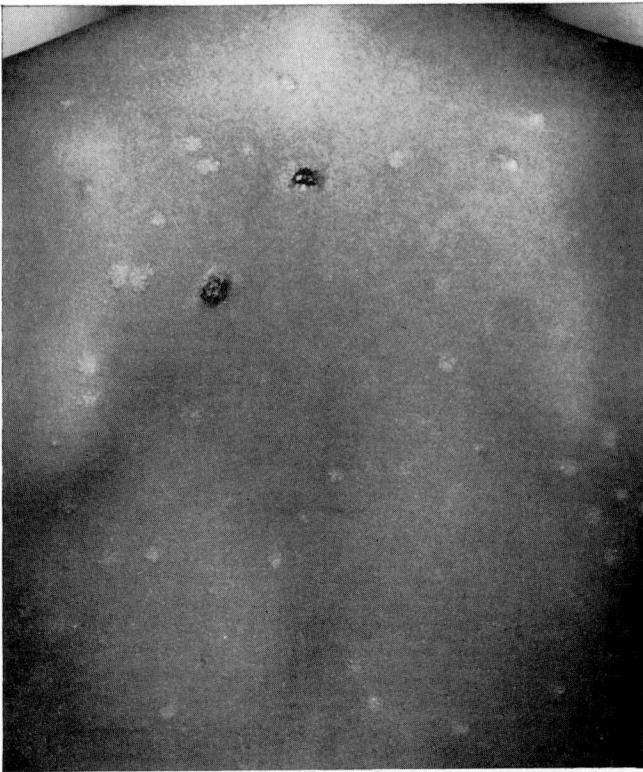

Fig. 147. Early yaws (occurring in the U.K.): secondary lesions on the body.

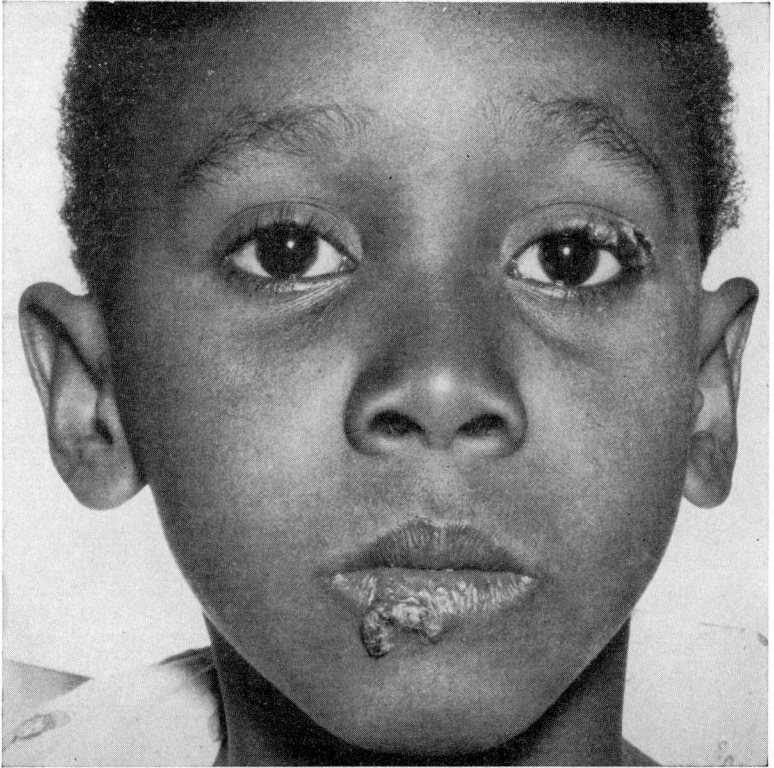

Fig. 148. Early yaws (occurring in the U.K.): secondary lesions on the face.

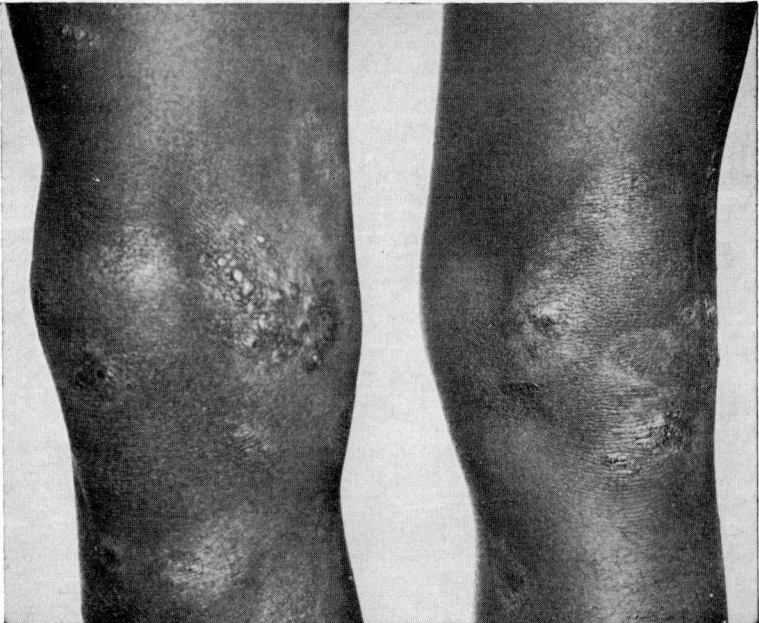

Fig. 149. Early yaws (occurring in the U.K.): secondary lesions on the knees.

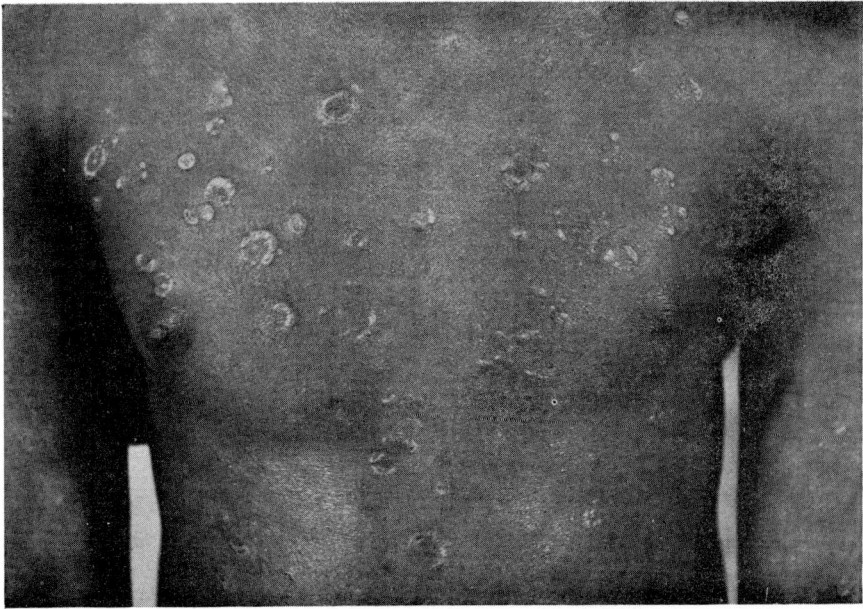

Fig. 150. Early yaws: secondary lesions.

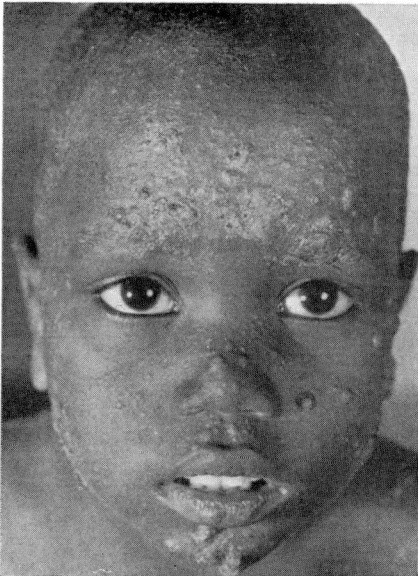

Fig. 151. Early yaws:
secondary lesions.

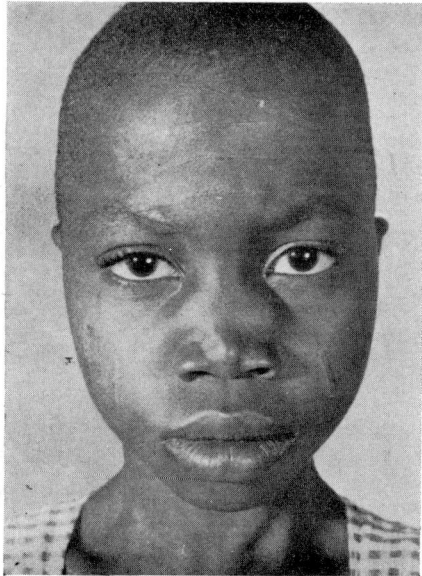

Fig. 152. Early yaws:
goundou.

2. *Squamous macular rash* presents with macules which are discoid, annular, crescentic or serpiginous in shape, and show fine desquamation on the surface.

3. *Squamous maculopapular eruption* is a later stage of the squamous macular eruption in which some of the macules are becoming papular.

4. *Simple papular eruption* is analogous to the papular rash of syphilis. The papules may or may not develop into papillomata.

5. *Umbilicate papular eruption* presents as hyperkeratotic papules with umbilication of the summits. They are usually found around knees and elbows. They do not develop into papillomata.

6. *Micropapular eruption.* In this, the papules are smaller and may be pointed, the so-called 'acuminate micropapular rash'. They do not usually develop into papillomata, although papillomata may also be present. In other cases the rash may be of the desquamating type, called squamous micropapular rash, in which the desquamation and abundance of lesions may produce a scurfy appearance.

7. *Plaque-like eruptions.* These are larger papular lesions which are fewer in number. They may be indurated, but heal without visible scarring.

8. *Nodular eruption.* This consists of rounded lesions deep in the skin and covered by unbroken epidermis. The nodules are found most frequently in front of the knees. They do not develop into papillomata.

9. *Papillomatous eruption.* These are the characteristic lesions of early yaws. They are large, hypertrophic and granular in appearance, and they may have wide distribution on the skin surface. In the moist regions of the body they can closely resemble the *condylomata lata* of secondary syphilis. They may be annular or serpiginous in outline with hyperpigmentation of the skin within the area of the lesion. Sometimes the lesions appear in clusters, called 'corymbiform papillomata'. Occasionally serpiginous erosion of the surfaces of the papillomata occurs, especially in children.

10. *Mucosal papillomata.* These are similar lesions which occasionally appear on mucous surfaces. They occur independently and not by extension from surrounding skin.

11. *Early lesions of the palms and soles* are of three varieties:

(a) *Palmar or plantar papillomata.* These are usually found towards the end of the early stage of the disease and they may be the only visible lesions.

(b) *Squamous macular palmar or plantar lesions.* These are erythematous macules which may be discoid, annular, crescentic or serpiginous in outline. They are superficial, well-defined and symmetrically distributed. They may closely resemble the palmar or plantar syphilide of secondary syphilis. As the name suggests, they show some scaling on the surface.

(c) *Hyperkeratotic macular palmar or plantar lesions.* These are macules lying deeply in the normally thick epidermis, which becomes parakeratotic and is shed irregularly to produce variously shaped craters. The lesions may be discrete or confluent. They are not preceded by papillomata.

12. *Other lesions of early yaws*. Bones may be affected and be painful and tender. Osteoperiostitis with focal destruction and new formation of bone from the periosteum affects chiefly the long bones. At this stage destruction is usually more evident than new bone formation but ulceration through the skin does not occur with the bone lesions of early yaws and the condition usually heals without sequelae. Hypertrophic osteoperiostitis of the nasal processes of the maxilla may give rise to a characteristic facial appearance called *goundou* (Fig. 152). This is common in Africa and also occurs in Haiti, Jamaica, and Venezuela. It does not occur in Brazil or in South-East Asia. It is not universally accepted as being caused by yaws. Polydactylitis, involving the phalanges of the fingers and sometimes the toes, is not uncommon in children. All the bones of the hands except the terminal phalanges and the carpus may be affected. The radiographs show spindle-shaped enlargement due to periostitis, and areas of osteoporosis in the bone substance. Sinus formation does not occur. There may be ganglion formation, especially about the wrists, generalized enlargement of lymphatic nodes and hydrarthrosis, especially of the knees.

During the first five years of the infection, there may be one or several relapses of cutaneous lesions of early yaws, or of lesions of mucous membranes or bones, separated by periods of latency of varying duration.

Late Yaws

(Figs. 153–155)

After five to ten years, or more, late lesions develop in some cases, although the condition remains latent in the majority.

Cutaneous Lesions

These are of four kinds:

(a) *Plaque-like lesions* are papulo-erythematous areas which sometimes show squamous changes. They are often found about the hands and feet, and may be associated with hyperkeratotic palmar or plantar lesions of late yaws.

(b) *Nodular late yaws*. The nodules may be cutaneous or subcutaneous. They may break down to form ulcerative nodular late yaws.

(c) *Ulcerative nodular late yaws*. The ulcers may be superficial or deep, the former giving rise to crusted, circinate ulcers which may be discoid or serpiginous. The coarsely granular floor of the ulcer is characteristic, and it may show healing in one place and extension in another. The deep lesions are very destructive and large areas of skin may be involved. The floor of such an ulcer is likely to be sloughing and irregular. The ulceration is very like that of the gummatous lesions of late syphilis. On healing there is much scarring, which may be of the 'tissue-paper' variety, but contractures are

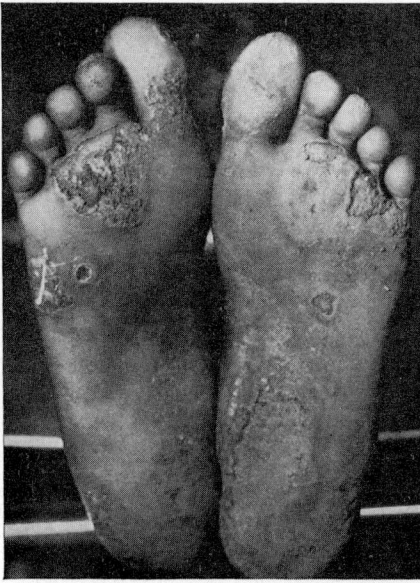

Fig. 153. Late yaws: plantar hyperkeratosis.

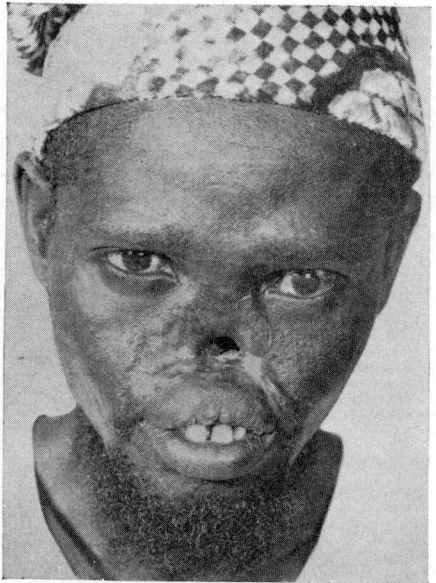

Fig. 154. Late yaws: gangosa.

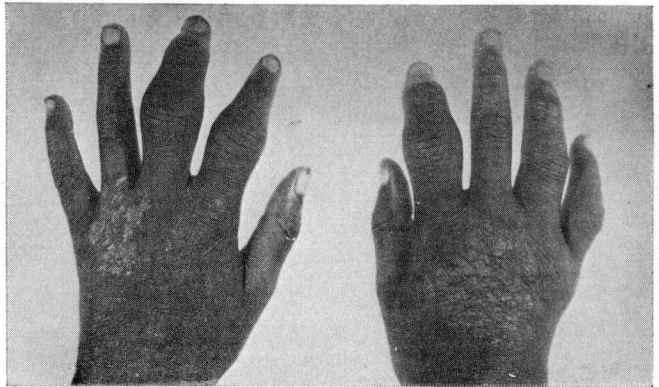

Fig. 155. Late yaws: dactylitis.

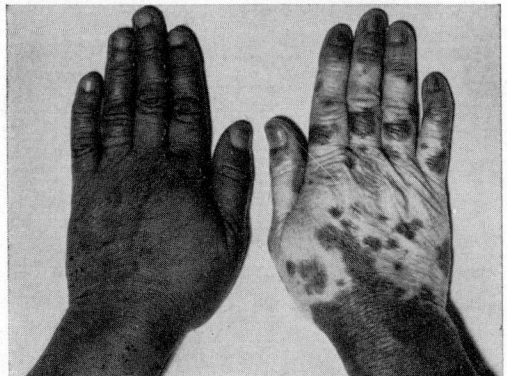

Fig. 156. Pinta: depigmentation of right hand.

not uncommon and there are likely to be pigmentary changes. On the face, destruction of the nose and palate may occur.

(d) *Hyperkeratotic palmar or plantar lesions of late yaws*. These are lesions with ill-defined margins of which the changes extend more deeply into the skin than those of early yaws. They are more polymorphic and less typical. They tend to leave scars or changed texture of the skin of the palms and soles, with loss of pigment on healing ('leucomelanoderma' or 'pintid yaws'). Ultimately, the skin may show atrophy and dyschromia, with contractures of the medial digits. The lesions usually start on the palms but may extend beyond them.

Other Lesions

Other late lesions include osteoperiostitis of bones in which the changes are indistinguishable from the gummatous lesions of bones of late syphilis, both clinically and radiologically. Ulceration may follow extension to the subcutaneous tissues and skin. There may be dactylitis (Fig. 155), involving the proximal phalanges of one or more fingers. Shortening of the digit may occur owing to partial destruction of a phalanx. Bones of the skull are not infrequently involved. Involvement of small joints may lead to deformities of fingers and toes, and of large joints to hydrarthrosis. Subcutaneous juxta-articular nodules, like those occasionally found in late syphilis, occur fairly frequently. Lesions may involve and destroy the palate, with extension to and destruction of the nasal septum and of the nasal bones, a condition called *gangosa* or *rhinopharyngitis mutilans* (Fig. 154). Bursitis, particularly round the knee, may occur and is usually bilateral.

Latency and Placental Transmissibility

Like late syphilis, late yaws may have long periods of latency.

The general experience has been that the disease is not transmitted from an infected pregnant woman to the fetus in utero even when she is suffering from early yaws, but there is some evidence that it may be transmitted in this way.[4]

Diagnosis[5]

The lesions are often highly characteristic. The diagnosis made on clinical grounds may be confirmed by finding the *T. pertenue* in the surface lesions of the early stages, and by positive serological tests in all but the very earliest stage. In Great Britain the distinction between latent yaws and latent syphilis, in immigrants from countries where yaws is endemic, is a considerable problem. In general, quantitative serological tests seem to be less strongly positive with latent yaws than with latent syphilis. Some patients are aware that they have suffered from yaws in childhood, and sometimes characteristic scars are present on the legs. X-rays may show evidence of old periostitis, which is more common in cases of yaws than of syphilis. In cases of doubt radiological examination to exclude aortitis and also tests of the cerebro-spinal fluid should be done. The presence of aortitis or involvement of the central nervous system is generally held to indicate that the patient is suffering from syphilis. It has been the general experience that yaws does not affect the cardiovascular or nervous systems, but patients who have suffered from yaws in the past may contract syphilis in later life. However, Lawton Smith et al.[6] in a cooperative study of 71 cases of late yaws in Venezuela, especially directed to neuro-ophthalmological investigation, found 'light-near dissociation' of the pupils, perivascular pigmentation, vascular sheathing in the optic fundi and moderate disc atrophy in several cases and attributed these findings to late yaws. In some cases there were abnormalities in the cerebrospinal fluid. Six had cell counts of 5 to 10 per ml and three of these had positive V.D.R.L. tests in the cerebrospinal fluid. Elevated levels of immunoglobulin G were found in 11 cases even though the total protein levels in the fluids were normal. In 2 cases trepo-nemata were found in the aqueous fluid and these organisms stained with the fluorescent antibody stain for *T. pallidum*.

Treatment

Penicillin is the drug of choice. Single doses of PAM, from 1·2 to 4·8 mega-units, have proved successful in campaigns organized by the World Health Organization against the disease. In Great Britain, where most cases of yaws are latent, it is customary to treat these patients as though they were suffer-ing from syphilis because of the difficulty of differential diagnosis (see Chapter 8).

ENDEMIC NON-VENEREAL SYPHILIS

In certain areas of the world, usually in primitive communities, syphilis is endemic and spread by non-venereal contact. Infection is generally trans-mitted from mouth to mouth, either directly or indirectly. The disease is common in infants and children and also in adults of infected families. Possibly because of the small inocula involved, primary lesions are not often seen, but they may occur in or around the mouth sometimes as the result of using communal drinking vessels. A previously uninfected mother may develop a chancre of the nipple from suckling an infected child. Because of the early age at which infection occurs, late manifestations are commonly seen in younger people. Congenital infection is rare because women of childbearing years have usually reached the late stages of the disease. Cardiovascular and neurological involvement are also said to be rare. The condition was widespread in the Bosnia-Herzegovina area of Jugoslavia after the Second World War. It was estimated that 120,000 people, amounting to 6 per cent of the population, were infected. As the result of mass campaigns by teams from the World Health Organization, commencing in 1949, there is good reason to suppose that this form of the disease has been eliminated in this area.[7] A further assessment in 1968[8] confirmed the conclusion that transmission of endemic syphilis had been completely interrupted. In most cases a single injection of 4·8 mega-units of PAM was given intramuscularly. The disease had also been described many years earlier in other parts of Europe, including Scotland where it was known as 'sibbens' and Ireland where it was known as 'button scurvy'.

BEJEL

This is probably a variety of non-venereal syphilis. It has been studied by Hudson[1] and Csonka.[9] It occurs among Bedouin Arabs in the Upper Euphrates Valley, and is also known elsewhere in the Middle East under the names of 'firzal' and 'loath'. Sixty per cent of the population are said to be infected before puberty, and those adults who escape infection in childhood may be infected by their children. A similar or identical disease has been described in Bechuanaland under the name of 'dichuchwa'. Overcrowding and unhygienic environment are factors in the spread of this infection.

Usually no primary lesion is seen. Lesions of the secondary type consist of generalized papular, annular papular, and papulo-squamous eruptions. Perianal and genital condylomata and mucous patches are common and are frequently seen without obvious rash. Generalized enlargement of lymphatic nodes is common. Patients often complain of hoarseness, due to laryngeal involvement, and nocturnal bone pains. X-ray examination may reveal localized periostitis. After a period of latency, there may be lesions of the tertiary type in subcutaneous tissue, skin and bones. The nasopharynx and larynx are often involved. Trauma and superinfection may predispose to the development of gummatous lesions. Depigmentation of the skin and hyperkeratosis of the palms and soles may also occur. Involvement of the nervous system, of the cardiovascular system or of other viscera is exceptional. There is very little evidence of transmission in utero.

Diagnosis

Diagnosis from syphilis is made on clinical grounds. The causative treponeme is indistinguishable from *T. pallidum* and serological tests for syphilis, both specific and non-specific, are positive.

Treatment

A single dose of 1·2 mega-units of PAM appears to be effective, but dosage may be doubled if bones are involved.

PINTA

This is a non-venereal treponemal disease which is endemic in Central and South America. One estimate puts the number of cases in that area as one million. Infection usually occurs in childhood, through skin contact. The cause is *Treponema carateum*, which is morphologically indistinguishable from *T. pallidum*. Serological tests are positive as in cases of syphilis.

Symptoms and Signs
(see Fig. 156, p. 340)

Although after experimental inoculation in man a primary lesion appears within 20 days, the incubation period of naturally acquired infections seems to last for several months. The initial lesion is commonly found on the legs, arms or face. It commences as a papule, but soon forms a circular, scaly patch termed a 'pintid'. The regional lymphatic nodes are often involved. After a further interval of several months a papular, annular papular, or papulosquamous rash appears on face and limbs. These lesions may last for years and be dark-ground positive throughout. Many years later lesions on the face, hands and feet produce first hyperpigmenation then atrophy and depigmentation which may cause psychological distress. Hyperkeratosis of the palms and soles and juxta-articular nodes has been reported, but aortic lesions and bone lesions are rare and nasopharyngeal ulceration is not seen. It is doubtful whether neurological involvement ever occurs and the disease is said not to be transmitted to the fetus. This is a relatively mild chronic disease and the prognosis is good.

Treatment

Penicillin is effective, especially in the early stages. Single doses of 1·2 mega-units of PAM have been used in mass campaigns with success.

REFERENCES

1. HUDSON, E. H. (1958) *Non-venereal Syphilis*, p. 189. Edinburgh: Livingstone.
2. HACKETT, C. J. (1957) *An International Nomenclature of Yaws Lesions*. Geneva: World Health Organization.
3. OVČINNIKOV, N. M. and DELEKTORSKIJ, V. V. (1970) *Br. J. vener. Dis.*, **46**, 349.
4. ENGELHARDT, H. K. (1959) *J. trop. Med. Hyg.*, **62**, 238.
5. HACKETT, C. J. and LOEWENTHAL, L. J. A. (1960) *Differential Diagnosis of Yaws Lesions*. Geneva: World Health Organization.
6. LAWTON SMITH, J., DAVID, N. J., INDGIN, S., ISRAEL, E. W., LEVINE, B. M., JUSTICE, J. Jr., McCRARY, J. A. III, MEDINA, R., PAEZ, P., SANTANA, E., SARKAR, M., SCHATZ, N. J., SPITZER, M. L., SPITZER, W. O. and WALTER, E. K. (1971) *Br. J. vener. Dis.*, **47**, 226.

7. GRIN, E. I. (1953) *Epidemiology and Control of Endemic Syphilis*. Geneva: *Wld Hlth Org. Monogr. Ser.*, No. 11.

8. GRIN, E. I. and GUTHE, T. (1973) *Br. J. vener. Dis.*, **49,** 1.

9. CSONKA, G. W. (1952) *Med. Ill. (Lond.)*, **6,** 401.

27

Other Lesions of the Genitalia

Patients present at venereal disease clinics with genital lesions of all kinds; many are not caused by venereal infection but, since they enter into the differential diagnosis, the venereologist must be familiar with them. For convenience of description the lesions may be divided into ulcerative and non-ulcerative lesions.

ULCERATIVE LESIONS

In preceding chapters, seven ulcerative manifestations of sexually transmitted infections have been considered:

1. The primary chancre of syphilis (p. 16).
2. Eroded papules or condylomata lata of secondary syphilis (p. 28).
3. Gummatous ulcers of tertiary syphilis (p. 47).
4. Chancroidal ulcers (p. 252).
5. Lymphogranuloma venereum: (a) primary lesion; (b) ulceration associated with elephantiasis of the genitals (pp. 258, 260).
6. Granuloma inguinale (p. 268).
7. Herpes genitalis (p. 325).

The following diseases must also be considered in differential diagnosis:

Malignant Neoplasms

AETIOLOGY. Carcinoma of the penis (see Fig. 157) very rarely occurs in circumcised persons; chronic or recurrent balanitis may occasionally play some part in its causation, particularly in the presence of a predisposing factor such as balanitis xerotica obliterans, a penile manifestation of lichen sclerosus et atrophicus (see p. 359). The erythroplasia of Queyrat and leucoplakia of the penis and vulva may also be pre-cancerous conditions.

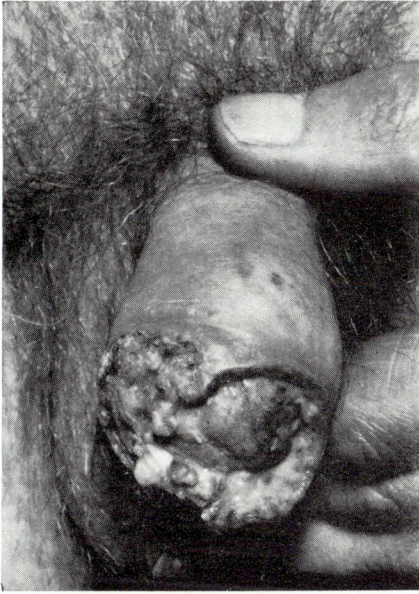

Fig. 157. Carcinoma of penis.

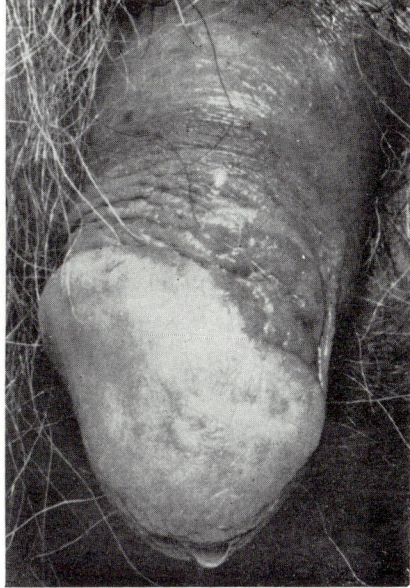

Fig. 158. Bowen's disease (intra-epidermal carcinoma) of penis.

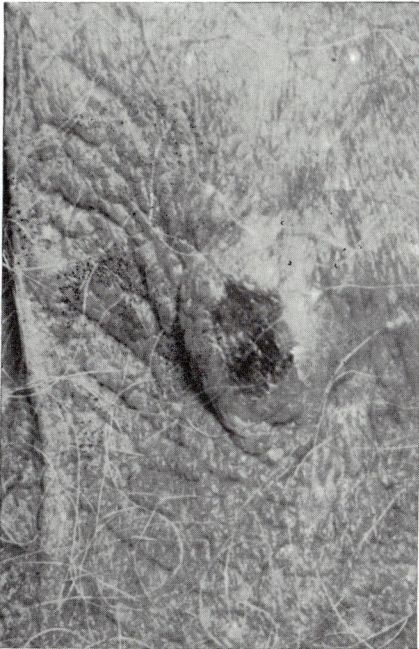

Fig. 159. Carcinoma of scrotum in a chimney sweep.

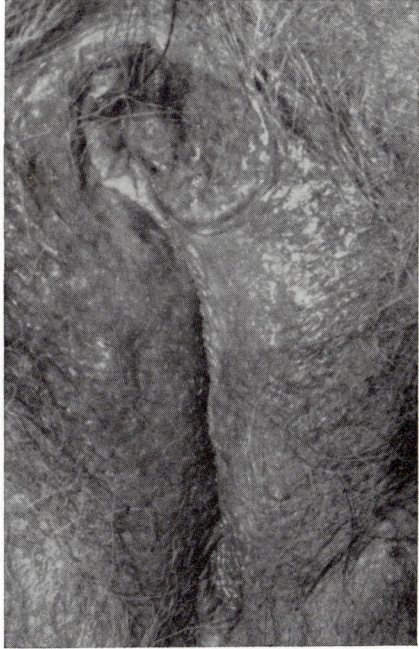

Fig. 160. Carcinoma of vulva developed on leucoplakia.

Bowen's disease (Fig. 158) and Paget's disease, both of which occur on the penis, are usually regarded as malignant neoplasms in themselves. Very rarely malignant transformation of genital warts may occur. The occupational hazard of the chimney sweep, epithelioma of the scrotum through constant irritation by soot, is now very rarely seen (Fig. 159). Basal-cell carcinoma (rodent ulcer) is rare on the genitalia.

Squamous-cell Carcinoma of the Penis

Patients are usually over 50 years of age, but the condition has been known to occur in the 20s. The malignant lesion usually develops under a tight prepuce. It is painless and starts as a small warty nodule or ulcer; it increases in size and may ulcerate through the prepuce as a fungating mass. A purulent or blood-stained subpreputial discharge may be the presenting symptom or a hard mass may be palpable below a phimotic prepuce. Some lesions are infiltrating and spread into the shaft and the glans penis; others soon ulcerate and present as infiltrative masses with ulcerating surfaces and raised, rolled, everted edges. The inguinal lymphatic nodes become involved in due course.

Squamous-cell Carcinoma of the Vulva

This is most likely to affect patients who have passed the menopause, but carcinoma of the clitoris has been reported in younger people. The condition often arises from a patch of leucoplakia, and is likely to be found on the inner surface of a labium majus (Fig. 160). The lesion starts as a nodule but soon breaks down to form an ulcer, with an infiltrated base; in other cases a papillary growth appears, which may resemble a vulval wart. Spread to the regional lymph nodes is likely to follow.

Early cases may be treated by radiotherapy. Otherwise these neoplastic conditions require surgical excision together with removal of the regional lymphatic nodes in most cases. Radiotherapy may be required after operation.

Balanitis and Vulvitis

AETIOLOGY. These conditions may be due to bacterial infection, for which anaerobic organisms may be responsible, or, more commonly, to non-specific treponemata or to Vincent's organisms. Sometimes *Trichomonas vaginalis* (see p. 312) or *Candida albicans* (see p. 321) may be the cause; in such cases there may or may not be associated urethritis. *Candida* infections are common in patients with diabetes mellitus and it is especially important to test the urine for sugar in any case of *Candida* balanitis, vulvitis, or vaginitis. Circinate balanitis may be found as a manifestation of hitherto undiagnosed Reiter's disease (see p. 299). Ulcerative lesions may also be seen with the Stevens–Johnson syndrome, fixed drug eruptions, contact dermatitis and erosive lichen planus. Lesions due to the bacillus of diphtheria are very rarely found on the male or female external genitalia. Balanitis is much more common in the uncircumcised when the prepuce is generally involved and the condition is properly called balanoposthitis. It is more likely to occur when there is phimosis so that the prepuce cannot be fully retracted and the area satisfactorily cleansed.

'Erosive Balanitis' (see Fig. 163)   *Borrelia vincenti (a spirochaete)*

This is an infection due to Vincent's organisms and it occurs only in patients with some degree of phimosis. Two to three days after sexual intercourse, a subpreputial discharge with some oedema of the prepuce is noticed by the patient. The discharge is purulent and foul-smelling. When the prepuce is retracted and the pus removed with a saline swab, the mucous surface of the prepuce and glans penis is seen to be reddened, with a number of small, round, superficial erosions over the surface. The erosions may fuse in the coronal sulcus forming an elongated lesion with serpiginous outline. The inguinal lymphatic nodes may be enlarged and tender. Destruction of tissue may be severe or extensive (phagedena or gangrenous balanitis), especially if drainage is not promptly established. The condition has to be distinguished from a severe primary herpetic infection and phagedenic chancroid. When the prepuce cannot be retracted the profuse discharge may resemble that due to gonorrhoea; smear and culture tests and examination of the urine after thorough subpreputial irrigation will clarify the issue.

TREATMENT. Saline washes or subpreputial irrigations at least twice daily are usually effective. Co-trimoxazole by mouth should be given in severe cases but treponemacidal drugs should be avoided. In the acute phase, dorsal slitting of the prepuce may be required, followed later by circumcision. Circumcision may also be indicated because of a tight prepuce or if balanitis is recurrent.

'Erosive Vulvitis'

This is less common, and care must be taken to differentiate it from herpes genitalis (see p. 326) and the acute vulval ulcers of Behçet's syndrome (see p. 350). The condition responds to local hygienic measures. If vaginitis is associated, treatment should be appropriate to the cause.

Herpes Zoster (Zona; Shingles)

AETIOLOGY. The virus, which is identical with that causing chicken-pox, attacks a posterior spinal nerve root, producing unilateral lesions of the skin in the distribution of the sensory supply of that root. Involvement of the third sacral root produces genital lesions. Most cases are due to re-activation of virus in later life after a childhood infection with chicken-pox.[1] The condition appears to be slightly commoner in men than in women (see Figs. 165 and 166).

CLINICAL FINDINGS. The first symptom may be burning pain in the skin of the area of involvement and there may be circumscribed patches of erythema. The patient complains of malaise, headache and mild fever. The typical large, grouped vesicles now appear over one side of the penis, scrotum, and a 'saddle area' of the buttock, which has the same sensory nerve supply. On the genitals, the vesicles soon break down and sero-sanguineous crusts may form on the surface of the lesions; or these crusts may separate, leaving shallow areas of ulceration. Secondary pyogenic infection may occur, with painful adenitis. The local pain may persist in the form of postherpetic neuralgia. The lesions heal in about two weeks, leaving scars which are anaesthetic to pin prick.

TREATMENT. Idoxuridine seems to be more successful in the treatment of herpes zoster than of herpes simplex infection. Good results have been obtained[2] in a double-blind trial of 5 per cent idoxuridine in 100 per cent dimethylsulphoxide applied four times daily for four days. Local antibiotics may be required for secondary infection and co-trimoxazole may be given by mouth, the dosage being two tablets twice daily for five days. If the vesicles are unruptured, local application of 2 per cent Ichthyol in collodion may give symptomatic relief. Calamine lotion may also be used.

Behçet's Syndrome

AETIOLOGY. This is a chronic, relapsing disease of unknown cause, giving rise to oral and genital ulceration often followed by inflammatory changes in the eye. It occurs most often in the Middle East and Japan, affects mainly young adults and is more common in males than in females. Sometimes several members of a family are involved. The main pathological changes are those of vasculitis with thrombosis and perivascular infiltration with round cells.

CLINICAL FEATURES. The earliest manifestation is usually oral ulceration but the patient may present with painful genital ulcers varying in diameter from a few millimetres to 1 cm. In males they occur most typically on the scrotum (see Fig. 161), but they may affect the penis; in females the lesions usually appear on the labia majora (see Fig. 162) but may occur on the vagina and cervix. The lesions may be destructive and scarring may follow. Some women suffer ulceration more often at the time of the menstrual period. The genital ulcers in the female have also been termed the 'acute vulval ulcers' of Lipschutz. In both sexes perianal and anal ulceration may occur. Painful ulceration of the aphthous type is seen in the mouth and may occur on the lips, tongue, cheeks or palate; deeper ulceration with subsequent scarring also occurs. A typical 'splash fibrosis' may be seen when the area is viewed under magnification. It is quite common to see patients with lesions restricted to the genitalia and mouth giving a history of recurrences dating back several years. It may be as much as 10 years before the eye lesions appear. The typical eye lesion is iritis with hypopyon

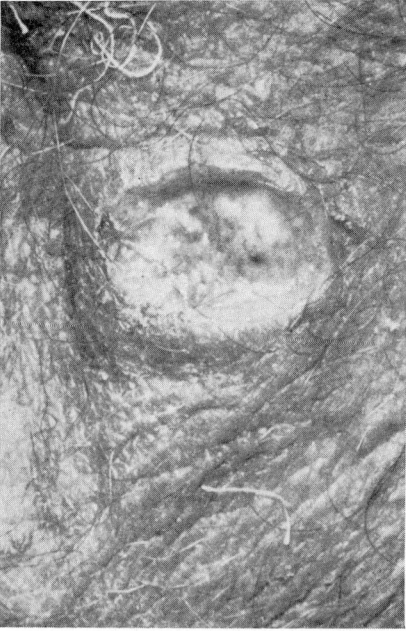

Fig. 161. Behçet's syndrome: scrotal ulceration.

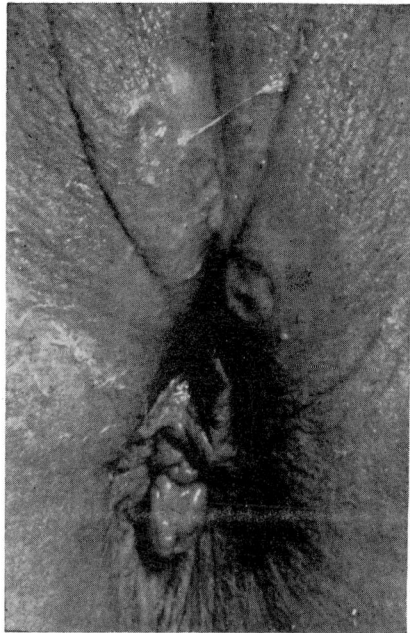

Fig. 162. Behçet's syndrome: vulval ulceration (acute vulval ulcers).

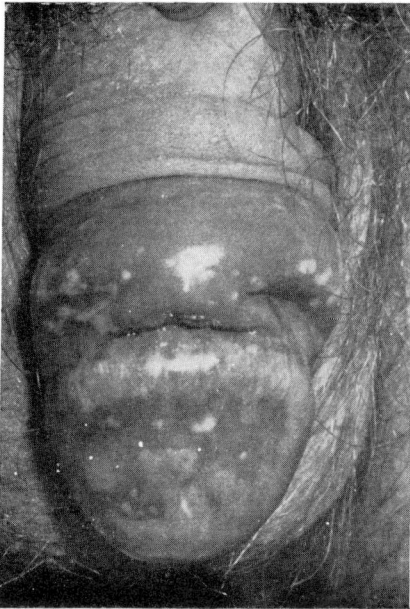

Fig. 163. Balanitis with erosion.

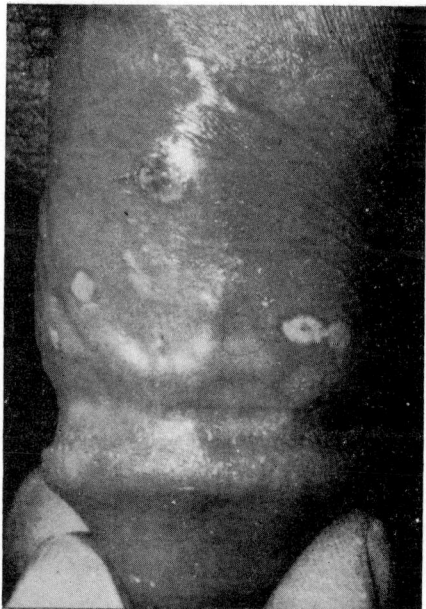

Fig. 164. Herpes genitalis.

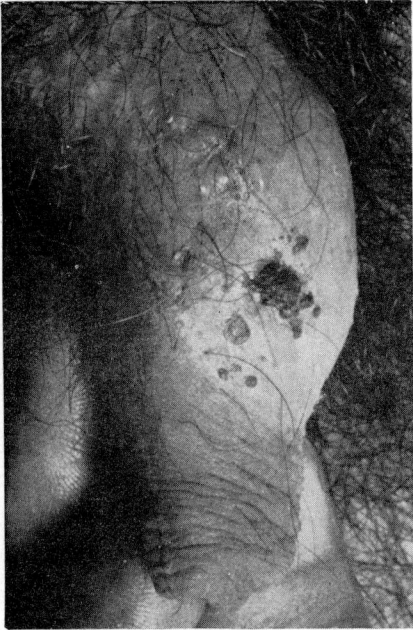

Fig. 165. Herpes zoster: penis, sacral 3 segment.

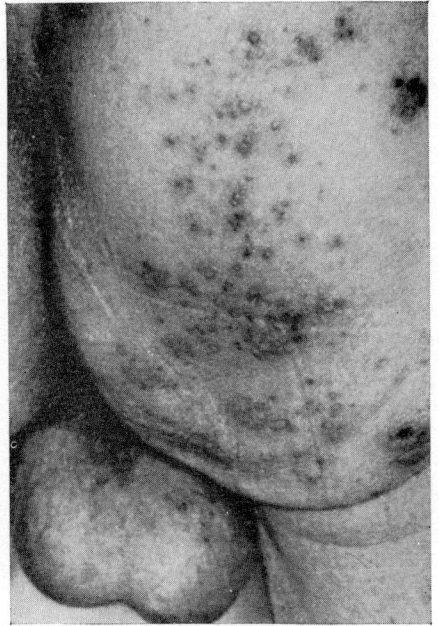

Fig. 166. Herpes zoster: buttock, sacral 3 segment.

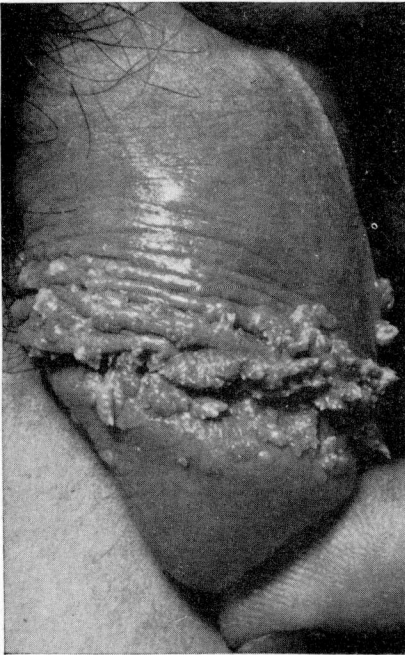

Fig. 167. Penile acuminate warts.

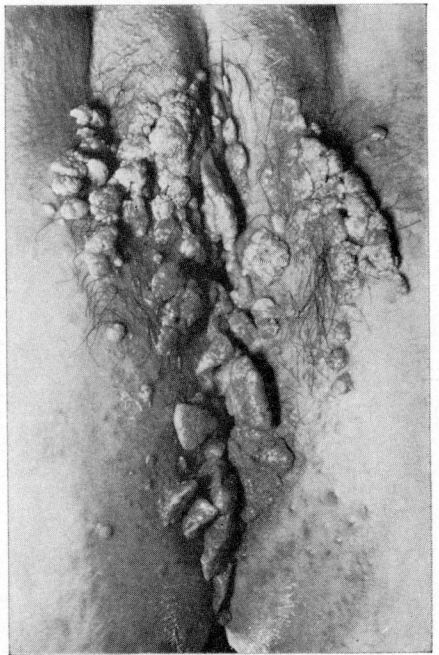

Fig. 168. Vulval acuminate warts.

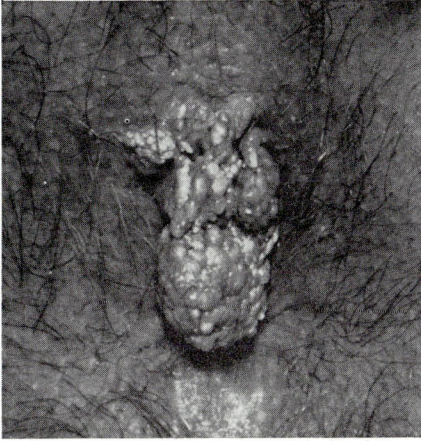

Fig. 169. Anal acuminate warts.

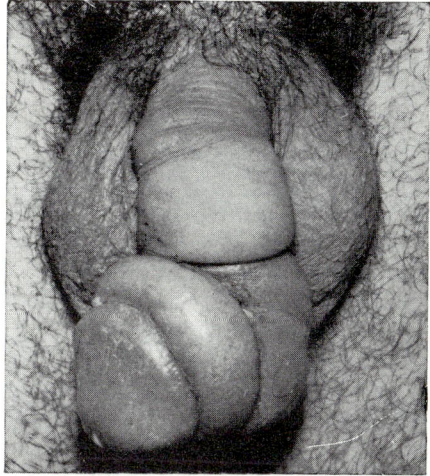

Fig. 170. Paraphimosis.

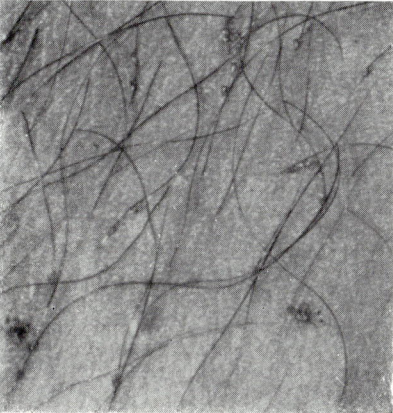

Fig. 171. Pediculi and nits in pubic region.

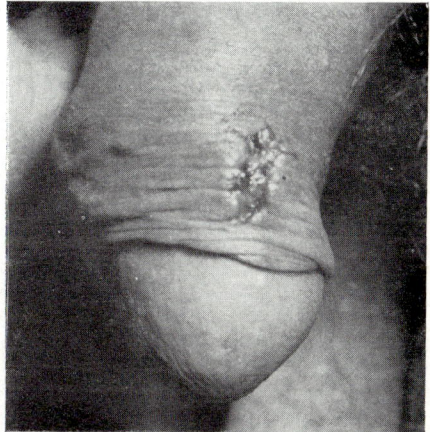

Fig. 172. Trauma to prepuce.

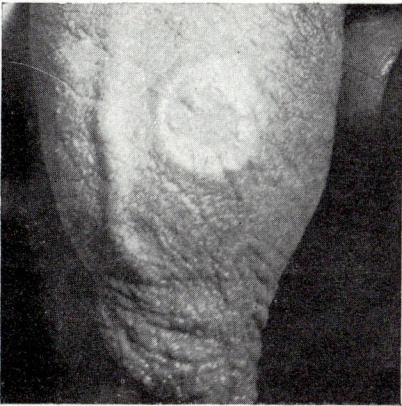

Fig. 173. Lichen planus, prepuce (annular type).

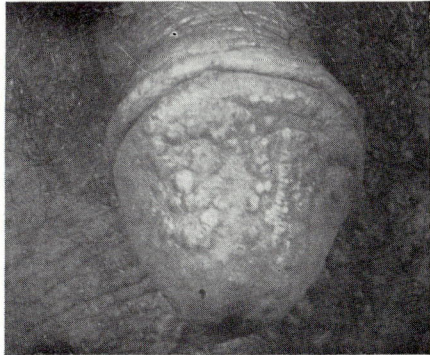

Fig. 174. Lichen planus, penis (papular type).

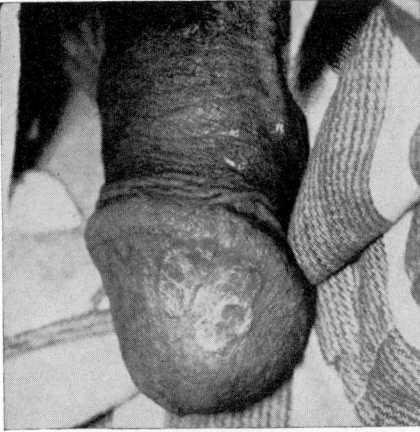
Fig. 175. Psoriasis, penis.

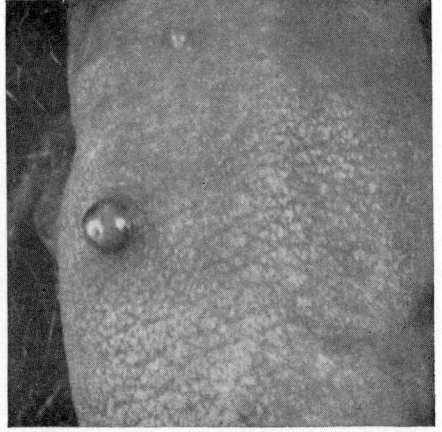
Fig. 176. Molluscum contagiosum, penis.

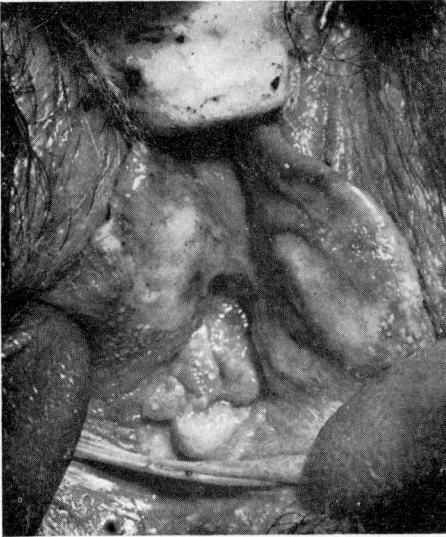
Fig. 177. Potassium permanganate ulcers of vulva.

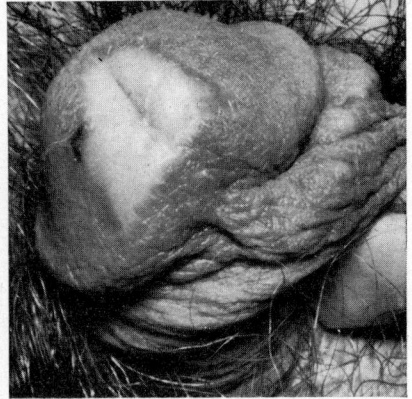
Fig. 178. Balanitis xerotica obliterans causing meatal stricture.

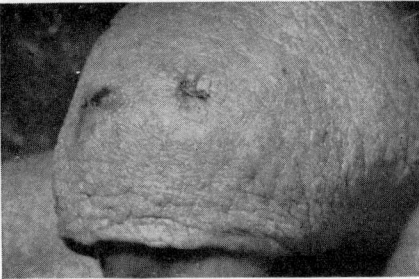
Fig. 179. Scabietic lesions of prepuce.

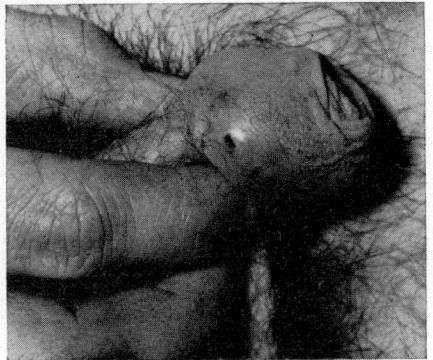
Fig. 180. Penile furuncle.

which frequently leads to blindness; conjunctivitis, scleritis, keratitis, retinitis and optic neuritis may also occur. Very occasionally lesions of the eye may precede other manifestations. Pustular lesions and lesions resembling erythema nodosum may occur on the skin; papules and pustules may develop after pricking with a sterile needle or injection with sterile saline. Arthritis and recurrent superficial or deep vein thrombosis occur fairly frequently. Intestinal ulceration, epididymitis, aortic aneurysm, aortic regurgitation and cerebral involvement have also been reported. In spite of remissions, the disease is likely to be progressive and may ultimately be fatal; however, in some cases it tends to become less troublesome in middle age.

TREATMENT. No specific treatment is known. Triamcinolone acetonide 0·1 per cent in Orabase may give relief when applied to oral and genital ulcers. Topical and, often, systemic corticosteroids are used for iritis. A systemic corticosteroid is used when the sight is threatened or when there are other serious manifestations. In such cases doses as high as 60 mg of prednisolone daily may be required at first. The dosage is gradually reduced, but relapse is common and it may be necessary to maintain a small daily dose of, say, 5 to 10 mg for a considerable period. Immunosuppressive treatment with azathioprine or chlorambucil has also been advocated and one of these is sometimes combined with a corticosteroid which can then be used in smaller dosage. Other drugs claimed to have therapeutic value are the immunostimulant levamisole (used after initial immunosuppression has controlled any activity) and penicillamine. Fibrinolytic agents have been advocated for patients who suffer venous thrombosis.

Scabies

AETIOLOGY. Infestation with Sarcoptes scabiei is generally the result of close bodily contact,[3] so that it is not surprising that transmission between adults often occurs during sexual contact. Other members of a family are likely to be affected, particularly when there is sharing of beds.

CLINICAL MANIFESTATIONS. In first attacks of scabies, itching does not occur for three to six weeks until the individual becomes sensitized to some product of the mite.

The patient may present with the classical features of the disease: irritation, chiefly at night, associated with the finding of typical burrows between the fingers, on the palms and wrists, the elbows, at the anterior axillary folds, the breasts in females, the genitals in males, and on the buttocks, umbilicus and feet. In some cases, however, lesions may be seen only on the genitals (see Fig. 179). In most cases only 1 to 10 adult female Sarcoptes, and therefore burrows, are present. Burrows on the genitals have a rather different appearance from the classical greyish sinuous scaly lesions on the hands and wrists. They are raised, slightly elongated, nodular lesions with the burrow tracks each seen as a thin, black, irregular line. Very often scratching by the patient removes the top of the burrow, leaving a small, shallow, longitudinal ulcer. The lesions are commonly seen on the prepuce, shaft of the penis, and scrotum; they may also occur on the glans penis. They are rarely seen on the female genitalia. By the time the patient presents there is often a generalized eruption on the trunk and limbs, but the head is not involved except in infants. The generalized eruption takes the form of excoriated papules and urticarial lesions and is thought to be produced both by the presence of immature mites in the hair follicles and by an allergic reaction to the contents of the burrow. Because of the scratching, secondary bacterial infection is common, resulting in impetigo, boils and loss of the typical appearance of the burrows. A certain diagnosis can be made, by demonstrating the mite in scrapings from a burrow mixed with potassium hydroxide on a slide and examined with the low power of the microscope; in practice, however, the diagnosis is often made on clinical grounds.

TREATMENT. Many treatments have been advocated for the condition but the following is a method conveniently used in clinical practice. Benzyl benzoate application (25 per cent benzyl benzoate with emulsifying wax and water) is applied with a brush or cotton wool to the whole of the skin surface from the neck downwards. It is allowed to dry, and the patient is advised not to take a bath and especially not to wash his hands. The treatment may be repeated on the following day and the patient allowed to take a bath and change the underclothes 24 hours later. Disinfection of clothing and bedding is unnecessary. Good results have also been obtained with local application of one per cent gamma benzene hexachloride as a cream (Lorexane) or lotion (Quellada) used in the same way, although one application is usually sufficient; most patients find this more acceptable and less irritating than benzyl benzoate. A single application of 0·5 per cent malathion solution (Prioderm, Derbac) may also be used but so far experience with this is limited. Whichever treatment is used, the patient should be warned that itching may persist for a week or two, otherwise he may continue to apply the remedy and produce an iatrogenic eczema, particularly if benzyl benzoate is used. The penile lesions may also take several weeks to resolve. It is important to examine and treat sexual contacts and also other members of the family.

Trauma

This may be physical or chemical.

Physical

Physical trauma of the genitals may happen during sexual intercourse. Often the only evidence of this is abrasion and bruising. In more severe cases there may be bleeding of the traumatized area, which the patient notices immediately after intercourse. In the male the prepuce (see Fig. 172) or its frenum may be injured. In a virgin female the hymen may be torn at the first intercourse. Traumatic lesions may become secondarily infected which may lead to persistent ulceration and painful enlargement of the lymphatic nodes. Self-inflicted genital trauma has been reported in mentally disturbed patients. Sometimes penile oedema without obvious external injury occurs after prolonged sexual intercourse,[4] especially if the partner has little vulval and vaginal lubrication. The condition is said to be more common in circumcised men and it should not be confused with para-phimosis or angioneurotic oedema.

TREATMENT. Most traumatic lesions of the genitals require only local hygienic measures to facilitate healing. If there is severe secondary infection co-trimoxazole by mouth may be given. Patients with self-inflicted injuries should be referred to a psychiatrist.

Chemical

Chemical trauma may result from the application of any irritating chemical substance to the genitals. This may have been applied by the patient as an ill-judged measure of prophylaxis, or by a psychotic patient or a malingerer with the purpose of inflicting damage. It may also be iatrogenic, particularly from podophyllin or trichloracetic acid used for treatment of warts. Chemical trauma may result in deep necrotic ulceration (see Fig. 177). In the past a method used by pregnant girls who wished to simulate mis-carriage, and thus persuade a gynaecologist to evacuate the uterus, was to insert tablets of potassium permanganate into the vagina. This preparation produces tissue necrosis and results in the formation of circular ulcers at points of contact. If the tablet has been placed high in the vaginal fornix the ulceration may involve a blood vessel and bleeding may be so severe that transfusion may be necessary. If the tablet slips down between the labia, it may be retained in situ by a vulval pad applied in anticipation of bleeding. It is then likely that the patient will present with two contact ulcers on the vulva, and these may be difficult to distinguish from contact primary chancres. Black debris of potassium permanganate may be seen at the vaginal introitus. Acute chemical urethritis sometimes results from strong antiseptics introduced into the urethra for the purpose of prophy-laxis. Severe and extensive stricture formation may follow.

TREATMENT. Once the cause of the chemical trauma has been assessed, no special treatment is necessary. Local saline washes and, if there is secondary infection, co-trimoxazole may be given and will not interfere with the diagnosis of syphilis.

Paraphimosis

This is a condition in which a phimotic prepuce has been retracted and cannot be replaced. The narrow opening of the prepuce acts as a con-stricting ring round the shaft of the penis, and the terminal part of the penis, especially the retracted prepuce, becomes grossly oedematous (see Fig. 170). If paraphimosis remains uncorrected for several days, linear ulceration develops along the constricting band. Paraphimosis gives rise to considerable pain and anxiety and requires prompt relief.

TREATMENT. Paraphimosis can usually be reduced by compressing the end of the penis with pads soaked in cold saline, and then pulling gently on the swollen prepuce with the fingers of both hands whilst pressing with both thumbs on the glans penis to bring the constricting ring over the corona glandis, thus relieving the constricting pressure. A general anaesthetic is sometimes needed, for it may be a very painful procedure. If reduction of the paraphimosis is not possible by this method, surgical division of the constricting band may be required. In most cases patients with severe phimosis should be advised to be circumcised to prevent recurrence.

Pyogenic Infection

Small furuncles resulting from staphylococcal infection of hair follicles may be found on the penis (see Fig. 180), the scrotum, the labia majora or the pubic region. The lesions discharge pus, which may be examined by smear and culture. When the pus has been evacuated from the lesion, a small, shallow ulcer remains, and there may be inguinal adenitis with local tenderness. The possibility of an underlying scabies or pediculosis should be considered. Occasionally a more widespread pus-coccal infection of the Bockhart type may affect the genitals and it might complicate hidroadenitis.

TREATMENT. Most cases require no treatment but co-trimoxazole may be given if indicated. Treponemacidal antibiotics should be avoided until the diagnosis of syphilis has been excluded. Attention to local hygiene may be required.

Tuberculosis

Tuberculosis of the external genitalia is generally regarded as a rarity. The decline in the incidence of other manifestations of tuberculosis in developed countries makes it now a very unlikely occurrence. The most likely manifestation is that of a discharging sinus from tuberculous epididymitis, which has not been recognized as such and has led to involvement of the overlying scrotal skin. Infection spreading from the bladder down the urethra has presented at the external meatus as irregular, spreading, painful ulcers on the glans penis; ulceration of the vulva has also been reported. It also appears from the literature that primary tuberculosis of the genitalia can be transmitted by sexual intercourse. Diagnosis depends on isolating the tubercle bacillus by smear and culture. There may be other lesions of tuberculosis elsewhere, especially in the lungs and kidneys.

TREATMENT is outside the scope of the venereologist. Admission to hospital at first together with long-term antituberculous drug therapy will be required.

Other Conditions

Other rare causes of genital ulceration have been reported including: (a) accidental vaccinia; (b) pemphigus vulgaris; (c) diphtheria (see pp. 288 and 348); (d) filariasis; (e) amoebiasis; (f) cutaneous leishmaniasis.

NON-ULCERATIVE LESIONS

In previous chapters, three non-ulcerative conditions due to venereal infection have been described as affecting the genitalia:

1. The very early stage of the primary chancre of syphilis (p. 16).
2. Papular and papulosquamous lesions in the secondary stage of syphilis (pp. 28 and 35).
3. Nodular gummatous lesions of the genitals in tertiary syphilis (p. 47).

As described in the preceding section, certain of the ulcerative conditions may be non-ulcerative at some stage in their course. The following additional non-ulcerative conditions must be considered in the differential diagnosis of lesions on the genitalia due to venereal infection:

Premalignant and Malignant Conditions

Balanitis Xerotica Obliterans

There is some controversy as to whether this is truly a premalignant condition, but there are several reports of cases in which carcinomatous change has apparently occurred.[5] It is believed to be a genital manifestation of *lichen sclerosus et atrophicus*. Most of the affected men are aged 20 to 40 years but it can occur earlier or later. It is usually non-ulcerative and commonly involves an area round the external urinary meatus, the glans penis, the skin of the terminal part of the prepuce but only very rarely the scrotum. There may be mild irritation. The skin becomes depigmented and atrophic, with some contracture of the tissues, so that meatal stricture or phimosis may occur (Fig. 178, p. 354). Sclerosis may extend for several centimetres up the urethra. There may be a urethral discharge, difficulty with micturition and even retention of urine. Beyond the margins of the atrophic areas, small petechiae and telangiectasiae are usually to be seen in the skin. In a few cases *lichen sclerosus et atrophicus* is found elsewhere on the skin. A similar condition may affect the vulva, perineum and sometimes anus in the female; irritation can be severe and narrowing of the vaginal introitus may follow, making intercourse difficult. The condition is most common at or after the menopause, but may occur at any age. These women have been shown to have a high frequency of auto-antibodies[6] but preliminary observations on men with *balanitis xerotica obliterans* seen at the London Hospital have not shown this finding. *Balanitis xerotica obliterans* is usually diagnosed on the clinical appearances, but biopsy shows a variable degree of hyperkeratosis, thinning of the epidermis, flattening of papillae, loss of elastic tissue, hyalinization of collagen and infiltration of the mid-cutis with lymphocytes.

TREATMENT. Local applications of hydrocortisone (one per cent cream) usually relieve irritation and the active inflammatory process in the earlier phases. Sclerosis may also be lessened in some cases, but it must be re-membered that more potent steroids may themselves lead to atrophy of skin and mucous membrane and they should only be used if hydrocortisone is unsuccessful. Meatal stenosis will require regular dilatation; in more serious cases lessening of the degree of stenosis has been reported following dilatation after infiltration of the tissue with hydrocortisone by injection.[7] Meatotomy is best avoided as stenosis may recur[7]; meatoplasty may be required but again there is a risk of recurrence of stenosis. Urethroplasty has proved successful in some cases of extensive urethral involvement.[8] Circumcision may be indicated when the prepuce is involved.

Erythroplasia of Queyrat

This usually involves the glans penis and coronal sulcus and occasionally the vulva. Men affected are nearly always uncircumcised. The appearance is that of a slightly raised bright-red moist area with a characteristically velvety surface; the lesion is soft and bleeds easily. It slowly increases in size but may then remain unaltered. The histological changes are those of intraepidermal carcinoma. Invasive change is indicated by induration, verrucosity or ulceration.

Bowen's Disease

This also is an intraepidermal carcinoma which may precede a squamous-cell growth (see Fig. 158, p. 347). The lesion appears as an elevated, irregular, reddish-brown, scaly plaque and may occur on the penis, vulva or in the perianal region, where it may persist unchanged for several years. It is sometimes associated with internal cancer.

Paget's Disease

Like Bowen's disease this may also affect the genitalia and is an intra-epidermal carcinoma. The lesion appears as a reddish scaly plaque with weeping and crusting resembling eczema.

Squamous-cell Carcinoma

Epitheliomata of the penis or scrotum may first appear in a non-ulcerative state as small nodules or plaques, or may have a wart-like appearance, but most of them ulcerate very quickly.

Balanitis and Vulvitis

The aetiology has already been discussed on p. 348 and many of these causes may also produce superficial or non-erosive changes. In the male this condition is often associated with some degree of phimosis; in both sexes there may be neglect of personal hygiene, with accumulation of secretions. Simple hygienic measures are usually sufficient treatment in such cases but circumcision may be indicated if there is phimosis or the balanitis recurs. Tight-fitting underwear which prevents evaporation, particularly nylon, should be avoided. Treatment of other cases depends on the underlying cause. Psychological factors should not be forgotten in patients with genital pruritus for which there is no apparent cause.

Plasma-cell Balanitis of Zoon

This is a rare form of chronic balanitis usually seen in the middle-aged or elderly. Moist shiny red patches resembling the erythroplasia of Queyrat occur on the glans or inner prepuce (Fig. 182). Sometimes there is a characteristic 'cayenne pepper' stippling due to haemosiderin. Biopsy is required for diagnosis and shows marked plasma-cell infiltration of the upper cutis. The condition may persist for years but is benign. There is no really satisfactory treatment but fluorinated corticosteroids sometimes help.

Herpes Simplex and Herpes Zoster

These may present for diagnosis in the early stages when the vesicles are intact.

Contact Dermatitis

Contact dermatitis may be the result of direct irritation from or sensitization to chemicals used in pessaries, deodorants and other applications, or to the material from which condoms or cervical caps are made. Dettol and other antiseptics added to bath water, 'bubble-baths' and scented soap are other causes. It may also follow the application of mercurial preparations (e.g. 'blue ointment') (see p. 362).

Pyogenic Infection

Unruptured pustules of folliculitis or of furunculosis may be seen.

Scabies

Scabies also may be seen in early stages before the lesions have been scratched.

Pediculosis Pubis

This is an infestation of the pubic and perianal hair with the pubic crab louse, usually, but not always, transmitted by sexual contact. From these areas the lice may spread to any other hairy parts of the body, even occasionally the eyebrows and eyelids but with the exception of the scalp. Typically the adult pubic louse clings to the adjacent hairs with its mouth parts buried in the skin where it feeds on blood. It is 1 to 2 mm in size and may appear as a bluish or brownish-grey dot or like a small blood crust. The female louse lays her eggs at the bases of hairs and each egg or nit has a chitinous envelope by which it is attached to a hair. As the hair grows the nit moves further away from the skin. It takes about a week for the egg to hatch, when the larva descends to the bottom of the hair where it matures after another week or so. The patient complains of itching of varying degree, and there may be evidence of scratching in the affected areas. Sometimes the patient notices tiny blood spots on the underwear. Pediculi and nits (see Fig. 171) can be seen with the naked eye but, in cases of doubt, a hair to which a suspected nit is attached should be removed and examined under the low power of the microscope, when the structure of the growing organism can be seen within its chitinous envelope.

TREATMENT. One per cent gamma benzene hexachloride may be applied in the form of a cream (Lorexane) or lotion (Quellada), rubbed with the fingers into the hair and the roots of the hair. One thorough application is usually sufficient, but with a heavy infestation the treatment may be repeated after an interval of three days, and, if necessary, on a third occasion. Good results are also obtained with a single application of 0·5 per cent malathion lotion (Prioderm, Derbac), which kills both adult lice and nits. Shaving of the hair is uncomfortable and unnecessary. In the past, mercurial ointment (ung. hydrarg. B.P., containing 30 per cent of mercury, 'blue ointment') was a popular application: if the patient uses it he may sustain severe contact dermatitis of the genitals and lower abdominal wall and only then may attend a clinic for advice.

Genital Warts (Condylomata Acuminata)

AETIOLOGY. Warts are caused by a virus and may occur on any part of the body surface. However, there is some evidence that the viruses of genital warts and common skin warts are antigenically and biologically different. Warts on moist surfaces, such as the genitalia, are less keratotic than those on dry surfaces; they are probably usually transmitted by sex contact, although auto-inoculation from the hands may sometimes occur. According to Oriel,[9] who studied a large number of cases of this condition, a very small number of patients with skin warts elsewhere than on the genitalia also had genital warts of distinctive appearance, resembling verruca vulgaris, and he thought it possible that transfer to the genitalia from other sites may have occurred. However, the frequency of warts elsewhere on the skin of patients with genital warts was no greater than in a control group without genital warts. He also found that 53 (60 per cent) of 88 people who had had sexual intercourse with individuals who were known to have had genital warts at the time subsequently developed genital warts. The incubation period ranged from three weeks to eight months, the average being 2·8 months. Warts in the genital area are common in both sexes (see Figs 167–169). In the year ending June 30, 1977, 14,648 males and 7737 females attending the venereal disease clinics in England were found to have genital warts. Many cases in women are also treated by gynaecologists. Perianal warts in males suggest the possibility of homo-sexual practices but are not proof of this; they are considerably more common than penile warts in homosexuals.[10] In the past, genital warts were termed 'gonorrhoeal' or 'venereal' warts. These terms are misleading and should not be used, although such patients quite often have associated venereal disease and should be examined and tested for this.

CLINICAL FEATURES. Warts are seen most often in young adults. They may occur on any part of the male or female genitalia, but are commoner on moist surfaces. In males they are often present in the subpreputial sac, but in general they are only slightly more common in uncircumcised compared with circumcised men.[9] They may also occur in the terminal urethra, usually near the meatus but occasionally more proximally. They are uncommon on the scrotum. In passive homosexuals they may be peri-anal in position, or may be found on the wall of the anal canal. However, subsequent spread to the perianal area from other sites occurs in about 10 per cent of heterosexual males suffering from this condition and perianal warts alone are sometimes found in men who deny homosexual activity.[10] In females they are commonly seen on the vulva, particularly the posterior part of the introitus, and may spread on to the perineum and perianal area in about 20 per cent of cases; they may also occur on the vaginal wall and on the vaginal portion of the cervix. In both sexes involvement of adjacent thigh or trunk is exceptional. The warts commence as minute swellings which rapidly grow into grouped, pedunculated, filiform lesions (hyper-plastic warts). A number of lesions may fuse into a cauliflower-like mass, appearing as a tumour, ranging from the size of a pea to that of a cricket ball. Extensive warts are more common in the uncircumcised and anal warts can become massive. The growth of warts is facilitated by sub-preputial or vaginal discharges due to *T. vaginalis* or non-specific spiro-chaetes, and also by sweating and faulty personal hygiene. Under these conditions the surfaces of the lesions may become macerated and mal-odorous. Warts tend to enlarge considerably during pregnancy, possibly due to depressed cellular immunity, but are quite likely to regress after delivery. Smaller, discrete sessile warts are sometimes seen on the shaft of the penis, somewhat resembling plane warts on the non-genital skin. They are more common in circumcised men in whom warts on the glans penis are rarer.[9] As already mentioned occasionally warts with the appearance of *verruca vulgaris* are seen on the shaft of the penis or the outer vulva or perineum. Warts are very occasionally seen in the mouth as the result of orogenital contact. It is possible that laryngeal papillomata in infants may be due to virus from genital warts in the mothers.[11]

Giant *condylomata acuminata* have been described on the penis which, although causing extensive destruction, are mostly histologically benign (Buschke–Loewenstein tumour). They are seen rarely on the vulva and in the anorectal region. True malignant change in giant condylomata has been described and, very rarely, malignant transformation of ordinary genital and anal warts. The matter is reviewed by Oriel.[12]

TREATMENT. It is essential to treat any predisposing cause, such as urethritis, balanitis, proctitis or vaginitis and to keep the area clean. The warts themselves, if not too large, may be treated by the application of 10 to 25 per cent podophyllin in spirit or tincture of benzoin. Podophyllin, which is a cytotoxic agent, irritates skin and mucous membrane and may produce chemical burns, so it is important to apply it accurately to the lesions; it should be allowed to dry and then the area lightly dusted with talc. Some patients react excessively to podophyllin and it is a wise precaution to begin treatment with an application of the 10 per cent strength to a small trial area. It should be washed off after four hours, but if there is no reaction this interval may be extended to 24 hours with successive applications. Patients should never be permitted to treat themselves with this remedy. Several applications of podophyllin at twice-weekly intervals may be necessary. Hyperkeratotic warts and intrameatal warts do not respond well to podophyllin. Concentrated trichloracetic acid, locally applied with a pointed orange stick, is a very effective remedy but requires great care in its use and is not suitable for large warts. If the warts recur, or if the warty mass is very large, electrocautery or diathermy under local or general anaesthesia may be necessary. Cryosurgery may also be used[13] and does not generally require any anaesthesia. Thomson and Grace[14] have described a technique for the scissors excision of large perianal warts which has given excellent results without scarring. They carried out the procedure under general anaesthesia but Russell[15] found that local anaesthesia is adequate in most cases.

In recent years the antimetabolite 5-fluorouracil has been claimed by some to give good results when applied as a 5 per cent 5-fluorouracil cream for a period of 2 to 4 weeks. With further experience results have been variable and the optimum frequency of application is uncertain, although twice-daily application seems to be more effective than once-daily.[16, 17] However, irritation and painful ulceration may be troublesome even after use once daily.[17] Van Krogh[16] obtained good results in the treatment of intrameatal warts and Dretler and Klein[18] also found it to be successful for more proximal urethral warts. Care must be taken to avoid contact of the cream with other mucous or skin surfaces and the eyes.

Autogenous vaccines have been used and excellent results have been reported by Powell[19] who treated 35 patients by this method. Nel and

Fourie[20] used a similar method and observed regression in 7 of 10 women. The place of vaccines in therapy is undecided but caution is advised before the systemic administration of a virus with possible oncogenic potential.

Even large warts occurring during pregnancy do not usually obstruct delivery. As already stated, they are quite likely to regress after delivery. If treatment is given during pregnancy it should be very conservative; Ghosh[13] recommends cryosurgery. Certainly podophyllin or 5-fluorouracil should not be used. A report[21] of severe peripheral neuropathy, followed by stillbirth, after treatment with podophyllin adds point to this warning, although a large quantity (7·5 ml of 25 per cent solution) was used. Severe toxic effects have also been reported in non-pregnant women and in men; podophyllin should never be applied to extensive areas of warts, particularly when they are congested, haemorrhagic or friable.

Sexual contacts should be examined.

Molluscum Contagiosum

This condition is caused by a virus, and lesions may occur on any part of the body surface. When lesions occur on the genitals, transmission has usually resulted from sex contact, and similar lesions may be found in the sexual partner. The incubation period is from three weeks to several months. In males lesions are seen on the penis (see Fig. 176) and scrotum, and in the female on the vulva; in both sexes lesions may also be seen on the thighs. The lesions vary in size from 2 mm to 1 cm. They may occur in groups or present individually, and are seen as wax-like pinkish-white papules, each with a central depression, which is filled with a white plug. When expressed, this material can be spread on a slide and stained with Giemsa's stain, when large, swollen 'balloon' cells can be seen to contain virus-inclusion bodies. Lesions may become secondarily infected to form pustules.

TREATMENT. Lesions may resolve if they are opened and the contents expressed. They may also be destroyed by applying pure phenol or concentrated trichloracetic acid on the point of a sharp orange stick. The papule will turn white and a crust form before healing occurs. The electro-cautery may also be used.

Lichen Planus

The cause of this eruption is unknown, but psychogenic factors are said to be contributory. It has nothing to do with venereal infection but sometimes appears on the genitalia in men and occasionally on the vulva or anal region in women. Lesions occurring on the prepuce, glans penis, or scrotum are either papular (see Fig. 174) or annular (see Fig. 173). The papules are small, shiny, flat-topped polygonal lesions of a violet colour sometimes with white striae (Wickham's striae); the annular lesions are of similar colour. In the moist subpreputial area the lesions may be white. The patient usually complains of itching. The eruption may also affect the legs, forearms or wrists. Quite often the diagnosis may be confirmed by the presence of typical silvery lesions on the mucous membrane of the inner surface of the cheeks and sometimes on the tongue.

TREATMENT. There is no specific treatment; local corticosteroid preparations may relieve the itching and sometimes accelerate healing, but the lesions tend to disappear without treatment after several months.

Psoriasis

This is another dermatological condition of obscure cause, in which the initial lesions may appear on the genitalia. They may be found on the penis (see Fig. 175) or scrotum in the male, on the vulva in the female, and also in the pubic region in the groin and on the perineum in both sexes. Lesions may be of the acute papular type, or more commonly they appear as plaques; these are dull red or purplish red in colour, covered with silvery scales, but on moist surfaces the scales may be absent and the surfaces red and shiny. Subpreputially the lesions may closely resemble circinate balanitis of Reiter's disease. Lesions may also be present on the knees, elbows, sacrum, along the hair margin or on the scalp, but sometimes the only confirmatory evidence is pitting and irregularity of the nails, due to involvement of the nail beds in past attacks. In about 5 per cent of cases the patients develop polyarthritis ('arthropathic psoriasis'). It is of interest that the microscopical appearances of psoriasis are very similar to those of keratoderma blennorrhagica (see p. 297).

TREATMENT. There is no specific therapy. Many forms of treatment have been tried with varying success. The management of these cases should be in the hands of dermatologists.

Seborrhoeic Dermatitis

The genitalia and perineum of either sex may be involved. The condition is usually generalized, and associated with pityriasis capitis (dandruff) and involvement of the ears and eyelids; the presternal and interscapular areas are often affected. Flexures such as the groins and intergluteal cleft are commonly involved. On the penis, the lesions are red and scaly, with a rather indefinite edge. Sometimes they may be very extensive.

TREATMENT. In the acute stage, lotions such as 1 per cent hydrocortisone may be used. In the more chronic stage, 1 per cent sulphur and salicylic acid ointment in an emulsion base may be applied to all areas involved, including the scalp. The latter should also be shampooed regularly with cetrimide or selenium sulphide.

Tinea Cruris

This is more common in males than females. Irritating lesions develop in the flexures of the groins; they tend to heal centrally and spread at the

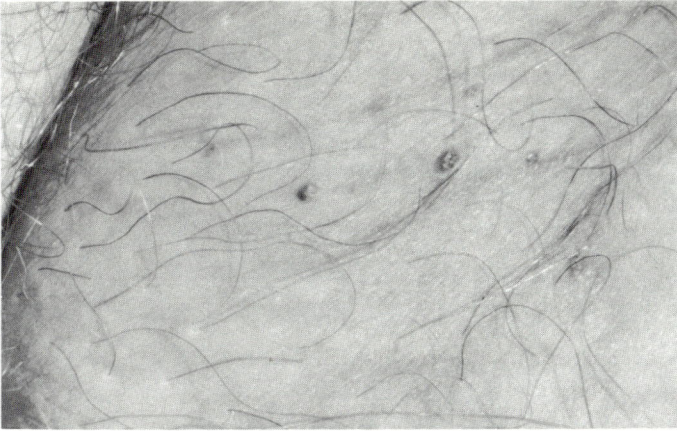

Fig. 181. Angiokeratoma of the scrotum.

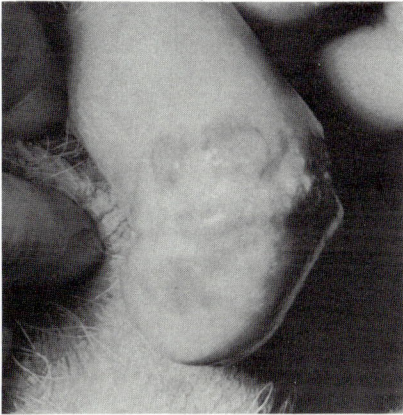

Fig. 182. Balanitis of Zoon.

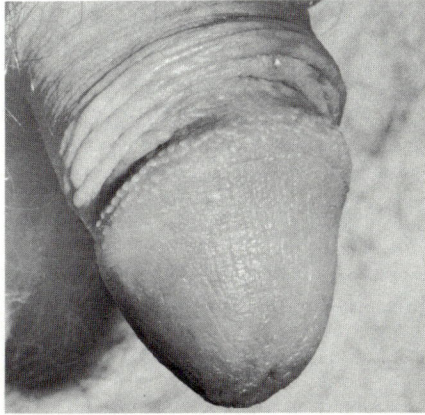

Fig. 183. Coronal papillae.

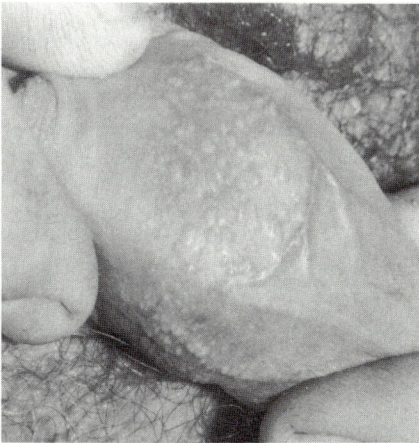

Fig. 184. Fordyce spots.

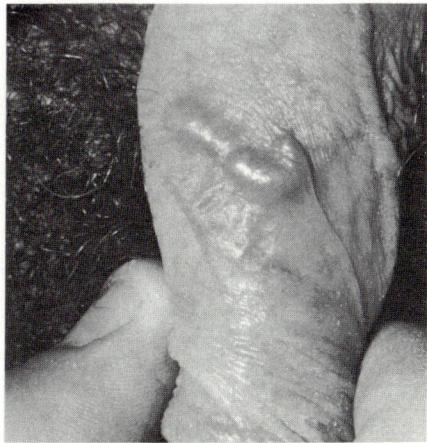

Fig. 185. Lymphocele.

periphery. The lesions are scaly and at the spreading edge vesicles or pustules may be seen. A scrape on a slide dissolved in liquor potassae shows the typical strands of mycelium of *Epidermophyton* or *Trichophyton*. The feet should be examined as tinea pedis may be associated.

TREATMENT. The lesions heal rapidly when a suitable fungicidal ointment is applied. Occasionally oral treatment with griseofulvin is also required. Tight-fitting undergarments should not be used.

Benign Tumours

Non-malignant tumours are occasionally seen on the genitalia; there may or may not be similar tumours on other parts of the body surface. They include fibromata, lipomata, haemangiomata, follicular cysts, and pigmented naevi.

Fibromata appear as firm painless lumps, which may become pedunculated. They may be seen on the scrotum or labium majus. If the lump is sensitive to pressure or if typical 'café au lait' lesions are present elsewhere, it may be a neurofibroma.

Lipomata are soft, slowly growing, painless lumps, which occur very occasionally in the subcutaneous tissue of the scrotum or vulva. They may be semifluctuant but have a definite edge.

Haemangiomata of all types occur on the penis, scrotum or vulva and may extend into the vagina or rectum. Angiokeratoma of the scrotum is the commonest of these lesions (see Fig. 181, p. 367).

Follicular cysts are retention cysts of sebaceous glands which appear usually in the scrotal skin. They form small, rounded swellings containing yellow material, which may be gritty due to calcification.

Pigmented naevi (moles) are brown or black, circumscribed lesions which are quite often seen on the skin of the genital region.

Biopsy may sometimes be needed to confirm the exact diagnosis of benign genital tumours.

TREATMENT. In certain cases excision or other methods of destruction may be indicated.

Peyronie's Disease (Induratio Penis Plastica)

This disease is of unknown cause and takes the form of fibrous infiltration of the septum between the corpora cavernosa of the penis, generally following an inflammatory process in the areolar connective tissue between the tunica albuginea and the corpora cavernosa. It occurs most commonly in middle-aged men. The fibrosis may extend into the tunica albuginea and corpora cavernosa on either side of the septum, giving rise to a firm plaque of varying extent; calcification and even ossification may occur. On erection the penis may be bent, usually dorsally but sometimes laterally or downwards, and coitus may be difficult or impossible. There may be considerable local pain, especially on erection, and the affected area may be tender at first. Dupuytren's contracture is also present in about 10 per cent of cases. Recently[22] an association between beta-adrenergic blocking agents, used for treating hypertension and ischaemic heart disease, and Peyronie's disease has been described. Smith[23] has found evidence of subclinical Peyronie's disease at autopsy in 23 out of 100 males aged between 17 and 78 years.

TREATMENT. According to Byström et al.,[24] in the absence of treatment spontaneous improvement is likely to occur in 50 per cent of cases and complete cure in 20 to 30 per cent. Thus claims made for the efficacy of any treatment must take this into account. Various treatments have been recommended, including excision of plaques, irradiation, ultrasound, vitamin E by mouth, injections of hydrocortisone, and potassium para-aminobenzoate (Potaba). Very often the results are difficult to assess because of the small numbers of patients treated. However, in selected cases partial removal of a well-defined fibrotic plaque, in patients with residual deformity preventing sexual intercourse, may correct the curvature sufficiently for successful intercourse to take place.[25]

MINOR ANOMALIES

Patients who are worried about the possibility of venereal infection may closely inspect the genitalia and notice for the first time certain conditions of no clinical significance and for which they require only reassurance.

Papillae of the Coronal Sulcus or Glans Penis (Hirsutes Papillaris Penis)

These tiny swellings, which are congenital anomalies, look like very early acuminate warts, and may be arranged in rows round the coronal sulcus or be scattered over the glans penis (see Fig. 183). They are merely hypertrophic papillae with normal epidermal covering.

Fordyce Spots

This condition arises from the presence of ectopic sebaceous glands; it may be found under the prepuce (see Fig. 184) and on the vulva. The lesions appear as multiple small, white or yellow spots in the submucosa.

Lymphocele (Benign Transient Lymphangiectasis)

In this condition the lymphatics in or near the coronal sulcus may become temporarily blocked and appear as worm-like translucent masses of cartilage-like hardness (see Fig. 185). Some cases follow prolonged or frequent intercourse or are associated with a genital lesion, but in the largest series reported[26] the majority were unexplained although the patients had had coitus. The condition resolves within a few weeks and no treatment is necessary.

REFERENCES

1. HOPE-SIMPSON, R. E. (1965) *Proc. R. Soc. Med.*, **58**, 9.
2. DAWBER, R. (1974) *Br. med. J.*, **2**, 526.
3. MELLANBY, K. (1972) *Scabies*, 2nd ed. Hampton: Classey.
4. CANBY, J. P. and WILDE, H. (1973) *New Engl. J. Med.*, **289**, 108.
5. BINGHAM, J. S. (1978) *Br. J. vener. Dis.*, **54**, 350.
6. GOOLAMALI, S. K., BARNES, E. W., IRVINE, W. J. and SHUSTER, S. (1974) *Br. med. J.*, **4**, 78.
7. CATTERALL, R. D. and OATES, J. K. (1962) *Br. J. vener. Dis.*, **38**, 75.
8. STAFF, W. G. (1970) *Br. J. Urol.*, **43**, 234.
9. ORIEL, J. D. (1971) *Br. J. vener. Dis.*, **47**, 1.
10. ORIEL, J. D. (1971) *Br. J. vener. Dis.*, **47**, 373.
11. COOK, T. A., COHN, A. M., BRUNSCHWIG, J. P., BUTEL, J. S. and RAWLS, W. E. (1973) *Lancet*, **i**, 782.
12. ORIEL, J. D. (1977) *Sex. transm. Dis.*, **4**, 153.
13. GHOSH, A. K. (1977) *Br. J. vener. Dis.*, **53**, 49.
14. THOMSON, J. P. S. and GRACE, R. H. (1978) *J. R. Soc. Med.*, **71**, 180.
15. RUSSELL, R. C. G. (1978) *J. R. Soc. Med.*, **71**, 460.
16. VON KROGH, G. (1976) *Acta derm.-vener.*, **56**, 297.
17. WALLIN, J. (1977) *Br. J. vener. Dis.*, **53**, 240.
18. DRETLER, S. P. and KLEIN, L. A. (1975) *J. Urol.*, **113**, 195.
19. POWELL, L. C. (1972) *Clin. Obstet. Gynec.*, **15**, 948.
20. NEL, W. S. and FOURIE, E. D. (1973) *S. Afr. med. J.*, **47**, 45.
21. CHAMBERLAIN, M. J., REYNOLDS, A. L. and YEOMAN, W. B. (1972) *Br. med. J.*, **2**, 391.
22. PRYOR, J. P. and KHAN, O. (1979) *Lancet*, **i**, 331.
23. SMITH, B. H. (1969) *Am. J. Clin. Path.*, **52**, 385.
24. BYSTRÖM, J., JOHANSSON, B., EDSMYR, F., KÖRLOF, B. and NYLEN, B. (1972) *Scand. J. Urol. Nephrol.*, **6**, 1.
25. POUTASSE, E. F. (1972) *J. Urol.*, **107**, 419.
26. HUTCHINS, P., DUNLOP, E. M. C. and RODIN, P. (1977) *Br. J. vener. Dis.*, **53**, 379.

28

Psychological Aspects of Venereal Disease

Any patient attending a doctor has some degree of apprehension and this will also apply to those who seek advice for venereal disease, particularly as it involves discussion of the patient's sexual activity. The attitude of doctors and other staff in clinics can have a profound effect on the patient who may already have strong feelings of guilt and fears regarding the consequences of his condition. A moralizing or patronizing attitude should never be adopted. Unfortunately the high pressure of work in venereal disease clinics has meant that often there is not adequate time to deal with the varied psychological aspects, but it is likely to save time in the long run if they are recognized and dealt with before anxieties and misconceptions become firmly established and difficult to remove.

Kite and Grimble,[1] using special interviews for patients attending a venereal disease clinic who were suspected of psychiatric disorder, found that 5 per cent of 887 consecutive new patients could be classed as 'psychiatric cases'. Principal symptoms were those of anxiety, phobia, genital pain or itching without organic cause, and depression. Of the main factors immediately related to breakdown, fear arising from some types of anti-venereal disease propaganda seemed to be the most prominent. It was therefore important to make any discussion about venereal disease as clear, straightforward and factual as possible and without implicit moral overtones; presentations which inspire shame, doubt or fear of dreadful consequences should never be used.

Pedder and Goldberg,[2] using a questionnaire in a series of new patients attending consecutively a venereal disease clinic in London, found that 30 per cent of 219 patients were probably 'psychiatric cases', which was a similar figure to that found in general practice and in a medical out-patient department. This finding contrasted with a rate of referral for psychiatric investigation of only 0·3 per cent previously experienced in the same clinic[3] so that for each patient referred there were likely to be many others for whom help was not sought.

Mayou[4] interviewed 100 first attenders at a venereal disease clinic in London, using a semistructured method. He found a considerable amount of psychosocial morbidity and rated 20 per cent as 'psychiatric cases'. There was no specific psychiatric pattern, but rather mixed neurotic symptoms. Whilst the majority reported anxiety about their possible illness, in a quarter the anxiety appeared to be of long standing and related to chronic social and psychological difficulties.

Personality Patterns

The personalities of patients attending a venereal disease clinic in Glasgow were studied by Wells.[5] He used Eysenck's psychoticism, extroversion, neuroticism (PEN) inventory on 199 men and 127 women. Males differed from the normal population in that they tended to be more extroverted. Females were substantially more neurotic than the normal population, with scores approaching those of clinical neurotics; they also had high scores for psychoticism which approached those of psychotic in-patients. Women infected by their husbands also had a marked degree of introversion. Extroversion declined with age, and middle-class people tended to score lower in PEN than those from the lower social classes. Women with the higher extroversion scores tended to default, but there was no correlation with default and the degree of neuroticism and psychoticism. However, male defaulters had significantly higher neuroticism and psychoticism scores than those who completed their surveillance, but there was no significant relation to degree of extroversion. He considered that it was women who most needed to be understood and communicated with, in view of their high levels of neuroticism and psychoticism, if venereal disease was to be controlled. A later study of homosexual patients in Glasgow,[6] using the Eysenck Personality Inventory (EPI), showed them to have lower scores for extroversion than heterosexual males, but they were significantly more neurotic than the general population. Fluker,[7] however, found little evidence of severe personality disorders among his homosexual patients; those who were exclusively homosexual seemed better adjusted than bisexuals, and readily cooperated in persuading their contacts to attend the clinic.

Promiscuity

The factors which determine promiscuity of individuals are complex. The truly promiscuous female is prepared to have sexual intercourse on scant acquaintance and is unable to form lasting relationships. Paradoxically she often has weak sexual drive and mostly fails to achieve orgasm. It is often said that these girls are searching for love but feel unworthy and have little hope of attaining it. It is not surprising that they are commonly depressive and sometimes suicidal. Often they have run away from home, and sometimes deliberately become pregnant, hoping to receive the desired love from the child. They are also more liable than others to become alcoholics or take drugs.

The truly promiscuous male also has difficulty in forming lasting relationships with women, of whom he may well be fundamentally afraid. His need is to dominate and humiliate the woman and to him copulation is a means of achieving this. If ever he does fall in love he may well become impotent.[8]

The above type of true promiscuity should not be confused with bouts of periodic promiscuity which may occur in otherwise non-promiscuous persons, for example when they are away from home.

Psychosexual Problems

At first sight it might seem that, apart from any discomfort of the disease, people who come to venereal disease clinics should not have sexual problems. On closer inspection, however, it becomes obvious that these most certainly exist, either at the patient's first attendance or arising later for various reasons. For example, a married man may have sought other sexual outlets because of an unsatisfactory sexual relationship with his wife; if he acquires an infection as a result of this and passes it on to his wife, this can only make matters worse. If the underlying psychosexual problem is not dealt with the whole process is likely to be repeated. Perhaps even more disturbing is when a moment of weakness results in the same course of events in someone who primarily had a satisfactory relationship with his wife. In some cases the wife's pregnancy may have resulted in a transient loss of attraction, or restriction of sexual intercourse may have been advised by the obstetrician. Although in the past long periods of abstinence were required before cure of many of the sexually transmitted diseases could be demonstrated, with modern treatment the periods required are much shorter, so that in general fewer problems arise from this.

A genital condition may cause pain or discomfort during intercourse or it may remove the desire for intercourse by the fear or shame that it produces, particularly when it is thought that the condition might be venereal in origin and that the regular sexual partner might become affected. Those conditions which are persistent or recurrent put most strain on a sexual relationship, especially when there is a fear (justified or not) that intercourse will produce a relapse.

In particular the management of non-specific urethritis requires a close observation of the patient's psychological reaction to his condition, especially when there is difficulty in eradicating it or when the patient believes he is not better although there is no evidence of disease. The latter often has a fear of infecting others together with guilt over having acquired the disease in the first place, so it is easy to see how sexual problems can arise. It may require much reassurance and persuasion to get these patients to resume intercourse.

Where there has been difficulty in eradicating the infection, it is often of value to see both sexual partners together. In this regard non-specific urethritis is more likely to throw great strain on a marriage than gonorrhoea, which can be more easily and rapidly eradicated. Even though married men generally get non-specific urethritis as a result of extra-marital intercourse, this is not invariably the case, and it can be helpful to point out to a suspicious wife or fiancée that the disease is not 'VD'. It is obviously helpful to be able to see such contacts in clinics held apart from the VD clinic; if this cannot be done the patients must be told that so-called VD clinics also deal with other conditions. If psychosexual problems are to be avoided, tactful and sympathetic handling of patients with non-specific urethritis is essential. All too often, repeated courses of antibiotics are given, sometimes on doubtful evidence of non-specific urethritis, with scant attention being paid to the patient's increasing anxiety and sometimes depression, which may result in impotence or premature ejaculation and consequent damage to present and future relationships. There are some patients, however, who will use a recurrent, often mild, non-specific urethritis, as an excuse not to have sexual intercourse for extended periods, if at all. They commonly have added symptoms, obviously unrelated to their non-specific urethritis but attributed by them to it. These patients are difficult to help and may need to be seen by a psychiatrist. In others all evidence of urethritis disappears but the patients have persistent symptoms for which there seems to be no organic cause. In some cases the symptoms may be attributed to 'chronic non-specific prostatitis,' as judged by examination of the prostatic fluid. However, as the changes indicating chronic prostatitis can be found in a fifth of otherwise healthy men, it is very difficult to interpret the findings in the individual case and to decide whether the symptoms are primarily psychogenic or physical. The same problem arises in men with discomfort in and around the genitalia who do not have, and have never had, urethritis. Certainly, in most of these the symptoms are psychogenic.

Symptoms Used as an Excuse to Avoid Intercourse

As already noted, some patients are seen in venereal disease clinics who complain of symptoms which, after careful assessment and full investigation, cannot be explained on any physical basis. A few of these patients will fall into the category of venereophobia, but others have no worries about venereal disease and seem to need their symptoms as a reason for not having sexual intercourse. Although seen in both sexes, it is more often found in women, and most of these patients find their way to gynaecologists rather than venereologists. However, if the underlying psychosexual problem is not recognized by the doctor or not accepted as being significant by the patient, she may attend several hospitals and different departments, including the venereal disease clinic, with symptoms such as vulval soreness and irritation, or abdominal pain, made worse by intercourse. *Candida* may well be found by chance and be offered as the cause of the vulval symptoms or dyspareunia, but the symptoms are out of all proportion to the physical signs, and persist after the candidal infection has been eradicated.

Nocturnal Emissions, Prostatorrhoea and the 'Bangladeshi Syndrome'

Sometimes adolescents and young men attend a venereal disease clinic in a state of great anxiety after experiencing a nocturnal emission. Others, especially if they have no outlet through masturbation, may notice a discharge when straining at stool or at the end of micturition—prostator-rhoea. These events are physiological and reassurance is all that is needed. They may also happen to married men when deprived of a regular sexual outlet during a wife's illness or by separation. This is well exemplified in the 'Bangladeshi Syndrome'. This may be defined as a chronic psychosexual problem arising in Bangladeshi men living in England. Language, cultural and socio-economic factors are implicated. A similar syndrome has been described in Indian immigrants.[9] Most of the Bangladeshi men are in their twenties and thirties and are Muslims. They are generally married but leave their wives and children in Bangladesh while they come to this country for several years to earn money, by doing semi-skilled or unskilled work. These men often live together in overcrowded all-male communities. One of the many problems they face is that of lack of a satisfactory sexual outlet. Because of their limited English and lack of social poise such outlets are mainly with prostitutes, and some thus acquire sexually transmitted diseases. However, a complaint of urethral discharge and penile pain may bring the patient to the clinic, but no evidence of sexually transmitted disease is found. Careful questioning reveals that the urethral discharge mostly occurs at the end of micturition, or whilst straining at stool. This picture points to prostatovesicular overflow as a consequence of sexual continence. Another complaint may be of 'weakness' which is regarded as due to 'too much night pollution' (nocturnal emission). Sometimes the genital symptoms are subordinate to various others such as chest or abdominal pain or 'pain all over', so that the patients may attend various other departments and have numerous investigations before the underlying psychosexual problem is discovered. Those men who have had sexual experience with prostitutes may be no better off. This is generally too infrequent to act as a satisfactory outlet, and when attempted is often unsuccessful, with premature emission or impotence. Cultural and religious taboos seem to dictate that masturbation, like frequent nocturnal emissions, is harmful. It is therefore not practised.

Treatment of this complex problem is difficult. The patient has little insight into his conflict. At the root of the problem is his sexual continence. This could be resolved by rejoining his wife, but by so doing he would have to abandon his money-raising enterprise and failure in this would have its own psychological repercussions. Bengali-speaking doctors in the area will be an obvious asset by rooting out depressive or other treatable psychiatric problems in the patient's illness. It is difficult to get the patients to accept that their symptoms are functional; they are loth to use masturbation as a sexual outlet so that nocturnal emissions are likely to continue. Treatment, especially by injections, is often requested by the patient for his supposed illness, and should be declined.

Sexual Dysfunction Presenting as Such to the Venereologist

Apart from men with the 'Bangladeshi Syndrome', few patients are either sent to or attend venereal disease clinics of their own accord, primarily because of overt sexual difficulties such as impotence or premature ejaculation. Sadly, these complaints are not always dealt with sympathetically elsewhere, and much more needs to be done to help couples with psychosexual problems. Unfortunately, this is not easy to do in hard-pressed venereal disease clinics, but it is important to lend a sympathetic ear and to examine the patients thoroughly so that they can be reassured regarding the absence of general illness or venereal disease as a cause of their problem. If prolonged counselling is required, and the time or expertise of the venereologist too limited to provide this, then arrangements can be made for the couple to be seen elsewhere.

Men with sexual problems may well increase in number because of the greater demands of and greater proficiency expected by their now more sexually aware partners. The ready availability of most venereal disease clinics may prompt some of these men to attend there rather than elsewhere. In some cases they may have previously attended a venereal disease clinic for other reasons and may relate their present problem to past sexually transmitted disease. Some patients are embarrassed to discuss the matter with their general practitioner, and prefer to do so with someone they do not know.

Homosexuals may, of course, also suffer from premature ejaculation and impotence. Most of those seen in clinics have accepted their homosexuality,[7] but occasionally a homosexual asks to be 'changed'. Others, whilst not wanting to change, become anxious or depressed about their orientation. Complicated psychosexual problems are likely to arise when a previously repressed homosexuality asserts itself in someone who has married, particularly when homosexually acquired disease is subsequently transmitted to the spouse.

Venereophobia

Venereologists commonly see patients who have a fear of venereal disease.

In most cases this is transient, being relieved by careful examination, tests and reassurance. The term 'venereophobia' is used only for those patients who persist in the mistaken belief that they have venereal disease, which is really more of a delusion than a phobia. They often attend several hospitals asking for further tests, insisting that their belief will eventually be shown to be true. In some cases the patient has, in fact, had a venereal disease but cannot accept that he has been cured. The condition may be part of an underlying depressive illness, anxiety or obsessional neurosis, paranoid state or schizophrenia. Not surprisingly, it is associated with impaired sexual function, and most of these patients have infrequent or no sexual intercourse and do not enjoy it when they do. The venereophobia might have arisen during a period of sexual inadequacy and serve as an excuse for curtailing further sexual activity. If there is obvious anxiety or depression, then tranquillizers or antidepressant drugs may help. Unhappily the condition is often intractable, but these patients may learn to live with their myth, which they presumably need to maintain. Such patients should, of course, be under the care of a psychiatrist, but they often fail to keep their appointments.

Because non-specific urethritis is now so common it may trigger the condition, and a relapsing non-specific urethritis may well confirm in the patient's mind that he has an organic cause for what are quite unrelated symptoms. Fortunately very few patients with relapsing non-specific urethritis develop full-blown venereophobia, although, as already mentioned, anxiety is common and depression may occur.

REFERENCES

1. KITE, E. DE C. and GRIMBLE, A. (1963) Br. J. vener. Dis., **39,** 173.
2. PEDDER, J. R. and GOLDBERG, D. P. (1970) Br. J. vener. Dis., **46,** 58.
3. PEDDER, J. R. (1970) Br. J. vener. Dis., **46,** 54.
4. MAYOU, R. (1975) Br. J. vener. Dis., **51,** 57.
5. WELLS, B. W. P. (1970) Br. J. vener. Dis., **46,** 498.
6. WELLS, B. W. P. and SCHOFIELD, C. B. S. (1972) Br. J. vener. Dis., **48,** 75.
7. FLUKER, J. L. (1976) Br. J. vener. Dis., **52,** 155.
8. CAUTHERY, P. (1976) In: Psychosexual Problems, ed. S. Crown, p. 178. London: Academic Press.
9. CLYNE, M. B. (1964) Practitioner, **193,** 195.

29

Venereal Diseases and the Public Health

The World Health Organization has in past years drawn attention to a rise in the incidence of venereal diseases which is almost world-wide.[1, 2] Reliable facts and figures are mostly impossible to obtain. In many countries neither syphilis nor gonorrhoea is notifiable; in others it has been shown that the actual incidence is several times higher than that indicated by the available statistics.[3, 4] Results of studies of the trends of incidence of early syphilis in 105 countries showed that in 76 (72·4 per cent) of them a persistent rise in incidence had followed an 'all-time low' in about 1955. In some countries the reported incidence had approached or even exceeded the maximum of the years immediately after the Second World War.

New problems of environment were creating obstacles to venereal disease control in both developed and developing countries. Modern methods of treatment were apt to engender a false sense of security, with indifference to the risk of infection and lessening of fear of the consequences of disease. Industrialization and the move from countryside to towns were breaking up the old social patterns, and the migration of workers and others contributed to the problem. In economically prosperous countries the number of sexually active young people had increased and so had the consumption of alcohol. Rapid movement of large numbers of people by land, sea and air and the increase in merchant shipping were additional factors. In some countries as many as 50 per cent of patients with early syphilis had contracted the infection abroad. Earlier maturity, freer association between young males and females, changing standards of morality and homosexual practices, all were believed to be contributory factors in many areas.

It had been suggested by some that the closing of licensed or tolerated brothels and the abolition of regulation of prostitution in countries ratifying, or adhering to, the United Nations Convention for the Suppression of Traffic in Persons and the Exploitation of the Prostitution of Others, had hindered control and contributed to the spread of venereal diseases. But the recent increase was similar in Scandinavian countries, where licensed brothels were abolished many years ago, to those in France and Italy, where they were suppressed more recently. In some countries prostitution remained a major problem; in others clandestine promiscuity seemed to be the major cause of spread of infection. Up to 1955, or so, the production and consumption of penicillin continued to increase and it seemed likely that many people received curative amounts of the drug during the long incubation period of syphilitic infection. After that time, reactions to penicillin became more common and production and consumption of the drug ceased to increase. From 1955 to 1960 the production and use of broad-spectrum antibiotics more than doubled and has since continued to increase; these remedies are ineffective or less effective against syphilis. Gonorrhoea was more often treated with remedies other than penicillin which are less likely to suppress incubating syphilis. Younger people, who are now increasingly exposed to risk of infection, are less likely to have had penicillin for the treatment of other diseases.

As regards gonorrhoea, a study by the World Health Organization[5] of long-term trends covering the period 1950 to 1960 showed that in some countries there was a more or less lasting fall in incidence by the middle of the decade; in others the incidence remained stationary; and in yet others an upward trend was evident after about 1955. Of 111 countries and areas surveyed, 53 (47·7 per cent) showed a persistent increase in the reported incidence after 1957. Annual rates in Europe varied from 100 to 500 per 100,000 adult population (defined as persons over 15 years of age). In several countries in the South East Asian, Eastern Mediterranean and Western Pacific Regions, the rates exceeded 1000 per 100,000 adults. Considerably higher rates were recorded in some countries of Africa and the Americas. There was known to be a large reservoir of infection in Africa, in some areas of which the disease appeared to be endemic. Many more cases were diagnosed in males than in females, the ratios varying from 2:1 to 4:1 or higher, depending upon local standards of facilities for diagnosis and treatment, case-finding and reporting, but suggesting a large reservoir of latent infection in females.

This problem was considered by an Expert Committee of the World Health Organization[6] in 1962 which concluded that the advent of antibiotic therapy had failed to influence the prevalence of gonococcal infection. The infectiousness of gonorrhoea, the short incubation period, the mode of transmission and other factors had made it impossible to evolve epidemiological methods effective against the very rapid spread of the infection. Nowhere had it been possible to bring a sufficiently large number of cases and contacts to treatment quickly enough to overtake the rapid spread of the infection in communities. Air travel allowed rapid transfer of infection between countries and continents. There were special itinerant groups, such as migrants, seafarers and the like, at particular risk of infection. Failure to interrupt transmission and to control gonococcal infection was world-wide and this should be recognized by public health experts, the medical profession and the public.

In a review of the problem of venereal diseases throughout the world, Willcox[7] pointed to the difficulty of obtaining accurate information. There had been a variable rise in the incidence of early syphilis in most countries, but late syphilis had declined in most countries and so had early congenital syphilis in practically all. Gonorrhoea was still increasing in most areas. Difficulties in control were exemplified by surveys which had shown that in the United States of America 7 out of 10 of all infections with gonorrhoea and infectious syphilis were not reported and thus escaped one of the main methods of control, namely contact investigation. He believed that, against the background of the likelihood of much greater mobility of populations, continuing permissiveness, more extensive use of oral contraceptives, increasing promiscuity and developing resistance of the gonococcus to antibiotics, the outlook for the successful control of the venereal diseases in the immediate future appeared to be bleak. In only a few countries in the world was there a case-finding organization and a comprehensive network of venereal disease clinics providing free treatment, and wherever these facilities existed they were being strained by increasing case loads. Much more money would have to be spent to provide facilities commensurate with the problem. The hopes for vaccines against the venereal diseases were still a long way from practical reality. In Poland some immunity had been established in rabbits by many intravenous injections of treponemes killed with penicillin, and in the United States of America by irradiated organisms, but such procedures were clearly impractical for use in men. Even if a vaccine became available it might raise many problems in interpreting the results of screening tests in expectant mothers and others. A successful vaccine for gonorrhoea seemed even less likely when many natural infections produced no immunity. There was also the possibility that successful immunization might do no more than result in the gonococcus being held in a carrier state. It was evident that the venereal diseases were here to stay and indeed they were likely to present an increasing problem in the foreseeable future.

Willcox[8] has also discussed the special problem of venereal disease control in developing countries; a lack of awareness of the extent of the problem and the presence of other more pressing medical problems lead to low budgets and poor facilities for diagnosis and treatment, with few cases being seen in official clinics and hospitals. Thus relatively small numbers of cases are reported and ignorance of the problem continues. The same could, of course, be said for several developed countries.

PREVENTIVE MEASURES

Facilities for Diagnosis and Treatment

The quality of medical and nursing care available to patients suffering from venereal disease is the most important factor in the control of these diseases. In Great Britain facilities for diagnosis and treatment were established by the Venereal Disease Regulations of 1916. The Regulations instructed the local health authorities to provide clinics for this purpose by arrangement with local hospitals and other institutions, in which diagnosis and treatment were to be confidential and free of charge. The National Health Service Act of 1946 brought the clinics under the control of the Regional Hospital Boards and Boards of Governors of Teaching Hospitals, from the appointed day in July 1948. Treatment continues to be free, and patients are not required to pay prescription charges. Patients are entitled to attend without letters from their doctors and, although in most clinics there is no regular system of appointments, the larger clinics in cities are usually open on weekdays for medical consultations continuously between 10 a.m. and 7 p.m. The local health authorities continue to be responsible for publicity relating to venereal disease, and for cooperation in the tracing of contacts and defaulters. At some hospitals, anonymous clinics are conducted on premises other than those of the venereal disease clinics and are not known by the patients to be concerned with venereal diseases. This gives the opportunity of examining patients from other departments of the hospital and contacts of patients with venereal disease, without necessarily disclosing in detail the purpose of the investigation. Countries with an established venereal diseases service, such as Britain and some in Eastern Europe, have suffered a less marked increase in venereal diseases than elsewhere.

Contact Tracing

Prompt and effective measures to identify the potentially infected and to induce them to accept diagnosis and treatment are the most important factors in control after the quality of medical care. 'Contacts' are of two kinds: a so-called primary contact is a source from which the patient contracts infection; secondary contacts are those to whom the patient may have transmitted infection before diagnosis and treatment. Primary contacts are often difficult to trace. They may be prostitutes, casual acquaintances or strangers, and if alcohol has been a factor in determining the association the patient may recollect no details. His distaste for the occasion and its outcome may make him loth to help. It is in these cases that the skill and persistence of the contact tracer are especially valuable. Most clinics in Great Britain have at least one such person who interviews patients in the clinic after they have been seen by the doctor and obtains information on which action may be taken. These people are chosen for personality rather than for qualifications on paper. They need to be persuasive, tactful, diligent and persistent. They need to be provided with transport to cover distances and bring in the contacts if necessary. Some of these interviews with contacts take place in public houses or cafés and they must have allowances for minor entertainment. In many areas their work has been highly successful. Secondary contacts are likely to be wives, fiancées or girl friends and about these most patients are conscientious and responsible. The contacts may be induced to attend with so-called contact slips issued to the patients at the clinic for transmission to the contacts indicating that they should attend the clinic of origin or some other clinic and giving the diagnosis in the form of a symbol recommended by the Department of Health. If the contact attends some other clinic, the latter informs the clinic of origin of the fact of attendance and the diagnosis. Patients may require the help of the contact tracers to put the matter tactfully to the secondary contacts and to persuade them to attend. The anonymous clinics already mentioned can be very useful for this purpose.

From time to time, during national emergencies, attempts have been made to secure, by legal compulsion, the attendance of individuals reported as sources of infection. In Great Britain the last of these was the war-time Emergency Regulation 33b; this was introduced in 1942 and allowed to lapse in 1947. Since then the procedure for tracing contacts has depended upon the voluntary cooperation of infected patients. In most countries in which legal compulsion may still be used, the full force of the law is seldom invoked.

Prenatal Investigation

Antenatal clinics perform blood tests to exclude syphilis as a routine precaution, but few take tests for gonorrhoea or other genital infection unless the patient complains of symptoms. For this reason it sometimes happens that genital infection is not diagnosed in a mother until her infant has developed ophthalmia neonatorum. There is need for more awareness of the problem in obstetric and gynaecological clinics, family planning clinics and those where specimens are taken for cervical cytology. All should play their part in the control of venereal diseases by learning to recognize the signs of infection and organizing the facilities for microscopical and laboratory diagnosis.

Suppression of the Quack and the Charlatan

In Great Britain the public is protected from quacks and charlatans by the Venereal Diseases Act of 1917, which imposes heavy fines or imprisonment on any unqualified person who gives advice on or offers facilities for the treatment of venereal disease. For the purposes of this Act, venereal disease is defined as meaning syphilis, gonorrhoea or soft chancre.

Control of Prostitution

Venereal disease is an occupational hazard of prostitutes, who can play an important part in the spread of disease. Of 478 prostitutes examined at Holloway Prison in London in 1967, seven were found to be suffering from infectious syphilis and 91 from gonorrhoea. Sixty-one of the prostitutes were between the ages of 15 and 20 years; three of them had infectious syphilis and 35 gonorrhoea.[9] With the sexually permissive society of recent years prostitutes have played a lesser role in the spread of infection in the western world, but they are still a major source of infection in some areas, particularly Asia. In the past, a prostitute who solicited in a public place in Britain was charged under the Metropolitan Police Act of 1839, and it was necessary for the police who brought the charge to give evidence of annoyance of passers-by. As the result of more recent legislation there is no longer need for the fact of annoyance to be established. In September 1957, the Report of the Committee on Homosexual Offences and Prostitution (Wolfenden Report) was published. As a consequence of the recommendations of that Report the Street Offences Act 1959 was passed and became effective on August 16, 1959. The Act makes the following provisions:

1. It shall be an offence for a common prostitute to loiter or solicit in a street or public place for the purposes of prostitution.
2. A person guilty of an offence under this section shall be liable, on summary conviction, to a fine not exceeding ten pounds or, for an offence committed after a previous conviction, to a fine not exceeding twenty-five pounds or, for a third or subsequent conviction, a fine of twenty-five pounds, or imprisonment for a period not exceeding three months, or both.

Under the heading of 'Punishment of Offences in Connection with Night Cafés', the Act fixes the penalties for allowing prostitutes to be in these establishments, as follows:

(a) In the case of a person not previously convicted of an offence . . ., twenty pounds (instead of five pounds); and
(b) in the case of a person previously convicted, fifty pounds (instead of twenty pounds).

An order for forfeiture of a licence may be made. Under the heading 'Punishment for Living on the Earnings of Prostitution', the Act increases the maximum term of imprisonment on conviction from two to seven years.

Health Education

Education of the public in matters concerning venereal disease is a difficult matter. It is, of course, linked with the even more difficult problem of sex education of children. Modern thinking rightly rejects the inhibitions of the past, as the result of which the problem was ignored or direct questions were answered by direct falsehoods. It is generally conceded that questions asked by children should be answered fully and truthfully, and that opportunities given by such questions should be taken to give useful additional information. Children should know about venereal diseases by the time that they reach the age of puberty. Information of this kind should be linked with advice on the value of self-restraint and should stress the idealistic view of the union of man and woman in marriage. The child should never be forced to obtain information on sex from ill-informed and prurient-minded street companions. Many parents shirk their responsibilities in these matters, and it is of the utmost importance that religious authorities, school teachers, organizers of youth clubs, and all others concerned with the welfare of the young should be aware that their responsibilities in the matter of imparting correct information are secondary only to those of parents. It is unfortunately true that the most admirable advice is hardly likely to be fruitful if the home background is unstable and unhappy. The example of parents is of paramount importance; all too often it leaves much to be desired.

In England, publicity concerning the venereal diseases is mainly the responsibility of local health authorities. The Department of Health and Social Security provides help in the form of advice and suitable posters; the Central Council for Health Education has issued pamphlets providing information for the lay public, and has assisted with lectures and film strips when required. The responsibilities of this organization have now been taken over by the Health Education Council. Instructional films and film strips are available through the Central Office of Information, and in recent years some television programmes on this subject have reached large audiences. Editors of newspapers and magazines have published many articles of varying quality on the subject.

Diagnosis and Treatment

The venereal disease service plays its part in the campaign to prevent the spread of venereal diseases, but this is a matter in which the whole medical profession and, in particular, the general practitioner have an important rôle. A number of points in the diagnosis and treatment of venereal diseases require special emphasis, because failure to observe fundamental rules may result in harm to patients and spread of infection. First, the practice of giving antibiotics to patients with genital infections before performing diagnostic tests is likely to prevent accurate diagnosis and raises considerable difficulties in dealing with potentially infected contacts. Second, it is important to bear in mind that the complement-fixation test for gonorrhoea is not a substitute for examination by microscopical smears and cultures; the fact is that, under modern conditions, this serological test is of little value. Another possible danger, of a different kind, comes from the widespread criticism of the requirement under the Adoption Agencies Regulations (1959) that the medical report on a child who is to be adopted must include the results of serological tests for syphilis on serum taken six weeks or later after birth; the criticism is that such a test is unnecessary if tests on the mother or of the cord blood are known to have been negative. But it is well established that a woman can transmit syphilis to her unborn child during the incubation period or the seronegative primary stage of the disease, and antibiotics given for other reasons may suppress or delay serological reactions, though the patient remains infectious. It sometimes happens, also, that an infant whose serological tests are negative at the time of birth is nevertheless syphilitic. Disinclination for serological testing of small infants usually arises from the mistaken idea that the technique of obtaining blood is difficult. This is not so if the correct method is employed. (See the Appendix, p. 392.)

The facts that knowledge of venereal diseases has progressed in recent years and that there is evidence that the incidence of some of these diseases is increasing raise the question as to whether adequate time and staff are devoted to the teaching of this subject to undergraduates. An analysis of the teaching of venereology in 437 medical schools throughout the world conducted by the International Union against the Venereal Diseases and the Treponematoses, with the cooperation of the World Health Organization[10] indicated that the public health and epidemiological aspects of the venereal diseases were receiving a minimal amount of attention. Interest in the sociological phases of the question was not great. In 1971 a survey of several medical schools in the United States of America revealed that teaching on venereal diseases was inadequate and frequently non-existent.[11]

The technical standards of venereology in Great Britain are constantly under review by the Medical Society for the Study of Venereal Diseases, which, in conjunction with the *British Medical Journal*, publishes the *British Journal of Venereal Diseases*. The Society sponsors the British Co-operative Clinical Group, which initiates and coordinates conjoint research into outstanding problems. The British Medical Association plays its part in the control of venereal diseases through the Venereologists' Group. The British Federation against the Venereal Diseases (BFVD) deals with the social aspects of VD, and is affiliated to the International Union against the Venereal Diseases and Treponematoses (IUVDT), which in turn is closely associated in the work of the World Health Organization.

Arrangements relating to the treatment of venereal diseases in seamen were the subject of an International Agreement, signed in Brussels by the representatives of 42 countries in December 1924 and known as the 'Brussels Agreement'. The contracting parties undertook to establish and maintain, in each of their principal sea or river ports, clinics available to all merchant seamen and watermen. Responsibility for supervision of the working of the Agreement was taken over by the World Health Organization in 1946. WHO has contributed greatly to the effectiveness of the Agreement by encouragement, coordination and interchange of information.[12] It has published an international list of venereal disease clinics and issued a 'Personal Booklet' (with detailed instructions in French and English for its use) for documentation in cases of venereal diseases in seamen.

In 1972 the Regional Office for Europe of WHO published the report of a Working Group on the 'Inter-Country Spread of Venereal Diseases'.[13] There was unanimous agreement that the most effective method of limiting the spread of these diseases between countries was by their national control. Another recent WHO publication lists all the venereal disease clinics in the European region.[14]

REFERENCES

1. Chron. Wld Hlth Org. (1964) **18,** 451.
2. Chron. Wld Hlth Org. (1965) **19,** 7.
3. CURTIS, A. C. (1963) J. Am. med. Ass., **186,** 46.
4. FLEMING, W. L., BROWN, W. J., DONOHUE, J. F. and BRANIGAN, P. W. (1970) J. Am. med. Ass., **211,** 1827.
5. Proc. 12th int. Congr. Derm. (Wash.) (1963) In: Excerpta Med. (Amst.), Int. Congr. Ser. No. 55, vol. 2, p. 833.
6. Wld Hlth Org. techn. Rep. Ser. (1963) **262,** pp. 5 and 60.
7. WILLCOX, R. R. (1972) Med. Clin. N. Am., **56,** 1057.
8. WILLCOX, R. R. (1976) Br. J. vener. Dis., **52,** 88.
9. A.R. med. Offr Hlth (Lond.) (1967) p. 71. H.M.S.O., 1968.
10. WEBSTER, B. (1966) Br. J. vener. Dis., **42,** 132.
11. Pan-American Health Association (1974) Report of the International Travelling Seminar on Venereal Diseases in the United States, p. 28. Scientific publication No. 280. Washington, D.C.: Government Printing Office.
12. Wld Hlth Org. techn. Rep. Ser. (1958) No. 150.
13. Wld Hlth Org. Reg. Office Europe (1972) Euro 1101. Copenhagen.
14. Wld Hlth Org. Reg. Office Europe (1972) Euro 1101 (1). Copenhagen.

Appendix

Routine Investigation of New Patients

History

Special attention should be paid to the recent history of sexual contacts. If there are several, it is useful to identify them by their first names. The exact dates of exposure and particulars of the consort and other individuals concerned should be noted. The possibility of homosexual exposure should not be forgotten. The town in which intercourse took place, whether in the country of origin or abroad, should be recorded and also details of contraceptive or other precautions employed by either partner. If the consort is known to be attending another hospital, a confidential letter should be sent to the physician-in-charge, requesting a medical report. The duration and nature of symptoms should be noted, with special emphasis on those related to the genito-urinary system.

The patient should be asked if there is any past history of venereal or other sexually transmitted diseases, together with details of treatment given. The history of any other illnesses or operations with dates should also be noted. Women should be asked about menstrual periods, the number and dates of live births, stillbirths and miscarriages, and details should be recorded in the notes.

Examination

Men

The patient should remove all his clothes and lie on a couch in a warm and well-lighted examination room. The pubic region is inspected for lice or nits, and the inguinal region palpated for enlarged lymphatic nodes. The genitalia are inspected; if the patient is uncircumcised, the prepuce should, if possible, be retracted. Any oedema, sores or swellings should be noted and the penile urethra milked for urethral discharge. If discharge is present, a specimen should be obtained with a platinum loop or swab and spread on to a slide for staining. A loop is then inserted into the terminal urethra and a scraping taken from the wall of the urethra; this material is now mixed with a drop of saline for examination for *T. vaginalis*, and a similar specimen can be inoculated into an appropriate culture medium for *T. vaginalis*. Some urethral discharge is collected on a Stuart's swab which is put into Stuart's transport medium or directly on to a culture plate preparatory to cultural tests for gonorrhoea. A swab may need to be taken even when there is no evident urethral discharge if asymptomatic carriage of the gonococcus is suspected; very small swabs* which can be passed well into the urethra are best used in these cases and direct plating is preferable. Such swabs are also the most suitable for obtaining samples for culture of *Chlamydia*. Dark-ground examination of serum from a genital sore or obtained by lymphatic node puncture is performed if there are lesions which require this investigation. Culture tests for herpes simplex or *Haemophilus ducreyi* may be indicated. The scrotal sac is inspected and the testes and epididymes are palpated.

The perianal region is then examined. Careful examination for anal ulceration should be made in an admitted homosexual, and specimens for dark-ground examination should be obtained from any open lesion. A proctoscope should be passed and specimens for smears and cultures taken from any pus or mucopus on the rectal wall or from the mucosal surface if there is no obvious exudate. Urogenital examination is more satisfactory if the patient has not passed urine for two or three hours; it is sometimes necessary to examine the patient after he has held urine overnight. He is then asked to pass urine into two conical glasses, filling only a third of the first glass. The urine is inspected, and if hazy, the second specimen is tested with acetic acid for alkaline phosphates. If the haze persists the other specimen may then be centrifuged and examined microscopically for leucocytes, red cells, sperms and organisms, including *T. vaginalis*. Culture of the deposit of the centrifuged urine for *T. vaginalis* may also be indicated and culture of a mid-stream specimen if bacterial urinary infection is suspected. If the patient has a subpreputial discharge, smears for *Candida albicans* and Vincent's organisms may be examined, and a moist specimen may be taken for *T. vaginalis*. Culture for *C. albicans* may also be indicated.

Women

The genital examination should be performed with the patient in the lithotomy position with a cloth or towel across her thighs. It is desirable that she should not have passed urine recently. The abdomen is examined first and palpated for signs of tenderness; the presence of scars is noted. For the genital examination an Anglepoise lamp may be used for illumination.

* These swabs are marketed by the Medical Wire and Equipment Company Ltd and also by the Inolex Corporation, U.S.A. The former have cotton-wool tips and the latter (Calgiswab) have alginate tips.

First the pubic, vulval and perianal regions should be carefully inspected for lice, any dermatological condition, or areas of oedema or ulceration; serum for dark-ground examination should be taken if indicated. The inguinal regions are then felt, and any abnormalities of the inguinal lymphatic nodes are noted. The vulva is inspected and the glands of Bartholin palpated. Smears and cultures for gonorrhoea and *T. vaginalis* are taken from the duct openings if the glands are tender and swollen or if discharge from the duct is seen.

If the patient is not *virgo intacta*, a Cusco speculum is passed without lubricating fluid, and the vaginal portion of the cervix is manipulated into view; the characteristics of the vaginal secretion and the appearance of the vaginal wall are noted. A specimen of vaginal secretion taken with a platinum loop is diluted in a saline drop on a slide to be examined for *T. vaginalis*. A specimen is also taken for culture of *T. vaginalis*. Smear and culture may be taken for *C. albicans*. A good routine adopted in many clinics is to take an Ayres smear for cytological study. Vaginal secretion is then carefully removed from the region of the external os uteri with a dry swab in a holder, and the appearance of the cervix is noted. The character of the cervical secretion and the presence of cervical erosion or Nabothian follicles are points to be observed. Smear and culture for gonococci are taken from the cervical canal.

The speculum is now withdrawn and the urethra massaged with the finger forward along the anterior vaginal wall; any discharge from the urethra or from the paraurethral glands of Skene is noted. Urethral smear and cultures for gonorrhoea and sometimes *T. vaginalis* are taken, and similarly from the glands of Skene if these show signs of infection. A proctoscope lubricated with liquid paraffin is now passed and the appearance of the rectal mucosa and the presence of pus or mucopus are noted; smear and culture for gonorrhoea are taken. If proctoscopy cannot be carried out a satisfactory specimen for culture can be obtained by passing a swab for 2 or 3 cm into the anal canal, but direct plating is then advisable.[1] Bimanual palpation of the uterus and tubes is performed and any abnormality recorded.

Both Sexes

The patient should now have a full physical examination of all the systems and tests of the urine for albumin and sugar. Blood (7 ml) is withdrawn for routine serological tests. Temperature and pulse are recorded when indicated.

When any sexually transmitted disease is found to be present, the patient should be asked to assist in persuading his or her consort to undergo the necessary examination and tests.

Female Children

The method of examination is similar, but a vaginal speculum is not passed.

Vaginal tests are taken (smear, culture and fresh specimens for *T. vaginalis*) and then urethral tests, using platinum loops or culture sticks. Rectal tests are also taken with a platinum loop or swab passed through the anal orifice.

SYPHILIS
Dark-ground Microscopy
Equipment

An ordinary microscope has to be adapted by replacing the Abbé condenser by a dark-ground condenser with an opaque stop which cuts out the direct light rays, so that only the peripheral rays pass through and are reflected at an acute angle on to the slide. An ordinary 2 mm objective can be used, provided a funnel stop is inserted to reduce its numerical aperture to 0·95; or, alternatively, a special 2 mm objective with a built-in adjustable diaphragm can be employed. The source of light has to be brighter than normal and a special substage lamp or a 'bull's-eye' lamp may be used.

Method of Obtaining the Specimen

Wearing rubber gloves, the operator obtains serum from a suspected syphilitic chancre or from any surface lesion of the secondary stage, or by puncture of regional lymph nodes. If the lesion is moist the surface is cleaned thoroughly with swabs soaked in sterile normal saline, and the friction of cleansing is usually sufficient to produce an adequate flow of serum. If the lesion is dry, or if healing has commenced, it may be necessary to break the surface with a scarifier and squeeze the base of the lesion between finger and thumb to encourage a flow of serum. The surface should be scarified near the edge of the lesion, where the treponemes are likely to be present in greatest number. A cover slip held in a Cornet forceps or between the fingers is applied to the surface of the lesion so that a drop of serum adheres to it. If the specimen is obtained by needle puncture a drop of fluid is expressed from the needle on to the cover slip. The cover slip, with the drop of serum on the under surface, is now placed on to a thin glass slide. It is pressed down firmly with a piece of blotting paper. It is a disadvantage to dilute the serum with saline, however small the quantity. In inaccessible areas, such as the cervix or anal canal, it may be easier to collect serum into a capillary tube or by a platinum loop. When specimens are taken from the mouth care should be taken to remove any surface saliva or debris which may contain oral non-syphilitic treponemes (see p. 5).

Method of Examining Specimen

1. Adjust the lamp so that the beam of light is brought to a focus at the centre of the mirror; move the mirror so that the light is reflected up through the dark-ground condenser.

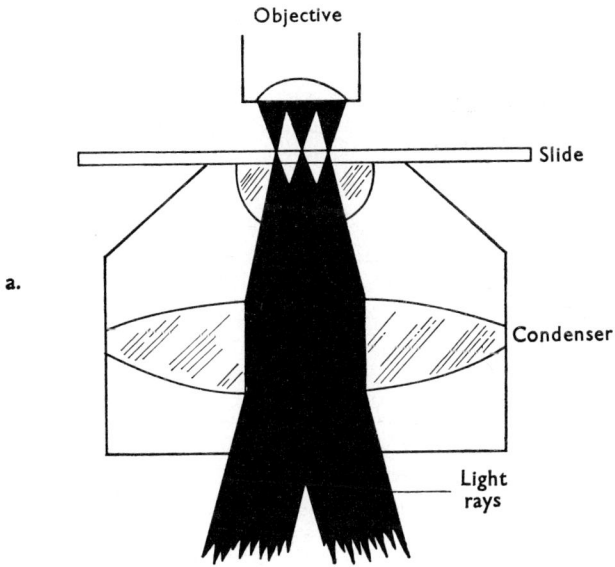

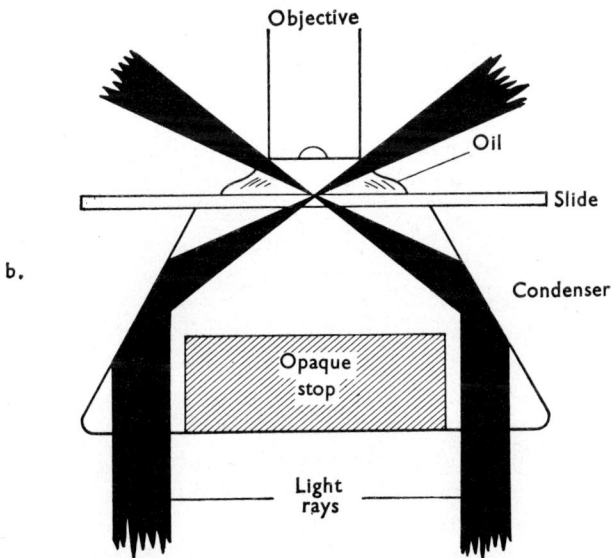

Showing Path of the Rays through the Condenser

a. Abbé condenser (bright-field).   b. Dark-field condenser.

(By courtesy U.S. Department of Health, Education and Welfare Public Health Service)

2. If the condenser has a centering circle engraved on its upper surface, focus this with the low-power objective and adjust the centering screws of the condenser until the circle occupies a central position in the field of view.

3. Put a drop of immersion oil on the upper surface of the condenser, and another on the under surface of the slide to be examined. Rack up the condenser until the two drops of oil coalesce without entrapping any air bubbles. Focus the slide with the low-power objective and adjust the height of the condenser until the spot of light is as bright as possible. Bring the spot to the middle of the field with the centering screws if necessary.

4. Put a drop of immersion oil on the cover slip and rack down the 2 mm immersion objective until it makes contact with the oil. Focus down carefully until the field comes into view. Adjust the mirror and the height of the condenser so that the field is evenly illuminated and the maximum contrast is obtained. The contents of the serum on the slide can now be seen as white objects on a black background.

If several specimens have to be examined in succession, it is most important to remove all the oil from the surface of the condenser each time, since the presence of too much oil may interfere with the optical system.

Serological Tests for Syphilis [2–4]

For full details see Chapter 7.

Method of Obtaining Specimen

ADULTS

Five to seven millilitres of blood are withdrawn from a vein in the antecubital fossa of the elbow; disposable syringes and needles are recommended. The needle is detached and the blood is emptied slowly into a sterilized screw-capped bottle which is correctly numbered and dated.

INFANTS

The simplest and safest way of obtaining blood is by stabbing the heel by the following technique:

The child's foot is immersed in warm water for a few minutes. It is dried and a light tourniquet is applied round the lower leg. The skin of the fleshy part of the heel is cleaned with 70 per cent alcohol. After a few minutes the heel is stabbed with a Hagedorn needle or a small snick is made through the skin with a sterile safety-razor blade or sharp scalpel. The blood flows freely and can be collected in a small test-tube or a Wright's capsule. The latter is a small glass tube the ends of which are narrowed to capillary diameter, one end being curved to a U shape. The curved end is applied to the drop of blood, which enters by capillary attraction. When full, the ends are sealed with candle grease or paraffin wax. One to two millilitres of blood should be collected. The cut made by the blade should be practically painless; bleeding stops when the tourniquet is removed and healing is prompt. Blood may also be obtained from a vein in the antecubital fossa, from the external jugular vein, and from the anterior fontanelle; but the technique of obtaining blood in these ways requires experience and venepuncture at these sites should not, ordinarily, be attempted.

Colloidal-gold Test

A row of 11 tubes is set up in a rack; 1·8 ml of 0·4 per cent sodium chloride in double-distilled water is added to the first tube and 1·0 ml to the remainder. 0·2 ml of cerebrospinal fluid is added to the first tube, mixed, and 1·0 ml carried over to the second and subsequent tubes, 1·0 ml being discarded from the tenth tube. No fluid is added to the eleventh tube, which acts as a control. This gives a series of dilutions of spinal fluid from 1:10 to 1:5120. 4·0 ml of gold sol. is added to each tube and the results are read after the tubes have stood overnight at room temperature. The degree of precipitation is judged from the colour of the fluid, with the use of the following scale:

Red (no precipitation)	0
Reddish-blue	1
Lilac or purple	2
Blue	3
Almost colourless, trace of blue	4
Colourless (maximal precipitation)	5

The degree of precipitation varies at different points on the dilution scale, and Table 5 shows the types of curve that may be obtained.

TABLE 5

DILUTION OF CEREBROSPINAL FLUID IN COLLOIDAL-GOLD TESTS

	10	20	40	80	160	320	640	1280	2560	5120
Normal	0	0	0	0	0	0	0	0	0	0
Zone 1 ('Paretic' curve)	5	5	5	5	5	4	4	4	0	0
Zone 2 ('Luetic' curve)	0	1	2	3	1	0	0	0	0	0
Zone 3 ('Meningitic' curve)	0	0	0	1	3	4	4	2	1	0

The colloidal-gold test only reflects changes in the distribution of proteins in the cerebrospinal fluid, and is not specific for neurosyphilis. Typical 'paretic' or 'luetic' curves may, for example, be found in some cases of disseminated sclerosis.

It is imperative that all glassware used for performing the test is scrupulously clean, and it is best reserved for use in this test alone. After use, it should be washed with tap water, put through dichromate–sulphuric acid cleaning fluid and finally washed with redistilled water. This test has been abandoned in some clinics and replaced by tests for immunoglobulins in the spinal fluid, but it is too early to assess the value of the latter.

Lumbar Puncture

Cerebrospinal fluid is usually obtained by lumbar puncture. This can be done in an out-patient department, but it is advisable for old or very nervous patients to be admitted to hospital for this procedure.

The patient should be fully informed about what is to be done and should be assured that the procedure will be simple and virtually painless provided he or she keeps still. The patient undresses and puts on a gown and bed socks. He or she then sits on a couch, on the far side of which an assistant stands. The assistant gets the patient to flex the spine with elbows resting on knees and supports the patient in this position. The operator, having scrubbed up, cleans the patient's back with spirit and places dressing towels in position; he then paints some iodine over the 3rd–4th lumbar intervertebral space, which is the space just above the level of the iliac crests. It is usually best to mark this area with a skin pencil before scrubbing up.

A syringe is filled with 2 per cent procaine solution, and a drop of this solution is injected intradermally at the central point of the 3rd–4th lumbar space; the needle is then pushed into the space while further procaine is being injected. The operator waits for one or two minutes for the local anaesthetic to take effect, and then places the second and third fingers of the left hand on the 3rd and 4th lumbar spinous processes respectively, while with the right hand he takes an appropriate lumbar puncture needle (Howard Jones or Harris) and pushes it firmly through the skin and interspinous ligament in a slightly upward direction in the midline of the intervertebral space. The needle point should not meet any resistance until it reaches the theca, which it then pierces. The stylet is now withdrawn, and spinal fluid collected in three sterile, screw-capped bottles after the first two drops, which may be blood-stained, have fallen. It is usually sufficient to collect 30 drops in the first, 10 drops in the second and 40 drops in the third bottle, at the rate of one drop per second. The rate of flow can be controlled by partial withdrawal of the stylet. The needle is now withdrawn with a slight rotatory action and a collodion dressing applied.

The bottles are numbered and labelled and forwarded to the pathologist, with a request for Wassermann reaction, or other appropriate test, cell count, protein estimation, and Lange test (or immunoglobulin estimation). If possible the FTA-ABS test should also be done. The cell count should be performed within an hour of the specimen being taken, as the cells begin to disintegrate after this period.

The patient lies face down with the back hyperextended for five minutes and then dresses and goes home.

Certain points in technique are worthy of mention. The lumbar puncture needle should always be examined before use, to check that the stylet is flush with the needle end and that there is no obstruction. When the needle is being introduced into the intervertebral space it may meet bone. If this is very superficial, it may be due to a calcified interspinous ligament, or if deeper, due to fusion of the vertebrae as in ankylosing spondylitis; both these conditions can be checked radiologically. But more often the needle is off the midline and should be withdrawn and redirected. Sometimes a needle which has been directed a few degrees in a lateral direction may strike the spinal nerve roots, and the patient will complain of a sudden pain down the right or left leg; the needle should be immediately withdrawn and redirected accordingly. Care must be taken not to thrust in the needle further after piercing the theca, otherwise the vertebral body or intervertebral disc may be struck and bleeding may occur from the venous plexus covering the posterior surface of the vertebral bodies. If blood-stained fluid comes from the needle after the first few drops, the needle should be withdrawn and the test abandoned, and not repeated for at least two months. Prolapsed intervertebral disc has been reported following lumbar puncture. It must be emphasized that a thoroughly aseptic technique should be used, and the operator and all assistants should wear masks. Faulty technique in this respect may lead to infection of the intervertebral tissues, resulting in abscess formation or meningitis. The rate of flow of the spinal fluid can be controlled by the stylet. Spinal fluid should never be aspirated with a syringe.

LUMBAR PUNCTURE REACTIONS

BEFORE THE TEST. The patient may be very nervous, and in this case it is best to arrange admission to hospital and to give 10 mg of diazepam (Valium) by mouth half an hour before proceeding with the test. The test may be done with the patient lying in the left lateral position if he or she feels more secure in that position. Sometimes a patient may be known to be sensitive to the procaine used for local anaesthesia. If necessary, lumbar puncture can be done without the local anaesthetic, diazepam being given if indicated.

DURING THE TEST. If the patient shows signs of agitation or movement during the test, the needle should be immediately withdrawn, as there is the risk that a sudden movement may snap the needle shaft.

AFTER THE TEST. Severe post-lumbar puncture headache sometimes occurs. Within 12 to 24 hours the patient complains of severe headache and stiffness of the neck; vomiting may occur and the patient may collapse. This reaction is believed to be due to a marked fall in spinal fluid pressure, producing meningeal tension. The fall in pressure is due not so much to the amount of spinal fluid withdrawn as to the continued leak of fluid through the hole or tear in the theca after the needle has been withdrawn. The headache is relieved by the patient lying flat on a bed, the foot of which may be elevated on blocks. The main method of preventing this reaction is to use a fine-bore needle and to make only one hole in the theca; even so a few patients will get this type of reaction. The reaction is probably less likely to occur if the patient can be admitted to hospital for the test and kept flat in bed for 48 hours; but this is often impossible, either because of bed shortage or because the patient is unwilling to be admitted. When the out-patient technique described is used, the incidence of post-lumbar puncture reactions is less than 10 per cent, and that of severe reactions less than 5 per cent. If a severe reaction occurs the patient will have to be admitted to hospital or rest at home flat for several days or even a week. Plenty of fluids should be given by mouth, a light diet advised, and an analgesic may be prescribed.*

Tests for Mental Status

These are of considerable importance when the diagnosis of general paralysis of the insane is in question or has been made. The following schedule of tests has been adapted from that used for many years in Department Medicine I of the Johns Hopkins Hospital, Baltimore. The tests are not meant as a substitute for an adequate psychiatric examination. Emphasis is placed upon the sensorium since we are particularly interested in detecting organic brain disease. A diagnosis of paresis can be made only on a clinical basis coupled with the findings in the cerebrospinal fluid. The mental status could form part of the examination of all patients suspected of having paresis and of all late syphilitics in whose cases the examination of the spinal fluid is strongly positive.

I. General Appearance and Behaviour: Is patient neatly dressed? Does he comport himself well or are there peculiarities? Is he unduly antagonistic? Does he appear to be psychotic on simple observation? Is there a logical sequence to his conversation?

II. Mood: Is patient unduly depressed or euphoric?

III. Delusions or Hallucinations: Present or absent. If present describe. Are there any delusions of grandeur or paranoid trends?

IV. Sensorium.

1. Orientation (as to time, place and person).

2. Retention: Of digits, digits backwards, retention of words after a time interval.

---

*Peelen[5] has recommended the use of tolazoline (Priscoline or Priscol) in the treatment of headaches due to lumbar puncture. He gave 25 to 50 mg by mouth every 8 hours for 5 to 7 days, finding that the drug acted almost as a specific in 12 cases. If the remedy were discontinued too soon recurrence might follow.

3. Memory: Subjective and objective.

a. Remote: Date of birth, age, age at entering and leaving school, years of attendance at school. Age and date of marriage. Number and birth dates of children. Last job—dates and length of time employed.

b. Recent: Method of transportation to hospital, foods eaten for breakfast and dinner.

c. Information: Last three Kings of England. Three largest cities. Largest city in France. Date of beginning of World War II. Adolf Hitler. Note: Questions asked must be commensurate with schooling and general IQ.

4. Calculation: Subtraction of 7s from 100, serially (simpler calculation to be used in patients with little schooling).

5. Judgement: Difference between baby and dwarf, lie and mistake, tree and bush. Absurdity test, e.g., 'I found a way to go to town downhill and come back downhill too.'

6. Speech and Writing Tests: Test phrases to be repeated three times by patient. The following may be used: 'Methodist Episcopal', 'Third Riding Artillery Brigade', 'Massachusetts General Hospital'. If in doubt observe handwriting.

7. Insight: Is patient aware of any mental difficulty? Does he appear duly concerned about his condition?

V. On neurological examination make definite note as to presence or absence of tremors of tongue, lips or outstretched hands, hyperactive tendon reflexes and pupillary changes.

VI. A statement as to patient's education to serve as a yardstick for evaluation.

VII. A statement from relatives or friends if present as to any peculiarities of behaviour. This is most important and may throw light on a situation not uncovered by the formal mental status. Ask about incontinence, untidiness, ability to dress self, lack of normal modesty, change in disposition, insomnia, reason for loss of work, etc.

VIII. The impression of the examining physician as to whether or not there is sufficient change to justify a diagnosis of paresis.

GONORRHOEA

Staining Methods (Gram's Stain)

Methods employing a single stain, such as methylene blue, which indicates only the morphological appearance of bacteria, should never be used. Some modification of Gram's method is most commonly employed. The technique is as follows:

Spread a thin smear of the material on a glass slide with a platinum loop and fix by passing through a flame. Do not overheat the slide, which is then allowed to cool. Stain with 2 per cent crystal violet for 30 seconds; now add Gram's iodine, which acts as a mordant, and leave for a further 30 seconds. The slide is now decolorized with acetone or alcohol till the fluid which flows from the slide is practically colourless. When acetone is used, this usually takes only a few seconds. After washing with tap water the slide is counterstained with 1 per cent safranine for 10 seconds, washed with tap water, blotted and dried.

Culture Methods

The subject of media for the transport and growth of the gonococcus is discussed on pages 190 to 194. For precise details of the preparation of the media the reader is referred to publications on this subject.[6-8]

Media for Fermentation Reactions

Gonococci ferment glucose, with the production of acid, but not maltose or sucrose. These fermentation reactions are carried out on hydrocele agar containing the appropriate sugar with phenol red as indicator.

Melt 100 ml of McLeod base, cool to 55°C and add 6 ml of hydrocele fluid (sterilized by Seitz filtration), 10 ml of 10 per cent glucose or maltose or sucrose (sterilized by Seitz filtration), and 3 ml of 0·02 per cent phenol red. Pour slopes in bijou bottles and, when set, incubate overnight to check sterility. After inoculation with the strain being tested, the bottles should be incubated with loosened caps to allow the escape of CO_2. If this is not done, the CO_2 produced during growth may affect the indicator and give anomalous fermentation reactions.

Prostatic Massage

The object of prostatic massage is to express prostatic fluid from the gland into the posterior urethra, whence it will pass into the anterior urethra and can be collected at the urinary meatus. The index finger is protected by a glove or finger stall which is lubricated with jelly; the finger is now passed through the anal sphincter and the size, shape, and consistency of the prostate estimated. If there is no evidence of acute infection, then massage is undertaken. The finger is passed above the lateral edge of the right lobe, and gently but firmly brought down in a direction parallel to the midline; two further strokes are made with the finger more medially. The same procedure is used on the left lobe. As a result the prostatic secretion is expressed into the urethra. Finally the finger is brought down in the midline twice so as to express the fluid through the sphincter into the penile urethra. The seminal vesicles should be palpated and may also be emptied.

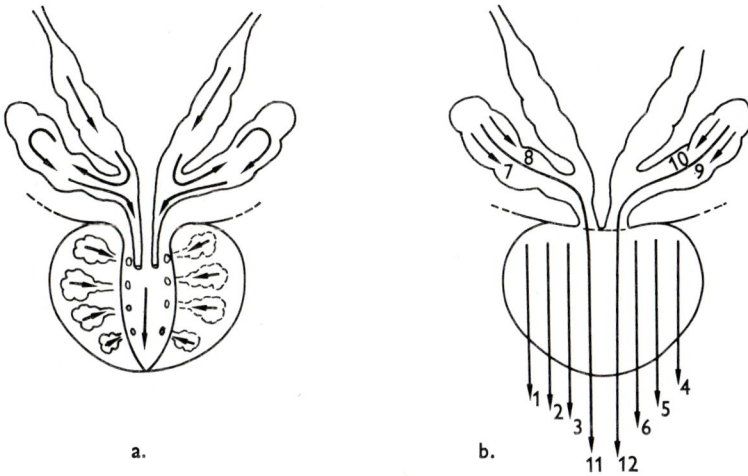

Prostatic Massage

(Redrawn from Burke's adaptation of Pelouze)

a. To illustrate normal direction of flow of fluids in prostate, vesicles and ampullae.
b. To illustrate prostatic massage and stripping of vesicles.

As the finger is being withdrawn the glands of Cowper should be palpated. It may be necessary to massage the prostatic fluid down the penile urethra till it appears as a slightly milky fluid at the external meatus. If there are several drops these should be collected on separate slides, on which cover slips are placed, for examination under the microscope. Smears stained with Gram's method may also be examined and culture medium may be inoculated.

Anterior Urethroscopy

This procedure does not require admission to hospital. A suitable instrument is the Harrison modification of the Campbell urethroscope with cannulae varying from 18 to 22 (special gauge). The examination should not be carried out if there is an acute urethritis, or following urethral trauma due to previous instrumentation. In the latter case air embolism may occur.

The usual precautions of asepsis must be observed. The patient lies on a couch and a towel with a central hole for the penis is placed over the genital area. The penis is cleaned by the assistant with 70 per cent alcohol. If the meatus is small and will not admit a size 18 cannula, dilatation with straight sounds may be necessary. A lubricated cannula of appropriate size is gently passed into the penile urethra and the obturator removed. Swabs on wooden sticks may be passed down the cannula to absorb any excess lubricant. The light is then introduced into the special aperture in the cannula and the

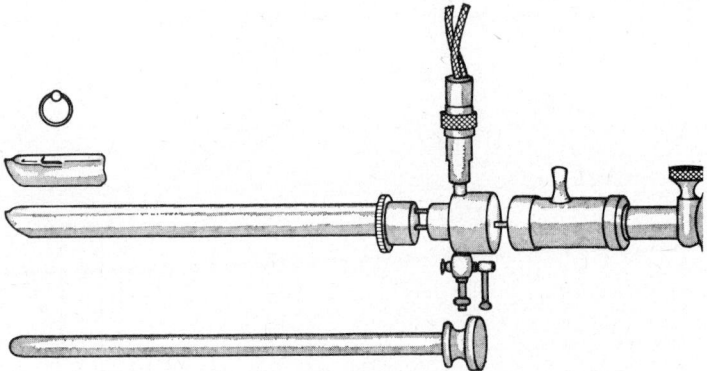

Urethroscope

(By courtesy of the Genito-Urinary Manufacturing Co. Ltd.)

eye-piece which is attached to it fitted firmly on to the top of the cannula. The assistant switches on the light while the operator looks into and focuses the eyepiece. The proximal penile urethra is seen to be closed off from the membranous urethra by the contraction of the compressor urethrae muscle, over which the mucous membrane appears in a star formation. Normally the mucosa is pink in colour. The rubber bag attached to the urethroscope is inflated, and the tap connecting it to the lumen is opened. Normally the walls of the anterior urethra should dilate; the openings of Cowper's ducts can be inspected and the cannula is slowly withdrawn while the assistant keeps the rubber bag inflated. The urethra should dilate symmetrically and the openings of the lacunae of Morgagni and of Littré's glands are seen, mainly on the dorsal aspect of the urethra. The mucosa of the penile urethra should be pink, though slightly paler than in the bulb. The cannula is finally withdrawn.

Urethral Irrigations

The patient should attend daily as an out-patient. The fluid may be either 1:8000 to 1:10,000 potassium permanganate or 1:8000 oxycyanide of mercury. The solution should be prepared in an irrigating can by adding (for concentrations of 1:8000) 15 ml of a 1 in 100 solution to 1150 ml of warm water (40°C). To the can is connected a rubber tube in which the flow of fluid is controlled by a clip. To the end of the tube is attached a freshly sterilized nozzle with shield. The pattern devised by Harkness is the best; it has different sizes of nozzle and various shapes designed to meet possible variation in the size and shape of the external meatus.

The procedure should be carried out by the physician or by a trained nursing technician, and not by the patient. Hand syringes are both ineffective and dangerous. The patient empties his bladder and the meatus and preputial sac are thoroughly cleaned with 70 per cent alcohol. The patient should preferably be lying on a couch, but sometimes it is more convenient to have him standing over a sink. The irrigator is raised to a level of 45 cm above the pelvis. The nozzle, previously sterilized, is attached to the rubber tubing and a small amount of irrigating fluid is allowed to run through the nozzle. Air is ejected from the tubing by squeezing with the hand from above downwards. The nozzle is then gently introduced into the external urinary meatus and the irrigating fluid allowed to run in and out of the anterior urethra, the nozzle being kept in place by gentle pressure and being frequently withdrawn slightly in a regular series of movements. The head of pressure is sufficient to irrigate the urethra as far back as the compressor urethrae muscle. If it is decided then to give urethrovesical irrigations, the irrigating can should be raised to not more than 75 cm above the patient's pelvis. The nozzle is held within the meatus firmly enough to prevent escape of fluid at the sides, and the patient is encouraged to relax the compressor urethrae muscle and so permit the fluid to flow back into the bladder. As soon as the patient begins to experience a sense of fullness in the bladder, he is asked to empty it in the normal way, and the procedure is then repeated until 1150 ml of fluid have been used. It is rarely necessary to give this treatment more than once a day.

If the patient finds it difficult to relax the sphincter in the early stage, the instillation of a local anaesthetic such as Xylocaine gel (lignocaine hydrochloride 2 per cent w/w in a water-miscible base) will often help to achieve the desired result. About 5 ml may be squeezed into the anterior urethra through the external meatus, gently massaged down into the bulb and left for a few minutes before irrigation is begun.

Culture Media for T. vaginalis

The media which have given the best results are the cysteine–peptone–liver–maltose (CPLM) medium by Johnson and Trussell[9] and the medium of Feinberg and Whittington.[10] These media have been compared by Rayner,[11] who found the former to be a more sensitive means of detecting *T. vaginalis*.

REFERENCES

1. KOLATOR, B. and RODIN, P. (1979) *Br. J. vener. Dis.*, **55**, 186.
2. Ass. Clin. Path. Broadsheet, No. 41. Serological notes for syphilis. (Whitechapel WR and RPCFT technique, VDRL.)
3. *Manual of Serologic Tests for Syphilis* (1964) U.S. Public Health Service. (TPI, FTA–200.)
4. DEACON, W. E., LUCAS, J. B. and PRICE, E. V. (1966) Fluorescent treponemal antibody absorption (FTA, ABS) test for syphilis. *J. Am. med. Ass.*, **198**, 624.
5. PEELEN, M. (1967) *New Engl. J. Med.*, **277**, 987.
6. REYN, A. (1965) Laboratory diagnosis of gonococcal infections. *Bull. Wld Hlth Org.*, **32**, 449.

7. Gonococcus—Procedures for isolation and identification. U.S. Dept. of Health, Education and Welfare. U.S. Publ. Hlth Service Publication, No. 499.
8. THAYER, J. D. and MARTIN, J. E. (1966) *Publ. Hlth Rep. (Wash.)*, **81,** 559.
9. JOHNSON, G. and TRUSSELL, R. E. (1943) *Proc. Soc. exp. Biol. (N.Y.)*, **54,** 245.
10. FEINBERG, J. G. and WHITTINGTON, M. J. (1957) *J. clin. Path.*, **10,** 327.
11. RAYNER, C. F. A. (1968) *Br. J. vener. Dis.*, **44,** 63.

Index

stigmata of congenital syphilis, 9, 126–31
Stokes' facies, 131
stomach, gumma of, 60
strawberry cervix, 313
Street Offences Act (1959), 383
streptomycin, in treatment of
  chancroid, 257
  gonorrhoea, 237
  granuloma inguinale, 271
  lymphogranuloma venereum, 265
  non-specific urogenital infection, 282
stricture of urethra, *see* urethral stricture
Stuart's medium, 191–2
subclavian artery, aneurysm of, 79
sulphamethoxazole–trimethoprim, *see* co-
    trimoxazole
sulpharsphenamine, 145
sulphonamides, in treatment of
  chancroid, 257
  gonorrhoea, 233–4
  granuloma inguinale, 271
  lymphogranuloma venereum, 265
  non-specific urogenital infection, 282
superinfection, 104
symptoms excuse to avoid intercourse, 374–5
synnematin B, in treatment of syphilis, 151
syphilides
  secondary
    annular, 28
    corymbose, 35
    destructive, 35–6
    follicular, 28–35
    framboesiform, 42
    macular, 28
    malignant, 36
    papular, 28–35
    papulosquamous, 35
    psoriasiform, 35
    pustular, 35–6
    roseolar, 28
    rupial, 35, 42
  tertiary
    nodular, 47
    psoriasiform, 47
    ulcerative, 47–52
syphilis, 1–132
  acquired, *see* acquired syphilis
  benign tertiary, 45–60
  blood tests, *see* serological tests for syphilis
  cardiovascular, *see* cardiovascular syphilis
  classification, 9
  congenital, *see* congenital syphilis
  definition, 1
  d'emblée, 16

syphilis (*continued*)
  diagnosis and diagnostic tests, 12–13, 390–7
  early, *see* acquired syphilis, early phase
  endemic non-venereal, 342–3
  epidemiology, 3–5, 12, 378–80
  follow-up after treatment, 162–3
  gummatous, *see* gumma
  history, 1–3
  in homosexuals, 5, 16, 378
  immunity, 8
  immunoglobulins in, 8
  incubation period, 15
  late, *see* acquired syphilis, late stage
  malignant, 36
  and marriage, 170
  maternal, 12, 19, 104–5
  nervous system, *see* neurosyphilis
  pathology, 9–12
  in pregnancy, 12, 19
  primary, 9, 16–23
    chancres, 16–19
    diagnosis, 19–22
    differential diagnosis, 22–3
  prognosis, 165–71
    treated, 166–70
    untreated, 165–6
  racial incidence, 12
  reactions to treatment, 158–62
  recurrent phase, 15, 42
  secondary, 11, 15, 23–41
    alopecia, 35
    arthritis, 40
    bursitis, 40
    cardiac involvement, 40
    choroido-retinitis, acute, 39
    constitutional symptoms, 26
    depigmentation, 36
    diagnosis, 40–1
    differential diagnosis, 41
    eruptions, 26–39
    gastric ulcer, 39
    haemorrhagic nephritis, 40
    hepatitis, 39
    infectivity, 40
    laryngitis, 36
    lymphadenitis, 39
    mucous membranes, 36–9
    nephrotic syndrome, 39
    neurological involvement, 40
    periostitis, 40
    pigmentation, 36
    signs, 26–40
    tendon sheaths, 40
    uveitis, anterior, 39